MADNESS, DISTRESS AND THE POLITICS OF DISABLEMENT

Edited by
Helen Spandler, Jill Anderson
and Bob Sapey

First published in Great Britain in 2015 by

Policy Press
University of Bristol
1-9 Old Park Hill
Bristol
BS2 8BB
UK
t: +44 (0)117 954 5940
pp-info@bristol.ac.uk
www.policypress.co.uk

North America office:
Policy Press
c/o The University of Chicago Press
1427 East 60th Street
Chicago, IL 60637, USA
t: +1 773 702 7700
f: +1 773 702 9756
sales@press.uchicago.edu
www.press.uchicago.edu

British Library Cataloguing in Publication Data
A catalogue record for this book is available from the British Library

Library of Congress Cataloging-in-Publication Data
A catalog record for this book has been requested

ISBN 978 1 44731 458 5 paperback
ISBN 978 1 44731 457 8 hardcover

Cover design by Policy Press
Front cover image kindly supplied by Jill Anderson
Printed and bound in Great Britain by Clays Ltd, St Ives plc
Policy Press uses environmentally responsible print partners

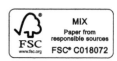

Contents

About the authors

Editors

Helen Spandler works as a reader in mental health in the School of Social Work at the University of Central Lancashire, UK. She has written extensively in the area of madness/distress including the books *Asylum to Action* (2006) and *Beyond Fear and Control* (co-edited 2007). She is also on the editorial collective of *Asylum: The Magazine for Democratic Psychiatry* (www.asylumonline.net).

Jill Anderson coordinates the national Mental Health in Higher Education project (MHHE), which aims to enhance networking and the sharing of approaches to learning and teaching about mental health. She has worked as a mental health social worker, has taught on qualifying and post-qualifying social work programmes and facilitates a national network (DUCIE) for service user and carer involvement workers based in UK universities. Jill is currently enrolled on the Doctoral Programme in Educational Research at Lancaster University.

Bob Sapey is a retired university lecturer who has written many papers on community care policy and practice, the role of technology in social care and more recently has challenged coercive social work practice with voice hearers. He is co-author of *Social Work with Disabled People* (1999, 2006 and 2012).

Contributors

Meg John Barker is a writer, academic, psychotherapist and activist specialising in sex and relationships. Meg John is a senior lecturer in psychology at the Open University and has published many academic books and papers on topics including open non-monogamies, sadomasochism, counselling and mindfulness, as well as co-editing the journal *Psychology and Sexuality*. They were the lead author of *The Bisexuality Report* and run many public events including Sense about Sex, Critical Sexology, and Gender and Sexuality Talks. Meg John is the author of the book and blog *Rewriting the Rules* www.rewriting-the-rules.com. Twitter: @megbarkerpsych.

Peter Beresford OBE is professor of social policy at Brunel University London. He is a long-term user of mental health services and co-chair of Shaping Our Lives, the independent service users' and disabled people's organisation and network. He has a longstanding involvement in issues of participation as an activist, educator, researcher and writer. He is author of *A Straight Talking Guide to Being a Mental Health Service User*, PCCS Books.

Shelley Briggs has a long history of working with trauma. Originally from Canada, she supported survivors of sexual abuse in the Scottish Highlands before completing her MSW in Dundee, and then worked with perpetrators and victims of sexual abuse in community and prison settings. Shelley went back to Canada and worked in mental health services in remote and northern communities for a few years and then returned to the UK to lecture in social work and social policy at the University of Central Lancashire, where she continues to be interested working with survivors, as well as looking at alternative practice with greater links to communities.

Fiona Cameron has worked in community mental health setting in the North West of England for a number of years. After training as an approved social worker (ASW) she was project manager of The Sanctuary, a residential crisis service run by Turning Point as an alternative to hospital admission. She has also worked as a mental health trainer with Richmond Fellowship; co-ordinator of an ASW training programme at Liverpool John Moores University; and a social worker at Guild Lodge, Forensic Unit working primarily with women. Fiona then worked for the Disability Advisory Unit at University of Central Lancashire where she is now a senior lecturer in the School of Social Work.

Kathryn Church is associate professor and director for the School of Disability Studies at Ryerson University in Toronto. For the past decade, she has been part of key initiatives that have brought the School's 'vision, passion, action' message to life across the university and in the public eye. As a researcher, Kathryn has been allied with the mad movement for 25 years. Author of *Forbidden Narratives: Critical Autobiography as Social Science* (1995) and co-editor of *Learning through Community* (2008) she wrote a dozen documents for psychiatric survivor-led organizations doing local economic development. She is an award-winning curator of arts-informed research and a dedicated instructor.

Bhargavi V Davar completed her doctoral research into the ethical and epistemological foundations of the mental and behavioural sciences in 1995. She is involved in the women's movement and is author of *Mental Health of Indian Women* (Sage 1999), editor of *Mental Health from a Gender Perspective* (Sage 2001) and co-author with Sundari Ravindran of *Gendering Mental Health: Knowledges, Identities and Institutions* (Oxford UP, forthcoming). She writes on the place of indigenous mental healing within public discourse, and on the colonial histories of psychology and psychiatry. She established the Bapu Trust for research on Mind and Discourse in 1999, a research and service provider devoted to social science, cultural and historical research on mental health practices and policies in India. Bhargavi Davar is a survivor of psychiatry, and is a trained arts-based therapist who works with people in crisis, particularly young people. She is global advisor to Human Rights Watch, a working group member of the UNESCAP on Incheon Strategy, Decade of persons with disabilities 2013-22.

Steve Graby is an autistic adult who was diagnosed at the age of 22, while in the final year of a politics degree. Coincidentally, he discovered the social model of disability around the same time, which led to involvement with the disabled people's movement, including the Disabled People's Direct Action Network and, more recently, Greater Manchester Coalition of Disabled People. He is now, after having been lucky enough to secure funding, working towards a PhD in disability studies at the University of Leeds, while hoping to find ways to fit some activism around the time constraints of this.

Kim Hopper is a medical anthropologist who works as a research scientist at the Nathan S Kline Institute for Psychiatric Research (USA), where he co-directs the Center for the Study of Recovery in Social Contexts. He also teaches at Columbia University's School of Public Health and Law and consults at the University of Alaska-Fairbanks. Since 1979, he has undertaken ethnographic and historical research on psychiatric care and homelessness, chiefly in New York City. For the last several years, he has co-directed a field school to teach research methods to persons with extensive mental health histories

Alex Iantaffi is a systemic psychotherapist, licensed marriage and family therapist, public health researcher and community activist. He is an assistant professor at the Program in Human Sexuality, University of Minnesota (USA) and is the editor-in-chief for *Sexual and Relationship Therapy*. Alex has researched and published on various aspects of gender, disability, and sexuality for the past two decades. His clinical work is focused on issues of human sexuality and gender identity across the lifespan. Twitter: @xtaffi

Nev Jones is a critical community psychologist and postdoctoral fellow in psychiatric anthropology at Stanford University (USA) with a background in continental philosophy. Her current research focuses on the phenomenology and sociopolitical context(s) of psychosis, early intervention in community-based settings, and identity development.

Frank Keating is a senior lecturer in health and social care in the Department of Social Work at Royal Holloway University of London (UK). His main research interests are ethnicity, gender and mental health, particularly focusing on African and Caribbean communities. He continues to advocate for racial equality in mental health services through his writing, teaching and public speaking.

Timothy Kelly is a PhD student in the Department of Rehabilitation and Counsellor Education with a minor focus in anthropology at the University of Iowa (USA). He is interested in transdisciplinary work focused on experiences often falling under the description of psychosis, attending to both sociocultural structure and lived experience, and bridging the gap between theoretical and applied work in community mental health and public advocacy.

Mick McKeown is reader in democratic mental health in the School of Health at University of Central Lancashire (UK). Mick has a strong commitment to equalities and critical perspectives in service provision and has been active at a professional and practical level around such issues as advocacy, service user and carer involvement and the complexities of addressing civil liberties within the constraints of secure units and wider mental health services. He has published widely and co-ordinated the production of the collectively written text: *Service User and Carer Involvement in Education for Health and Social Care* (Wiley-Blackwell). Mick has been a UNISON activist for all of his working life.

China Mills is a lecturer in critical educational psychology at the University of Sheffield's School of Education. She is the author of the book *Decolonizing Global Mental Health: The Psychiatrization of the Majority World* (Routledge 2014). China's research interests lie in the intersections and interconnections between psychiatry, colonialism, and the pharmaceutical industry. She is currently critically engaged in exploring how the psy-disciplines intervene into poverty at both national and international levels – or what might be called the psychiatrisation of poverty. China has previously worked alongside the hearing voices movement in the UK, and with non-governmental organisations doing mental health work in India.

Tina Minkowitz represented the World Network of Users and Survivors of Psychiatry in the drafting and negotiation of the United Nations Convention on the Rights of Persons with Disabilities (CRPD). She served on the steering committee of the International Disability Caucus and was a member of the 40-person drafting group that created the official text of the treaty for negotiation. She is credited with much of the paradigm-shifting character of the CRPD in the areas of legal capacity, liberty and respect for integrity of the person. Ms Minkowitz is an attorney admitted in the state of New York. She is a survivor of psychiatry and believes in the development of authentic user/survivor perspectives in human rights.

William J Penson is a disabled PhD research student at the University of Central Lancashire, an associate lecturer at Sheffield Hallam University, a part-time lecturer at the University of Bradford and a part-time trainer with Community Links, a mental health charity in Leeds (UK). In addition, he worked in mental health practice for 12 years before working as a senior lecturer and teacher fellow at Leeds Metropolitan University for nine years. His current research interests include postcolonial perspectives in mental health and disability discourse.

Anne Plumb identifies as a mental health system survivor. She has been a member of the former Survivors Speak Out in the UK, including two years as treasurer, and of a small training collective, Distress Awareness Training Agency (DATA). When domestic circumstances made such involvements difficult she began to organise material she had at home into two archives: one is that of grassroots disabled activist Ken Lumb, her late partner; the other is of mental health survivors and their allies. She is currently a member of a survivor history group. Anne can be contacted at anplumb.uncrpd@gmail.com.

Donna Reeve is an honorary teaching fellow at the Centre for Disability Research and the Division of Health Research at Lancaster University. Her publications and research interests are related to psycho-emotional disablism and the complex relationships between disablism, impairment, identity and culture. Rooted in disability studies, her theoretical work is interdisciplinary, drawing on fields such as feminist theory, sociology of the body, sociology of the emotions, phenomenology and political philosophy to extend understandings of the lived experience of disablism.

Jasna Russo comes from the former Yugoslavia and lives in Berlin, Germany. After emigrating in 1992, she joined the international user/survivor movement where she has remained active in different organisations and roles. Jasna has an MA in psychology and works as an independent survivor researcher and trainer. Her articles have been published in various anthologies and journals in Germany and the UK.

Debra Shulkes is a survivor of psychiatry from Australia. Based in the Czech Republic, she has been active as an organiser and editor in the European and world movements of users and survivors of psychiatry. She is especially interested in campaigns for human rights and social justice for people who have been psychiatrically labelled. She works as a writer and editor.

Jerry Tew is reader in social work and mental health at the University of Birmingham (UK). His professional background is mental health social work and he co-founded the Social Perspectives Network. He is currently involved in national research projects on recovery and on personalisation, and has led a national study evaluating 'whole family' approaches in mental health. Much of his research has been in collaboration with people with lived experience of mental distress as co-researchers. His recent book *Social Approaches to Mental Distress* (Palgrave Macmillan 2011) offers an analysis of the crucial role played by social factors and life events in bringing on (or averting) mental distress, and sets out a vision for mental health practice that emphasises the centrality of issues of social identity, participation and relationship.

Jan Wallcraft is a freelance researcher whose work is informed by lived experience as a mental health service user and activist. She has worked in service user involvement for a range of non-governmental organisations in England. She has a PhD from London South Bank University based on narrative accounts of first experiences with psychiatric hospitalisation. Currently she is a fellow of Birmingham and Hertfordshire Universities; she is also a research associate with

Wolverhampton University, looking at the role of creative education in supporting wellbeing and recovery.

David Webb completed what is thought to be the world's first PhD on suicide by a survivor in 2006, followed in 2010 by his book *Thinking about Suicide* (PCCS Books). After many years as a (psychosocial) disability advocate/activist, chronic illness has forced him into early retirement and he now lives quietly in Castlemaine (Australia), an old goldrush town near Melbourne.

Foreword

This is such an important book. Not only does it comprehensively address one of the most vexed issues concerning the social model of disability, but it also illustrates both the way in which the field of disability studies has developed extraordinary breadth and depth in the last decade or so, and the exciting potential for further research, analysis, policy and practice development.

It is a regrettable fact that, in the early days of the development of the social model, the emphasis (sometimes unspoken) was very much on physical impairment. Those of us with physical impairments who found the social model so liberating did so because it enabled us to move away from seeing our impairment as the problem and instead to focus on social, economic, attitudinal and environmental barriers. The social model gave us the possibility of changing things for the better – we couldn't change impairment but we could change society.

Over the last 30 years or so, the voices of a wide range of people who experience discrimination and exclusion, of those who use various forms of support, have got stronger. As disabled people's, and survivors' organisations, self-advocacy groups, coalitions and campaigns have become more prominent in public debate, more influential in driving policy and service improvements, we have also been in dialogue with each other – although we have sometimes not put as much effort into these dialogues as perhaps we should have.

It has taken this book to fully bring home to me why the terms 'disabled' and 'disability' can be so oppressive and frightening to some people who use mental health services And to understand that one of the problems with our use of the social model has been the tendency of some of us to take impairment for granted. For many people, as illustrated by some of the chapters in this book, 'impairment', 'illness', 'medical condition', 'disorders' are problematic terms in themselves. Can the social model encompass analysis, not only of disabling barriers, but also of 'impairment'? What are the implications when impairment ceases to be neutral, when the terminology associated with the social model can feel offensive and to belong to an oppressive social context instead of being a liberating way of describing one's place in the world.

If we have learnt nothing else over the last 30 years or so of disabled people's movements, it is that research, analysis and policy development will only be helpful, rather than harmful, if we start with people's lived experiences. This means creating spaces for voices to be heard in ways which set agendas, define problems, and determine not only the analytical frameworks required but also any resulting policy recommendations. This book is an admirable illustration of the value of starting from individuals' self-definitions and descriptions of their experiences, focusing not on individual pathology but on how people experience their place in the world.

Whereas the main focus of disability studies has been on the socio-economic context of disabling barriers, one of the things the book illustrates is the enormous potential for applying the social model to the creation and definition of 'impairment'. Such an approach challenges not only the norms applied to the way our bodies and minds work but also challenges the imposition of medical diagnoses on experiences which result from material conditions: as many of the chapters in this book illustrate, people who have been diagnosed with a disorder or 'disability' have in fact in many cases been disordered and disabled not only by the society in which they live but also by medical diagnosis and treatment.

Contributors remind us of increasing evidence that global capitalism creates impairment and distress; and how neoliberal economics promotes 'small states', the primacy of the market and profit motive for the production of goods and services, and the replacement of communities of interest with individual self-interest. Alongside all of this sit policies which insist that individual pathologies cause social problems, such as the current UK government's insistence that 'psychological barriers' cause long-term unemployment.

This book also teaches us that a number of countries in the global south suffer not only the consequences of 'psychiatric colonialism' but also the imposition of 'modern' social policies by current international ('western'-dominated) organisations. Meanwhile, in some countries of the global north we are struggling against the co-option and distortion of our most progressive ideas into policies which atomise us into isolated individuals, blame us for our own 'misfortunes', and throw us back onto nothing but our own resources. Yet as a number of contributors make clear, across the whole world self-determination and equal access to opportunities require collective and democratic action, and the building of alliances with workers and other groups negatively affected by global capitalism.

There are diversities of opinion throughout the book – for example on whether the UN Convention on the Rights of Persons with Disabilities is helpful or potentially harmful for people experiencing madness/distress. Yet this diversity, like human diversity itself, does not have to lead to conflict and can be accompanied by respect for each others' views and acknowledgement of each others' experiences. Our perspectives may differ but two fundamental principles enable our common enterprise: our commitment to full human rights for all; and that there must be nothing about us without us.

Jenny Morris
Previously policy analyst and researcher on disability issues, now retired
October 2014

Introduction

Bob Sapey, Helen Spandler and Jill Anderson

What are the consequences, for someone experiencing madness or distress, of being categorised as a disabled person? What are the benefits and limitations of adopting a disabled identity? Can disability policies benefit people with mental health problems (and what are some of the barriers preventing them from doing so)? Can the social model of disability apply to madness and distress (and if so, how)? How much can the mental health service user/survivor movement learn from the disabled people's movement, and vice versa? How do mad studies and disability studies connect, if at all? How can disabled people and mental health service users and survivors work together and form alliances to advance our collective interests? These are some of the pressing questions at issue in this book.

We decided to put this book together because we have struggled over these questions for a number of years. In particular, we have been worrying about the implications of the distress and/or disability conundrum for people with mental health problems; particularly as individuals who may be struggling for an identity that provides them with adequate support and protection, and/or those seeking a collective home in disability studies or the wider disabled people's movement. While there has been a long history of political activism and theorising, about disability on the one hand, and madness and distress on the other, these debates have tended to happen separately. Fifteen years ago Peter Beresford asked: what have madness and psychiatric system survivors got to do with disability and disability studies? (Beresford, 2000). He thought this question was, even then, in need of addressing urgently. Discussion about this issue has taken place over the intervening period, in academic journals, conferences, activist settings and – more recently – on social media. Yet the conversations and contributions have been scattered, making it difficult for disparate ideas to be placed in dialogue with one another.

Although there is much to gain from bringing together disability and madness/distress, as we do in this book, doing so reveals significant points of disjuncture: both political and conceptual. This disjuncture suggests that there is an unsettled relationship between madness and disability which has rarely been acknowledged. We think that there is something important to be gained from exploring and articulating these disconnections, but seeing them as a 'possibility rather than [as just] a complication' (Goodley, 2012, 66).

It may be that policy has 'jumped the gun' by framing madness and distress as disability without an appreciation of the myriad complexities involved. These complexities are not just evident at an abstract or theoretical level. They continually manifest themselves in practice; that is, within activism, policy, education, employment, health and welfare. For example, in an educational context, mad students – or students experiencing distress – may be required to identify as 'disabled' in order to access the accommodations they need. Some commentators see disabled and mad people as being increasingly 'lumped together' under a disability rubric in the administration of health and welfare services (Nabbali, 2009, 4) and some users/survivors have expressed misgivings about being positioned as disabled. At the same time, other mental health activists have strongly advocated for the application of disability legislation to gain human rights and social protection

Mental health has tended to be a side-issue within disability studies which, in the eyes of some, has failed to 'adequately conceptualise the experience, phenomenon and constitution of mental health in critical and politicized ways' (Goodley, 2012, 62). Some activists and researchers in the area of critical mental health have felt 'marginalised by disability theory' (Goodley, 2012, 62) and people with mental health needs have been peripheral to the wider disability movement, and may feel they don't belong there. Arguably, the disability movement has been slow to include mental health issues, and could even be said to have shown prejudiced attitudes towards madness and distress (Nabbali, 2009; Plumb, 1994). Yet, since the early 1990s, mental health problems have overtaken physical health problems as the most common reason why people claim welfare payments such as the incapacity benefit in the UK (Brown et al, 2009; Cattrell et al, 2011). Although this raises all kinds of tricky issues about the relationship between madness/distress, disability and illness, it does indicate an increasing mental health constituency who might be considered chronically ill or 'disabled'. Therefore, in this context, it is worth exploring whether models and policies developed to liberate disabled people have liberatory potential for those experiencing madness and distress.

Disability studies developed out of the disabled people's movement and focused on the relationship disabled people have with society. The social model of disability, which has dominated UK disability studies, has been primarily concerned with the discrimination and disadvantages people face because of social responses to impairment. The model was initially concerned with the position of people with physical impairments but, over time, attempts have been made to make it relevant to other groups, including people with learning difficulties, D/deaf people and those experiencing madness and distress. In one notable example, Liz Sayce (2000) examined different approaches to overcoming discrimination and social exclusion in mental health and concluded that the social model offers the best possibility of making progress. She is critical of three other approaches: 1) treating mental illness as a disease of the brain, in an attempt to put it on a par with physical illness; 2) viewing distress as part of a continuum of individual growth – that is, as a psychological response to life issues that affect us all, but sometimes at an extreme; and 3) a libertarian rejection of psychiatric diagnosis as an infringement of rights, in an assertion of individual freedoms. By contrast, she argues that a 'disability inclusion' model would help people develop a positive identity, rejecting shame as something imposed by others, while also providing rights by giving individuals recourse to the law through anti-discrimination legislation.

It is worth noting that the social model of disability has undergone significant modifications and revisions, most notably embodied in the 'relational' social model and the notion of psycho-emotional disablism (Thomas, 1999), which has particular resonance when applied to mental health (Reeve, 2012a). Despite these important developments, the social model has not proved easily transferable (Beresford, 2000; Beresford et al, 2010; Anderson et al, 2012). Application of the social model to the lives of people who use mental health services has been described as 'an area where little work has been done so far' (Oliver, 2010, 5) and, for some, there remains a 'pervasive divide between the social model of disability and mad activism' (Nabbali, 2009, 9). The social model has been described as 'pallid, even empty, when addressing the convoluted systems of psychiatry and mental health', such that its 'political practicality for mad people appears to be largely rhetorical' (Nabbali, 2009, 7).

While the place of 'impairment' in the politics of disablement has been hotly contested by disability scholars (Crow, 1996a; Shakespeare and Watson, 2002), for those engaged in the politics of mental health the concept has proved particularly problematic. No matter how far disability scholars may debate impairment in relation to physical disability (claiming, for example, that not only disability but also impairment is socially constructed), it would be rare for them to dispute the existence of impairment itself. In fact, we could say that the disability movement's demands – for equal access, participation and independent living support – *depend on the existence of impairment*. However, no such consensus exists in mental health. Indeed contesting the existence of mental illness (and thus of impairment) has been the *raison d'*être of radical sections of the psychiatric survivor movement (Plumb, 1993).

In addition, unless we take a purely bio-chemical view of mental illness (as brain disease), it may be impossible to disentangle the impairment in mental health from the disabling social conditions that may cause – or at least shape – mental health problems. Here, disablement isn't necessarily predicated upon a pre-existing impairment which is then oppressed or marginalised by society or social agents ('on top of' the impairment). Stigma and disadvantage are central issues in the field of disability, and while they are also important in mental health, critical work here has tended to focus on re-conceptualising the experience of madness or distress itself, and its *primary* origins in oppressive social relations. The worry has been that a main focus on social exclusion and discrimination might inadvertently 'bracket out' discussions about the nature of madness itself, conceding interventions to psychiatry and medicine and letting the dreaded 'medical model' in through the back door (Plumb, 1994). Therefore, while Sayce's (2000) model makes a detailed case for why and how the disability inclusion model can be made to work in mental health, it could be seen as ultimately endorsing what Lord et al (2001) described as a traditional paradigm. Here services may change location or style, but continue to defer to medicine's definitions and understandings of mental illness. Arguably then, the disability inclusion model glosses over the wider and deeper critique of the medicalisation of mental illness that has gained increasing momentum over recent years (for example, the rejection by voice hearers of psychiatry and its medicalisation of their experiences and their distress).

These questions prompted us to organise a two day symposium in November 2011, under the auspices of the Mental Health in Higher Education project, the Centre for Disability Research at Lancaster University and the School of Social Work at the University of Central Lancashire in the UK. We took as our starting point Anne Plumb's foundational document 'Distress or disability?' (Plumb, 1994). Anne wrote this for the Greater Manchester Coalition of Disabled People to highlight some of the difficulties of integrating mental distress within broader disability politics, and it remains one of the clearest articulations of the issues to date. The symposium brought together mental health and disability scholars (including academics, activists and research students) from the north-west of England, to explore the issues raised by situating distress and madness within a disability framework. We explored some possibilities and limitations of applying

4

the social model of disability to madness and distress; specifically, the extended 'social-relational' model of disability which incorporates the idea of 'psycho-emotional disablement' (we were privileged that Carol Thomas and Donna Reeve took part in the proceedings, two key proponents of that idea). We also included special themed sessions on recovery, trauma and abuse (see Anderson et al, 2012, for symposium proceedings).

Despite two days of lively debate and discussion, we realised it needed more thought and time and we wanted to see how we might process each other's ideas to develop our own thinking. So we invited people who had attended and presented at the symposium to further develop their ideas in the light of these discussions. We also invited users/survivors, disability and mad scholars, practitioners and activists from elsewhere in the UK, and internationally, to contribute specific chapters to this book.

Authors adopt common, different and sometimes conflicting positions on the issues we set out here; each contributing something new and unique. Some argue that we need to *apply* the social model of disability to madness and distress; others that we need to *extend* (and/or revise) the social model to help it fit madness and distress; others believe we should develop our own *separate* (and/or equivalent) framework, so we can have a dialogue with disability activists, on equal terms. Ultimately, although it seems that applying the social model remains problematic, such problems are not necessarily insurmountable. We think that, in different ways, all of the chapters in this book contribute to overcoming these difficulties and taking the discussions forward.

Many contributors refer to one particular development that is worth noting here: the United Nation's Convention on the Rights of Persons with Disabilities (CRPD). This Convention was adopted in December 2006 and has been signed by 155 countries, to date. It is noteworthy for a number of reasons. First, it is a wide-ranging framework for the provision of human rights for disabled people that specifically applies to people with mental health difficulties as well as to people with physical, learning and sensory disabilities. Second, it specifically enshrines the rights to equal recognition before the law (Article 12) and to liberty and security (Article 14), attracting the attention of those in the mental health survivor movement. The World Network of Users and Survivors of Psychiatry (2008) have described Article 12 as creating a paradigm shift in the attitude towards mental distress, as it entitles people to decide whether to receive treatment, go to hospital or access alternative settings. Furthermore, detention on the grounds of mental disorder is considered a breach of human rights under Article 14, because it states 'that *the existence of a disability* shall in no case justify a deprivation of liberty' (United Nations, 2006, emphasis added). If people with mental health problems are considered 'disabled' (as they are under the terms of the Convention) then this has wide-ranging implications for practice. For example, it potentially challenges the legitimacy of many mental health laws throughout the world and appears to conflict with other conventions; such as the European Convention on Human Rights, which permits certain human rights exceptions on the grounds of a person being of 'unsound mind'.

The UN Convention is often cited in support of the argument that disability policy can be of benefit to people with mental health problems. However, consideration of the Convention also highlights some of the complicated issues at stake. Within this book, the application of the Convention to madness and distress is both celebrated and questioned, reflecting not only the ideological stances of the authors, but also their geographical and political locations within different welfare systems (where the consequences of implementation may differ). While most authors are encouraged by the Convention, we think Anne Plumb's concerns about its application to users and survivors (set out in Chapter Thirteen) provide an important contribution to on-going debates.

As might be expected, definitional complications go to the very heart of the issues we grapple with in this book. If mental illness is considered a disability then what is the nature of the disability or the underlying (mental) impairment? 'Madness' is beginning to be reclaimed within the user/survivor movement, and a number of recent publications herald the emergence of 'mad studies' – alongside queer and disability studies (Curtis et al, 2000; Gray, 2006; LeFrançois et al, 2013). Like queer, and indeed disability, madness concerns itself not only with individual experience, but can be seen as a new critical field of enquiry. Indeed, while the term 'madness' is often used as shorthand for distress, mental illness or disorder, we are aware that some individuals reject the term as pejorative and stigmatising (Beresford et al, 2010). The word 'distress' is often preferred by many users/survivors, but is potentially too broad a term on its own to encompass the situation of people with very acute and long-term mental health difficulties, and it is these people who are more likely to be considered 'disabled'. In addition, we recognise that not everyone who is considered 'mentally ill' experiences distress (although other people may be distressed by their situation or behaviour).

Given the lack of consensus over terminology we have tried not to impose false certainty, but to reflect the diversity of opinion that exists among our contributors and elsewhere. We use the terms 'madness' and 'distress' to try to distance ourselves from the medicalised and sometimes pathologising categorisation of 'mental illness' and 'disorder'. We also avoid the term 'mental health', where possible, due to its frequent use as a euphemism for its opposite (a situation that has been described as a 'semantic paradox', Vassilev and Pilgrim, 2007). We could have adopted the term psychiatric or psycho-social disability, as some of our contributors do, but that would have perhaps pre-empted a consensus about the merits of framing madness and distress as a disability. In addition, we usually deploy the term 'disabled people' as opposed to 'people with disabilities'. That is because we generally adhere to social model of disability thinking which tries to locate the 'problem' of disability in the disabling relationships and structures of society, rather than in the individual disabled person.

In view of the above, it will come as little surprise that this has not been a straightforward book to write and edit. We have grappled with our understanding of the issues; our vision for the final product; and our role as editors. Alongside contributors, we have often struggled to voice thoughts and opinions which, in many cases, have not previously been articulated or appeared in print. We have learned a lot in the process, both about the issues and about how best to support the attempts of others to express them. For various reasons, some contributors were unable to write their chapters as planned and, rather than abandon these contributions, we took a different approach. For example, in two cases, we present an edited version of an interview conducted with the author and we think that these make a refreshing change from the more academic style of other chapters.

Throughout the editing process, we have tried to push our thinking, individually and collectively. We have aimed to achieve coherence, not through a consensus of views, but through encouraging reflection on the key concerns we set out here. The issues remain incredibly complex, but we hope that we have stimulated, and will continue to trigger, further thinking, reflection and action. We are grateful to everyone who has contributed to this publication for their insight, commitment and patience. We hope that the book will be a useful resource for individuals; for disability studies; for mad studies; and for the user/survivor and disabled people's movements.

The book is in five sections which reflect some commonalities in the way authors have tackled the issues. Part One includes chapters that foreground specific issues raised by madness and distress, which help us to make sense of the distress/disability conundrum. We start with a chapter from ourselves (Helen Spandler and Jill Anderson) which identifies and explores some underlying issues and tensions which might prevent people with mental health problems benefiting from disability policy and legislation. We then include a chapter by Jasna Russo and Debra Shulkes who chart the debates within the European Network of (Ex-)Users and Survivors of Psychiatry (ENUSP) about the disability question and the need for it to be tackled differently at three key levels: the individual, welfare policy and social movement/organisational. We follow this with a chapter by Nev Jones and Timothy Kelly from the US, in which they draw on their personal experience to explore the complications and heterogeneity of madness and distress, before considering interconnections with disability experience. Finally in this section, we include a chapter by Bill Penson, from the UK, who argues that the lack of evidence for a medicalised account of madness destabilises the idea that distress can be treated as disability/impairment.

Part Two includes chapters which utilise different, but complementary, social approaches to theorising madness, distress and disablement. Jerry Tew draws upon his extensive work in developing social approaches to understanding and working with distressing experiences, to shed more light on the disability question. Jan Wallcraft and Kim Hopper make the case for applying Amartya Sen's Capabilities Approach to support the rights and entitlements of people with mental health needs and disabled people. Finally in this section, Donna Reeve explores the relevance of psycho-emotional disablism for people experiencing mental distress and helps to disentangle the complex relationship between mental distress, disablism and impairment.

Part Three specifically includes chapters applying social models of disability to madness/distress. Shelley Briggs and Fiona Cameron, as social work lecturers from Canada and the UK, argue that women who have experienced intergenerational trauma can suffer additional distress through psycho-emotionally disabling reactions from family/ community and psychiatric services. This is followed by a chapter from Frank Keating who draws on ideas from critical race theory to explore the advantages and limitations of the social model for black and minority ethnic service users in the UK. Meg John Barker (from the UK) and Alex Iantaffi (from the USA) apply social model thinking to people deemed to be suffering from 'sexual disorders' and 'dysfunctions' (what they call sexual distress), arguing that dominant sexual norms effectively disable us all. Finally, an interview with David Webb from Australia explores his support for the inclusion of mental distress within the UN Convention on the Rights of People with Disabilities (CRPD) and his views on the value of the social model for people experiencing suicidal feelings.

In Part Four we explore some wider debates and issues relating to the universalising of disability policy. We start with an interview with Tina Minkowitz from the USA, focusing on the adoption of a disability and human rights framework for advancing the rights of users and survivors of psychiatry, especially through her input into the Convention on the Rights of People with Disabilities. In contrast, Anne Plumb, writing from a European welfare context in the UK, articulates her concerns that the approach taken in this Convention may not always be in the best interests of people experiencing distress/madness. China Mills, also from the UK, then draws on her research in India to question the way that the 'global mental health movement' is imposing particular medicalised ideas of disability and madness on the global south which may obscure the social causes of distress. This theme is continued by Bhargavi Davar, who argues that the colonial legacy in India has actually prevented individuals with mental health needs benefiting from disability identities and polices.

The final section, 'Meeting places', includes contributions which specifically suggest ways forward for alliances and working together across distress and disability. Steve Graby explores the ways in which the neurodiversity movement has specific commonalities with both the disability movement and the user/survivor movement and may help to 'bridge the gap' between the two. Peter Beresford draws on his own extensive experience of work in this area to point out the potential for working together across difference, and his hope for positive gains from mad studies. Kathryn Church, from Canada, explores some of the possibilities and challenges that she and colleagues encountered while incorporating mad studies within a school of disability studies in Toronto. Mick McKeown and Helen Spandler explore how individuals and groups might take part in discussions to arrive at a better informed politics of mental health and disability, in the context of UK trade union/community organising. Our final chapter draws the book to a close by reflecting on possibilities for joint work and alliances across madness, distress and disability and highlighting work that still needs doing to achieve this.

Part One
Disjunctures between disability and madness

ONE

Unreasonable adjustments? Applying disability policy to madness and distress

Helen Spandler and Jill Anderson

The rights of disabled people are now enshrined in law and reflected in policy at national and international levels. As a result, in many countries disabled people can access financial and social care support, through mechanisms like independent living payments. They are also entitled to reasonable adjustments or accommodations, to facilitate their access to education, employment and goods and services. Although the disabled people's movement still has some way to go to achieve its full demands, and recent advances have been threatened by reduced welfare spending, these measures have been very welcome. However, despite the fact that people with mental health problems are potential beneficiaries of these policy developments, as 'disabled people', application in a mental health context has not been straightforward. For example, the demand for 'reasonable adjustments' throws up specific challenges in the context of madness and distress.

In this chapter, we identify some tricky issues that may underlie difficulties in putting disability policy in to practice in relation to madness and distress. The first issue is that madness is, by definition, unsettling, especially as it relates to notions of *unreason* and *irrationality*. This throws up particular difficulties and challenges which relate to the second issue, the pathologisation of madness. As a result of their perceived unreason/irrationality, people with mental health problems are actively pathologised and socially excluded. In the light of these first two issues, individuals are then faced with a third: the problematic adoption of a 'mentally ill' and/or disabled identity. Taken together, these issues present major obstacles for people who experience madness and distress, preventing them from benefiting from wider disability policy.

Some disability activists, particularly advocates of the social model of disability, have been hesitant to discuss the personal difficulties and limitations which may result from an individual's impairment, and other 'impairment effects' (such as pain and discomfort). This arises from a fear of locating the 'problem' back with the individual, rather than locating it, where it is seen to belong, in discriminatory social relationships and structures. Similarly, some radical mental health activists have been reluctant to engage directly with the issue of *mental* impairment which cannot be simply reduced to disabling social arrangements. Some have argued that this silence has got in the way of people dealing with the difficult aspects, and effects, of impairment (Crow, 1996a). As such, this has been referred to as the 'elephant in the room'.[1] We use it here to refer to the tendency to ignore (or disavow) the tricky question of the nature of madness and distress.

These 'impairment effects' are especially hard to acknowledge and describe in relation to madness and distress. Yet some people may experience severe 'pain and discomfort', as a result their own distress or madness or that of others. The impact of unusual experiences – such as disorganised thinking, racing thoughts, feelings of paranoia and persecution, or feelings of being controlled by others – while glaringly obvious on one level, and the cause of genuine distress, may be difficult to talk about in certain settings (Mulvany, 2000). We believe, however, that acknowledging and exploring these issues is necessary if we are to understand the application of disability policy to madness and distress. Therefore, we start this discussion with the unsettling nature of 'madness', and how it might differ from disability in relation to physical impairment.

Madness as unsettling

Madness is thoroughly social and deeply relational. In other words, what is seen as mad behaviour manifests and plays out, in relation to others, in a social context: 'with mad people, very specific behaviours transgress cultural mores and *it is these behavioural disruptions which become their supposed impairment*' (Nabbali, 2009, 7, our emphasis). Whether or not such behaviour is put down to a brain disease, neurological dysfunction, social factors, or whatever, in the words of one survivor activist: 'it only exists through consensus and only persists by convention' (Nabbali, 2009, 7). Similarly, Pilgrim and Tomasini (2012) point out that whereas physical disabilities, like mental health problems, often involve cultural and normative judgements and social role failure (possibly due to disabling barriers), 'mental disorder... strongly implicates rule *infraction* as well' (Pilgrim and Tomasini, 2012, 632). In other words, mental disorder, by its very definition, implies behaviour that transgresses agreed social norms and 'emotion rules' (Pilgrim and Tomasini, 2012, 640).

We might wish to challenge these social rules, deeming them to be inflexible and harmful (as indeed the social model has done, in relation to the treatment of people with physical impairments). However, in the case of madness, it has been argued that without some social contract about acceptable behaviour 'social life as we know it would be impossible' (Shotter, cited in Pilgrim and Tomasini, 2012, 640). Put another way, it has been argued, 'if we were all mad there would be no functioning society, because there would be no implicit social contract that warranted any recurrent mutual accountability' (Shotter, cited in Pilgrim and Tomasini, 2012, 640). While this vision may seem overly bleak, it does signal something about the extent of the enduring problem with which psychiatry and allied mental health professions have been charged to deal. If it was merely a matter of rule infraction then why should mad people be treated any differently from anyone else who breaks social rules, norms or laws? Why are they considered in need of protection, as *disabled* people?

One of the trickiest issues in these discussions is that the 'impairment' in mental health, can profoundly affect, not only the person themselves, but also those around them. Whereas a person's interpersonal functioning is usually unaltered by a physical impairment per se (even if it might be profoundly affected by disabling social relations), madness is, by definition, deeply interpersonal (as well as intrapersonal). Indeed people are sometimes referred to as *psycho-socially* disabled, implying impairment at this level, that is, that people experience difficulties not only in relation to themselves (their 'internal world'), but also with people around them.

As Nev Jones and Timothy Kelly illustrate (in Chapter 3) there is an enormous heterogeneity of user/survivor experience. This may encompass, for example, people who feel victimised and damaged *by* psychiatric intervention – and there are a lot of instances of that in the radical psychiatry literature (for example, Breggin, 2007; Whitaker, 2010; Burstow et al, 2014). However, it may also include people who feel that psychiatry has failed to intervene, or has intervened ineffectively. For example, a child brought up by a parent struggling with complex mental health issues who either refuses any support, or is insufficiently supported by the mental health system, may feel inadequately cared for and neglected. They may even experience long-term mental health problems as a result, an issue highlighted in very different ways by Doe (2011) and Jones (2014). This illustrates uncomfortable issues that do not map neatly onto an overarching framework of *individual* rights, that is, the parent may have a right to refuse psychiatric treatment (and a right to parent); yet the child has rights too, to be loved and protected from neglect.

Pilgrim and Tomasini (2012) break down the complexity of mental impairment into: people whose behaviour is socially unintelligible; people who are so anxious or unhappy that they are unable to meet social obligations to others; and those who are have difficulty in maintaining mutually acceptable relationships with others. This is potentially useful because it provides a sociological, rather than a medicalised, codification which is probably more honest; though it perhaps rather too neatly maps onto the psychiatric categorisation of *psychosis, neurosis and personality disorder*, with all the pathologisation that entails. Their position is similar to that of Thomas Szasz (1960) who argues that psychiatry labels people whose behaviour offends *others* as psychotic, and those whose thoughts and feelings upset *themselves* as neurotic.

Pilgrim and Tomasini go on to suggest that the alignment of the user/survivor movement with the disability movement (and the social model of disability in particular) is fairly straightforward in relation to what is often called common 'mental distress', but more of a challenge in relation to what they call 'risky behaviour or incorrigible conduct' (Pilgrim and Tomasini, 2012, 642). It is, however, a challenge well worth engaging with. While people who experience 'common mental health problems' such as anxiety and depression are certainly stigmatised and oppressed, it is people with more 'serious' diagnoses (such as psychosis, schizophrenia and mania) who are more likely to experience on-going discrimination and social exclusion (Rose et al, 2011); and are, therefore, sorely in need of the protection and support of disability legislation. David Webb (Chapter 11) makes a compelling case for applying the social model to suicide/suicidal feelings which can certainly be seen as 'risky behaviour'.

In relation to a physically disabled person, there wouldn't usually be any issues regarding mental capacity and consent (although such concerns are more likely to be raised in relation to a person with learning difficulties). By contrast, whole legal systems have been put in place to assess, protect and sometimes override the legal capacity of those who are deemed 'mentally ill' or 'mentally disordered'. That, among other reasons, is why human rights protections (such as those enacted by the European Court of Human Rights) often exclude people who are subject to mental health laws, on the grounds of 'unsound mind' (Spandler and Calton, 2009). The person themselves may not accept that they have a 'mental health problem' even though people around them consider that they do (and may have concerns about the safety of the person, their own safety, or that of others). That is one of the reasons why mental health laws allow people to be detained and treated against their will. Regardless of whether we think these mental health laws are inherently discriminatory (see Chapter 12 by Tina Minkowitz) or justifiable on the grounds of medical paternalism, their continued existence underlines the enormous complexity of the issues we are grappling with. As has often been pointed out (although rarely in critiques of psychiatry) it is not always psychiatry or the 'psy professions' that labels people as mad or mentally ill; they usually rubber stamp (and specifically *medicalise*) decisions which have been *made already* in the lay arena by family, friends, neighbours or colleagues.

With this in mind, Pilgrim and Tomasini (2012) make the case that *reasonableness* is central to understanding the difference between disability and madness/distress: 'Although physically disabled people are disadvantaged in society, this is not about an attributed loss or lack of reason. By contrast loss or lack of reason is *at the centre* of the social reaction typically evoked by mental health problems...social exclusion is *actively justified* on grounds of un-reason' (Pilgrim and Tomasini, 2012, 634, emphases in the original).

While lack of reason is seen as intrinsic to the 'mental disorder', it is important to note that receiving a psychiatric diagnosis doesn't make someone necessarily or always unreasonable or an inherently unreasonable person. In the UK, the Mental Capacity Act (Department of Health, 2005) is interesting in this regard because it clearly states that: no-one should be automatically deemed lacking in capacity because of a disability or mental illness; that capacity should be assumed unless good evidence is given to the contrary; and that capacity should be assessed on a case-by-case basis (in accordance with the particular decision being made, not with the individual making it).[2] It is also worth bearing in mind that everyone's behaviour is context-bound, not just that of a person deemed to be mentally ill. Our behaviour may make sense only to ourselves, and sometimes not even to ourselves at the time; insight may come later, if at all. In addition, of course, there are people who might be considered 'unreasonable' or 'irrational' and are not psychiatrised. Politicians, bankers and chief executive officers are often given as examples (Babiak and Hare, 2006). Indeed, the attribution of 'madness' in these examples is often used as an (unsophisticated) critique and insult; witness recent discussions about Tony Blair's continuing 'irrational' beliefs about the merits of the Iraq War (for example, Humphreys, 2014).

Given these kinds of negative assumptions and stereotypes about mad people in society, reluctance to explore these issues openly and honestly may be understandable. Indeed, influential social theorists such as Foucault (1967) have argued that modern society has been established on the basis of the active identification and exclusion of unreason. Many subsequent critiques of psychiatry have built on this argument and, necessary though these critiques may be, they may have inadvertently served to marginalise more difficult discussions about madness and distress. Beyond the important work of deconstructing psychiatric discourse and classificatory systems (Parker et al, 1995), if disability policies are genuinely to benefit people with mental health problems, we need to find ways to address these uncomfortable issues.

There seems to be a paradox here: what sense can we make of the notion of things like *reasonable adjustments* or *accommodations* for a person whose behaviour, at the time, is deemed inherently *un*reasonable? One way out of this conundrum lies in positively reframing unreason. In this context, George Bernard Shaw (1903) famously said:

> The reasonable man [sic] adapts himself to the world; the unreasonable one persists in trying to adapt the world to himself. Therefore all progress depends on the unreasonable man.[3]

This quote aptly reminds us that adapting to seemingly 'unreasonable' demands might sometimes create better social conditions, and not just for the person deemed unreasonable. Meg John Barker and Alex Iantaffi's chapter (Chapter Ten) – which details the damage done to all of us by dominant sexual and gender norms – is a good example of this. Perkins et al (2009), in their report for the UK government on providing workplace support for people with mental health problems, make an important contribution to the tricky application of 'reasonable' adjustments in mental health. They draw a distinction between 'reasonable employer adjustments' and the provision of the 'more support' which may be required for some individuals, over and above the former.

In addition, it is harder to write off collective reflections on common experiences as irrational or unreasonable. It can be argued that the user/survivor movement has effectively advanced a form of 'collective reasonableness' by pooling experiential knowledge (Pilgrim and Tomasini, 2012, 642). Responses to hearing voices and self-harm are two examples of this. Before the development of the international Hearing Voices Movement in the 1990s, 'auditory hallucinations' were considered, by definition, a meaningless symptom of a brain disease such as 'schizophrenia'. In psychiatry, attempting to listen to, engage with, or respond to people's voices has historically been seen as irrational, and/or irresponsible and has been actively discouraged. Organisations like the Hearing Voices Network in the UK have helped us to see voices as meaningful to the person themselves, in the context of their own life; and have made strategies like 'voice dialogue' more acceptable and reasonable, at least in some contexts (Sapey and Bullimore, 2013). Similarly, before the development of the self-harm survivors' movement, self-harm was frequently seen merely as damaging and 'para-suicidal' behaviour. Self-harm organisations helped us to reframe self-harm as a valid coping mechanism, pioneering approaches such as self-harm minimisation that are now well respected (Spandler and Warner, 2007; and see Jerry Tew's chapter, Chapter Five, for more reflections on these issues). In addition, Mick McKeown and Helen Spandler's chapter (Chapter Nineteen) explores how good practical wisdom can emerge through collective discussion and deliberation about tricky experiential issues.

It is clear that a lot of supposedly 'mad' behaviour can be understood within the context of a person's life circumstances, or as a response to unusual experiences (such as hearing voices or seeing visions), and this can't always be appreciated by other people, or indeed by the person themselves, at the time. Arguably, once behaviour has been 'de-coded' or understood like this, it becomes, by definition, no longer unreasonable, irrational (or even 'mad') but *thoroughly reasonable* – as a rational and understandable response to difficult life events and circumstances. Some psychologists have argued that many 'mental illnesses' could actually be reclassified as responses to trauma (Johnstone, 2011). Indeed, this has been one of the aims (and successes) of the survivor movement. However, there are lots of experiences that haven't been re-framed or re-claimed in this way. For example, Nev Jones (2014) argues that positive re-framing has yet to be achieved with experiences like so-called 'thought disorder', which can be extremely disturbing. In other words, it is an *unfinished project*.

In addition, some people – especially those experiencing a 'first episode' crisis, for example – may lack the resources to understand and negotiate their distress with others. Jan Wallcraft and Kim Hopper (Chapter 6) and Anne Plumb (Chapter 13) explore this issue in different ways. Moreover, people without obvious trauma histories might find the idea that their madness is a response to trauma difficult to relate to. In these situations, where there is a need to accommodate difference and diversity, perhaps we can learn valuable lessons from the neurodiversity movement (see Steve Graby, Chapter 16). An acceptance of people's different 'ways of being' in the world potentially gets around the problem of entitlement to services and support. This is because it doesn't deny that some people may need accommodations; especially in a social world organised around a set of dominant norms and values which may be at odds with some other marginalised ways of being.

Indeed it may be that there is a failure of imagination when faced with envisioning reasonable adjustments to issues of madness and distress, and/or a lack of political will to address these issues. Arguably, this is likely to be the case when the 'bottom line' in prevailing society is economic profit rather than compassionate contexts and relationships (Spandler and Stickley, 2011). The development of societies which are more mentally (as well as physically) enabling is clearly a pressing issue here. Societies need to be organised in ways that are both less distressing for their members – in terms of combating abuse, neglect, poverty, oppression and inequality; all common predictors of mental distress (Bentall, 2003; Rogers and Pilgrim, 2010; Poole et al, 2013; Read et al, 2014) – *and* more accepting and tolerant of difference, diversity and madness.

We have spent some time discussing the unsettling nature of madness because we think it is particularly tricky to address and therefore requires careful articulation. However, we are acutely aware that it is difficult to create the kind of society described above without also addressing the issue of pathologisation.

The pathologisation of madness

The dominant societal response to expressions of unreason and irrationality is pathologisation; that is, individuals are described and/or treated as psychologically abnormal. The problem of pathologisation is well-rehearsed in the critical mental health literature, so we won't dwell on it too much here. Suffice to say that modern society, via psychiatry and medicine, has drawn (some would argue, artificial) distinctions between the sane and the insane; the normal and the abnormal; the rational and the irrational. In each case these distinctions have served to socially exclude the latter (Foucault, 1967). In contrast to physical disability, where a *part* of the person is considered 'impaired', in mental health the whole self is implicated and discredited. This has enormously damaging implications for the person, who can be seen as a 'non person' by others and can have their rights negated (see Bhargavi Davar, Chapter 15). Szasz described this as 'cruel compassion'; the idea that designating someone as 'mentally ill' and in need of help takes away their agency and disenfranchises them (Szasz, 1973). Rights-based legislation notwithstanding, mad people can still be legally detained and treated against their will, on the grounds of being of 'unsound mind'. Indeed radical mental health activists often point to the spectre of coercion and forced treatment of mad people which, they argue, can derail supposedly progressive social policies such as recovery and social inclusion and even trump human rights legislation. It is worth noting that David Webb (in Chapter 11) refers to forced treatment not as the 'elephant' but as the 'giant gorilla in the room' in human rights discussions.

This pathologisation of madness is often reduced to (but not fully captured by) the notion of *stigma*. Thus many mental health campaigns have set out to combat stigma, especially the public perception that associates madness with violence. However, by emphasising the notion that 'mental illness is an illness like any other', such strategies have arguably been counterproductive (Corrigan and Watson, 2004; Read et al, 2006). That may be because, while trying to remove blame from the individual and family, they simultaneously introduce, or reinforce, mystifying ideas of brain disease and biochemical imbalances. Perceived to be at the mercy of their neurochemistry, people may appear more, rather than less, frightening to others. Read et al (2006a) argue that explanations for madness and distress that are more social would result in less stigma and discrimination, because they enable people to understand, empathise and relate to a person's behaviour in the context of their life. A number of chapters pursue this logic (especially that by Shelley Briggs and Fiona Cameron, Chapter Eight).

If madness was not pathologised, and there was not the threat of coercion, it might be easier for a person to identify as having mental health problems. However, without this identification, and in the absence of some other physical impairment, it is difficult to see how one can logically identify as 'disabled'. Given such pathologisation, there is a price for adopting the identity of someone who is mad or mentally impaired, but also to electing *not* to. If we elect not to, then we may be excluded from the protection of certain policies, disability welfare payments and even mental health services, where some kind of diagnosis is usually a precondition. For example, people find themselves in danger of losing their welfare benefits and social care support, or discharged by a psychiatrist or community mental health team, if they are not seen as having a *legitimate* mental illness. Indeed employers have defended themselves against cases brought by people with mental health problems, by arguing that the Disability Discrimination Act (1995) or the Equalities Act (2010) did not apply because the person did not have, or did not disclose, a 'clinically well-recognised' mental illness. Employers might ask: how can we make *reasonable adjustments* if you don't tell us what it is that we need to adjust *to*? Ironically then, one could argue that people need to be pathologised before they can claim certain disability rights.

This Catch 22 situation places people with mental health problems in something of a double bind (Bateson et al, 1956). If they accept that they are mentally ill, it appears to discredit their selfhood and capacity (their reason, sanity and rationality) and they risk pathologisation. Conversely, if they resist this identity, they may be unable to get the support and protection they may need (and they are likely to be pathologised anyway). This conundrum is explored in Jasna Russo's and Debra Shulkes' chapter (Chapter Two) and Bill Penson's chapter (Chapter Four). It is also addressed by Tina Minkowitz (Chapter Twelve) and David Webb (Chapter Eleven) through their notion of 'perceived' or 'attributed' disabilities. Here it is possible to be considered disabled because of an attribution of impairment by others, even if that impairment is contested by the person themselves. This is a potentially important development because, where people are treated *as if* they are disabled and may be medically treated (often against their will), they may need disability protection, regardless of how they choose to see themselves. This raises the interesting question of whether it is disability, and not simply human rights, protections that are required. In the UK there is now one Equality Act which incorporates all previous equality legislation relating to, for example, gender, race and disability. However, the question still remains: should mental health be subsumed under disability within such laws (as it currently is in the Equalities Act)? If the United Nations were to follow the UK example, and have an overarching equality (rather than a disability) convention, would we still need a distinctive category to protect the rights of people labelled as mad or mentally ill (as well as provisions relating to race, gender, disability etc)?

Where does this leave people struggling with madness and distress? The final section explores the implications of these issues for individuals who have to navigate this tricky terrain.

Negotiating a mad/disabled identity

In the context of the above, there are numerous responses that an individual can make to the madness/disability conundrum. First, they can reject the notion that they have a mental health problem or 'impairment' entirely, and refuse to accept any attribution of this by others. This is a resistance stance of some power, which may work for an individual at certain times, and is supported by the notion of 'perceived' disability. However, this stance may still make it difficult for people to access support or services; or to benefit from disability policies, including the UN Convention which is still underpinned by some notion of underlying impairment.

Even if one identifies as distressed, mad or mentally ill, a number of factors may prevent one from taking the next step: identifying as disabled (or being identified by others as such). Whereas the critical mental health (and emerging 'mad studies') literature has quite a lot to say about the assertive ways in which users/survivors might dispute the relevance of impairment or disability to their situation (Plumb, 1994; Beresford et al, 2010), it has less to say about the deeply felt sense of diffidence or shame which can attach to making a disability claim that one believes may be illegitimate or rejected by others. Therefore, in the above scenario, I may assert – on the basis of arguments such as those rehearsed earlier – that it is illegitimate for you to label me as 'mentally ill' or 'impaired' and that I reject such a positioning *myself*. In the second, I may feel that any claim I make to being disabled will be deemed illegitimate *by others*.

In January 2014 a twitter chat took place, in response to the question, 'Why are people with mental health problems reluctant to describe themselves as disabled?'[4] This helped inform our understanding of the difficulties faced by individuals in the second scenario: that is, those who may feel that they need a disabled identity in order to access effective support, understanding and services. Contributors to this discussion described their fear of being deemed a malingerer by others. For example, one person said that they didn't identify as disabled because they have been told so often that they are lazy or attention seeking. Mental health services themselves may reinforce the need for such pretence. Another contributor suggested that, in an age dominated by 'recovery', it is not acceptable to have enduring mental health issues. Indeed, this was one of the drivers for the so-called recovery philosophy, the idea that if someone is told they are 'disabled', and as a result, receives long-term disability payments, then they have little incentive to, or belief that they will, recover. More broadly, within society, there can be a lack of awareness of the often debilitating impact of mental health issues, and how certain mental health difficulties can compound each other (hearing voices for example, can result in depression and anxiety). Chapters by Donna Reeve (Chapter 7) and Shelley Briggs and Fiona Cameron (Chapter 8) address the complex interrelationship between a person's social experiences, their mental health difficulties and the impact of disablement; all of which can reinforce each other.

The above concerns can result in a reluctance to assume a disabled identity, for fear of somehow *over-claiming*. The association of disability with serious, long-term, and permanent impairment, can result in a sense that unless one has a lifelong condition, one should not claim to be 'disabled'. One contributor to the twitter chat suggested that they don't always feel that the term mental health fits, and don't want to use the term in a way that seems flippant. It seems clear that these concerns relate to the (real and/or feared) attitudes of others, which can be internalised. This process was encapsulated by another contributor who suggested that she had, in the past, received the message from psychiatrists that she wasn't 'mad enough'. This internalisation is similar to *psycho-emotional disablism* described by Carol Thomas (1999), and see Donna Reeve's chapter (Chapter Seven), where people 'take in' other people's projections about their impairment, which can adversely affect their identity and sense of self.

This stance may include all kinds of assumptions and projections about disabled people by people with mental health problems, for example as being *necessarily* vulnerable and in need of care, an assumption long criticised by the disabled people's movement (Hunt, 1966; Finkelstein, 1980). However, the concerns expressed in this twitter discussion all relate to not feeling *legitimately* disabled and therefore not entitled to the protection and support one might (or should) expect if one were so. This is important to bear in mind, because it means that some people may feel that they are not *deserving* or worthy of support and rights. Here, it is difficult to disentangle an individual's own felt sense of (lack of) legitimacy and entitlement from that which is projected onto them by others.

Many of the barriers to identifying as disabled seem to link to two related issues, both of which concern understanding. First, understanding in the sense of comprehending the nature of madness or distress (that is, the fact that mental health is such a contested issue gets in the way of defining its relationship with disability). Second, understanding in the sense of sympathetic awareness, compassion and tolerance (of oneself and others).

In the meantime, it remains the case that in order for people with mental health problems to benefit from disability policies and legislation, they usually require some kind of identifiable 'impairment' with which to bargain. In the absence of alternative bargaining chips it seems that we may be stuck with the concepts of mental illness and/ or disability, however unpalatable they may be.

Conclusion

This chapter has explored disconnections between policy discourse that conceives of people with mental health problems as disabled, and the positions taken by individuals experiencing madness and distress. We have explored some potentially tricky questions about the nature of madness in relation to issues of reason and rationality; the pathologisation and social exclusion of mad people; and the negotiation of a disability identity in the context of questions of legitimacy and entitlement. We think it may be difficult to put radical ideas (and progressive polices) into practice unless we can more fully understand the issues set out here. Many academic and policy discussions in mental health, especially those framed within a social model of disability (for example, Sayce, 2000; Repper and Perkins, 2003; Slade et al, 2014), seem to side-step these concerns. Perhaps it can feel safer when a problem is ascribed to external, often abstract, factors such as social barriers, stigma and discrimination (or even mental health laws). However, issues relating to unreason, rationality and pathologisation are not easily reducible to stigma and discrimination, and highlight some key challenges in applying disability policy to mental health. More than this, they potentially highlight some fundamental tensions at the heart of radical mental health politics.

One thing seems clear: the tricky issues we have raised here are likely to remain with us for the foreseeable future, so we need to find ways to think about and address them. Although this chapter may have covered familiar territory, we have tried to shed new light on old issues in the context of the specific focus of this book. Some of these issues will be revisited, close up, in succeeding chapters; others, just glimpsed here, await further thinking and debate.

Notes

[1] For example, see http://makingrightsmakesense.wordpress.com/2014/06/02/we-need-to-talk-about-the-elephant-trap-in-the-room/.

[2] However, the Mental Capacity Act can be overruled by Mental Health law, meaning that it no longer applies when a person is subject to the Mental Health Act (for example, if they are detained).

[3] http://en.wikiquote.org/wiki/George_Bernard_Shaw.

[4] Hosted by the Everyday Ableism Project which aims to promote open discussion about 'all aspects of disability, illness, and mental health': @EverydayAbleism.

TWO

What we talk about when we talk about disability: making sense of debates in the European user/ survivor movement

Jasna Russo and Debra Shulkes

Introduction

The European Network of (ex)-Users and Survivors of Psychiatry (ENUSP) is the place where the two of us met. An independent, grassroots organisation, ENUSP is run by and for people who have experienced psychiatric treatment. It connects regional, national and local organisations and individuals across 39 European countries. We joined the network at different points in time and from different places. Like other participants, we brought in our personal experiences of madness and psychiatric treatment together with our own expectations and visions of political organising. What profoundly connects us is our interest in each other's experiences and opinions, a deep sense of solidarity, and also a desire to learn about and from other users/ survivors.

Our joint work on this text is an expression of this attitude. Rather than starting off with any imperative to resolve the dilemma – distress or disability?[1] – we want to bring our views into dialogue and explore where that leads us. We do not argue for one particular political strategy; our suggested way forward for organisations and networks of users/survivors is this very commitment to allowing the free communication of our convictions and also our doubts. Yet, we know from our experiences of international activism that achieving an atmosphere of respect for all our differences is not as easy and self-evident as it may seem.

Hoping to enlarge the space for freedom of thought in our movement, we will share our evolving personal perspectives about the controversial concept of disability. We will use our knowledge of key discussions and developments around disability within ENUSP as a frame of reference and explore how we can move from thinking as individuals or single organisations to taking international action. Our initial search of the network's records suggests three distinct levels on which users and survivors in Europe discuss the concept of disability. First, there is a personal level connected with the use of 'disabled' as a possible identity for people with psychiatric histories. Second, there is a socio-economic level, related to the fact that many users and survivors who receive state welfare support are classified as disabled. Finally, there is an organisational dimension concerning the adoption of a disability framework as a strategy for our political organising and advocacy. Problematically, these three levels are often blurred in heated discussions about disability in our movement. We believe, however, that they need to be distinguished so that we can reach a deeper understanding of what is at stake. We will therefore consider these different levels in turn. Before we do this, we want to share how we first responded to the framing of our experiences of madness and distress in terms of disability.

Reverberations of 'disability'

Our coming together and organising politically as people who have been subjected to psychiatric treatment is usually motivated by very personal experiences. Those experiences do not just concern things like diagnosis and treatment. When we gather together internationally, we also bring in our knowledge and experiences of the different contexts in which we live. These contexts are sometimes very far from each other in terms of politics, economy, culture, social and welfare systems, language, prevailing beliefs, and so on. However connected we may feel, the fact remains that words like *mental illness*, *patient*, *survivor* and *hospital admission* resonate with us in different ways and reflect different personal and social realities. *Disability* is one of these words. It has distinct meanings for individuals in the network, who inhabit different geo-political regions. Due to a considerable gap in economic development, there is a vast disparity in the impact of being classified as disabled in these places. While the status might allow people to live independently in some western countries, in many eastern European states, disability payments are so inadequate that their recipients cannot afford even the most basic independent accommodation.

The two of us also had our own initial reactions to the surfacing of a disability framework within ENUSP. These reactions mark key moments in our ever-shifting relationships to the concept of disability; they are part of our realities as people, necessarily imperfect and confined by our own histories. Though speaking about these realities can be surprisingly hard, we believe it is vital that everyone has the freedom to communicate them openly and honestly, without immediately being judged and corrected. This freedom is, we maintain, a precondition for individual and collective growth.

Jasna

Late 1996, Berlin. We are having the last Board meeting before the third ENUSP conference. Unexpectedly I learn that ENUSP has joined the European Disability Forum by a decision of the chairs. My world falls apart. The world that has just opened up for me two years earlier when I finally found all these people; people with whom I could share so much, feel so close to and work together against all the awfulness and injustice of psychiatry. I suddenly learn that I was wrong to believe that things are all right with me. I learn that, at the end of the day, I do have a disability. What for so long I invested in un-learning, I now have to learn again. Coming from my peers this hits me differently than when it came from a psychiatrist. Everything in me rebels and hurts at the same time.

I leave the meeting in a rage and sit myself in the bar next door. Berlin is where I live, I organised this meeting, and now have to wait for everybody so I can direct them to dinner. Drinking Southern Comfort, I think of my friend Jessie whom I met on the ward in my country of origin (the former Yugoslavia). At the age of 26, on the grounds of her psychiatric diagnoses, she was declared disabled and put on a pension. Unlike the situation in countries like Denmark and UK, the monthly sum she was assigned meant that she could never afford to move away from the horrors of her parents' house. Her new legal status was also not subject to revision. She was sentenced to life-long misery, which she escaped from by killing herself shortly after her 28th birthday. I think of her and remember her funeral. I feel so alone and miss her. I hate disability pension and the chairs of ENUSP. I hate the whole board and the whole world. Then I walk everybody to dinner and stay with them talking about other things.

Debra

March 2009, Brussels. I'm sitting in a hotel conference room at my first ENUSP meeting. I look around nervously at these 25 people I've just met: they are activists from all over the European Union. I stare down at the coffee mug in my hands, trying to find the words that will justify my presence here. I have never done this before, never been in a user/survivor group. I found ENUSP on the Internet where I spend so much time now searching desperately for something that may not exist: a place where I can talk freely about the psychiatric history that dogs me…I worry I am never going to be able to deal with any of it: my treatment in a mental hospital ten years ago on another continent: the label applied to me by psychiatrists and inscribed now on every health record. Worse, it exists inside me, stoking my deepest fear: there is something innately wrong with me. I am defective, dangerous, subhuman. Anger surges through me as I think about these things. This is what has brought me to this meeting. This, and the word 'survivor'. It is a beacon; it has real power and brings comfort.

I listen to what delegates are saying. Through all our different accents, I hear similar strains in people's accounts of what their lives are like and how they ended up in the mental health system. They use ordinary, human words: they had a crisis, they were stressed out, grief-stricken, abused, they were in the wrong place at the wrong time. I sit up when someone says it is devastating to be a psychiatric patient and that no-one would want the life you're left with.

I like this environment. Up to now, I have only attended a conference for professionals from which I came away feeling alone and violated. But this space is very different. It is strange and wonderful to be somewhere where the conversation is so crucial and pressing. For once, I am not frightened about the language that might be given to my experience.

Then someone mentions 'disability'. The word barely registers at first. It's ENUSP's representative from the European Disability Forum talking. He's showing us slides about user/survivor groups, pointing out our total lack of money and power compared with everyone else; he says we are not on the national councils of disabled people. I hear him say that we are all people with psychosocial disabilities. I opt out instinctively. I understand being disabled as a personal identification and I respect that others make it. But I can't bear to be told what I am. As it happens, I do not even try to access disability benefits because to do so, I would need to have a psychiatric assessment, and I feel that would kill me.

Later in the day, someone else describes a new human rights treaty called the Convention on the Rights of Persons with Disabilities. She says it absolutely covers psychiatric survivors. That it bans forced psychiatric treatment and even names it as torture. I don't know quite what to make of this, but it feels like a way forward. I sense the weight of the United Nations and the law behind her words, and I am hopeful and excited.

Three levels of disability debates

The background for our work on this chapter is the longstanding disagreement among members of ENUSP about the relevance of the concept of disability for users and survivors of psychiatry. This has been a point of contention since fairly early on in the network, and it has flared up periodically over its 22-year history. To get a better sense of vying opinions on the topic, we revisited the records available to us (ENUSP, 1994; 1997; 2009; 2010). This search was in no way an attempt to draw definitive conclusions about what is a rich and complex story, much of which remains within the memories of people, rather than in formal documents.

What our archival work made clear, however, is that there are several levels on which the concept of disability has been, and continues to be, debated among European users and survivors. They include what might be called a personal level, which refers to the place of disability in the self-understanding and self-identification of the network's members. In this regard, the majority of people see themselves as users or survivors of psychiatry, and not as people with disabilities. Some individuals strongly reject the application of a disability framework to their experiences, while a small number have started to identify as people with psychosocial disabilities.

Our search also uncovered a second level of discussion which connects disability with the dire socio-economic situation of many people with psychiatric histories. Many users and survivors in Europe are officially categorised as 'disabled' based on a psychiatric assessment that they have a serious medical condition (mental illness). This status entitles them to basic income or living support, usually in the form of disability benefits or a pension, and also includes some disability-based concessions (for example, with transport). This is a critical concern given the increase in poverty experienced by long-term psychiatric patients.

Finally, we encountered an organisational level of debate referring to the calls from part of our movement for the adoption of a disability framework as a strategy to increase the network's influence and achieve key human rights goals. This debate has intensified since the 2006 adoption of the United Nations Convention of the Rights of People with Disabilities (CRPD), a treaty created with vital contributions from international user/survivor activists. The convention opens up many opportunities to contest the abuses perpetuated against our people as violations of international human rights law. However, the question remains whether we must do so as 'people with psychosocial disabilities'.

Reflecting on these disability debates, which have often been highly emotionally charged and filled with antagonism, we noticed an almost continual blurring of these three levels as though they involve the same issues. We consider this situation to be detrimental both to the content and the culture of the debate around disability in our movement. Believing that all three levels – personal, socio-economic and organisational – are equally important, we maintain that it is possible to examine them separately without discounting the worth of any one of them. Further, we think this step is essential if we are to have an open and inclusive conversation about the disability framework within our movement. Though our reflections below took shape in the context of our involvement with ENUSP, our thinking about these issues goes beyond this particular network.

The personal level: the right to name our own experience

Many of us who identify as service users or survivors have experienced the imposition of a psychiatric 'expert' account over our own. This imposition may even lead to the complete loss of our own account and a long process of re-establishing the credibility of our own story and our views. Finding our own words again, reclaiming the right to say how it was for us, and finding others with whom we can share and think through that experience, without being assessed and diagnosed, are all crucial parts of our political organising. In her insider research into the US consumer/survivor/ex-patient movement, Linda

Morrison accurately observes that 'the power to name and define the experience of the self is at stake' (Morrison, 2005, xii). People with a psychiatric diagnosis know very well what it means to have a foreign, pathologising framework imposed on our experiences and our personhood. Reclaiming the authority to speak for ourselves, including the very act of acquiring an identity other than 'mentally ill', has huge emotional and political significance.

As survivor activists, we are convinced therefore that the matter of our name – what we are to call ourselves, and how we are to understand ourselves – is never 'just' a question of semantics. The decisive aspect of any act of naming is always the question of *who* is doing that naming. There is a world of difference between embracing an identity for yourself and having a label applied to you: 'Re-defining someone's reality for them is the most insidious and the most devastating form of power we can use. It may be done with the best of intentions, but it is wrong scientifically, professionally, and ethically' (Johnstone, 2013).

Knowing that peers can also re-define each other's realities, we really appreciate the efforts of our international movement to allow room for different standpoints and self-definitions. At the same time, we are aware that such room cannot be endless if we – different as we are – want to unite and act on issues of importance to us all. It may be that taking on a collective identity always compromises our personal one, and this is a price that everyone pays for involvement in political organisations. Even so, when we reflect on the difficult and delicate task that was undertaken by (former) psychiatric patients across Europe in finding a name under which we could all work together, we find great value in that process itself. The adoption of *user and survivor* identities has helped us to articulate and develop our own political agenda over the last two decades. However imperfect these terms may be, they also represent powerful and emancipatory acts of collective self-identification: 'For me, being able to choose what to call myself – and how to think of myself – was essential. I identified as a survivor, and in so doing, could finally explore and understand my experience. It was transformative to be in dialogue with others who were also doing this' (Shulkes, 2013 unpublished ms).

In contrast, *disability* identity has been introduced into our movement in Europe largely with the aim of achieving certain organisational and advocacy goals. Recently we have also come across an implicit, and sometimes openly stated, demand that we all adopt the disability framework. This has started to interfere with people's right to self-define. It is often accompanied by an insistence that a collective identification as disabled is essential if we are to succeed in pursuing human rights claims, or indeed to have any future at all as a political movement. These opposing opinions expressed in the ENUSP online discussion forum (February 2013) capture this debate:

> If we don't accept the concept 'disability', we have nothing to do with the CRPD anymore, and cannot claim any of the rights that the CRPD confers to us.
>
> If we are not allowed to question the concept of psychosocial disability unless we have an alternative model/framework to pull out of our pocket, I don't know how we are to work towards common understanding and define common goals in our organisations. Taking our thinking and our action forward requires open discussion, respect and interest in each other's lives, courage to unpack the taboos.

While acknowledging our alliances with the disabled people's movement as a valid possibility for mutual learning, exchange and joint actions – for all the reasons described above – we maintain that evangelism and ultimatums cannot be the way forward. Personal identification remains a vital ethical issue in our organisations precisely because so many of us were robbed of the right to find the meaning of our experiences. There can't be any right or wrong when it comes to self-definition. Instead, an open-ended exploration of what different terms and concepts mean to different people might be the only way to take our thought and action forward.

The socio-economic level: the price of subsistence

Many people with psychiatric histories in Europe are officially classified as disabled based on a psychiatric diagnosis, and they subsist on a disability pension or benefits. Discussions in our movement about whether users and survivors should accept the label 'disabled' cannot be separated from the reality that for many of us the options for economic survival are slim. This is especially true at a time of ideologically driven welfare cuts which are forcing people in many countries into unsafe and oppressive work conditions. In this situation, securing one's day-to-day existence is a more urgent concern than the right to self-define, or the rather theoretical question of what constitutes a 'psychiatric disability'. We are aware that many individual users/survivors are politically silenced and cannot challenge the concepts and systems on which their most basic needs depend. For all these reasons, it seems even more important that our representative organisations take a different approach. Unlike individual users/survivors, they are in a position not only to defend people's urgent rights and demand a social safety net, but also to challenge and examine the dominant concepts imposed on us. Furthermore, knowing the realities of madness, distress and psychiatry, our organisations are also equipped to develop alternative solutions. Writing about the importance of the language that we choose as thinkers and activists, Canadian activist, Bonnie Burstow, suggests 'that we look beyond survivors in the-here-and-now and ask how our language will affect the larger world, and what type of world it helps create' (Burstow, 2013, 89). So, with this in mind, we ask ourselves: what constitutes a psychiatric disability?

Officially, there is a diagnosis of 'mental illness', but we know that this has never been proven to have any valid biological basis. Even so, the emotional and other difficulties that many of us experience are real and can disrupt what is considered to be a normal life course. For example, it may be particularly hard to complete education or stay in employment in competitive settings that demand consistent performance. Continuing mental health difficulties, fluctuating crises or extreme states of mind can have similar effects to disablement. However, this doesn't mean that these phenomena are rooted in any kind of brain malfunction or mental impairment. A recent inquiry among UK service users into their attitudes around the social model of disability confirms that 'while many felt they were "disabled" as mental health service users, they did not necessarily see this as underpinned by some actual specific impairment' (Beresford et al, 2010, 26).

We maintain that the impact of psychiatric treatment may itself be intrinsic to what counts as 'psychiatric disability'. Psychiatric interventions can damage and jeopardise both physical health and people's capacity to think, feel and trust. We rarely become stronger and wealthier after psychiatric experience. Procedures such as electroshock and neuroleptic drugging can cause irreparable physical damage; diagnoses pathologise our experiences and our personhood, and mean that we are likely to face discrimination. Our self-esteem and self-confidence usually decrease after psychiatry and our social, work and love lives are more likely to worsen than to flourish. This 'iatrogenic disability' (disability caused by psychiatric treatment) disappears in the notions of both 'mental illness' and 'mental impairment'. Maybe in our day-to-day struggles, it really doesn't matter where all the difficulties come from once they are there. Nevertheless, we believe that it is important for our movement to carefully examine and address the exact nature of 'psychiatric disability' and to keep exposing the central role of psychiatric treatment in the process of our disablement.

Even though the disablement experienced by users/survivors might have similar or even the same effect as other kinds of disabilities, one fundamental difference remains: 'mental illness' cannot just be pronounced equivalent to physical or sensory impairment. Aware that the latter is also being challenged as a construct, we maintain that people with psychiatric experience cannot simply adopt the social model of disability one-on-one without further examining the nature of the 'impairment' in our case. This powerful, emancipatory model resulted from the efforts of disabled people themselves. However close these experiences are to our own, simple appropriation of this achievement cannot replace equivalent systematic work and effort needed from users/survivors ourselves. It remains our task to work towards a similarly comprehensive framework for understanding madness and distress which does justice to *our* experiences and *our* lives in the same way that the social model of disability captures the realities of many disabled people. Working towards our own framework is also likely to shed light on the struggle we often have in translating concepts that are useful to the disability movement like 'barriers' and 'reasonable accommodation':

> [W]e can claim that society is disabling us by not making space for us to be who we are and by not giving us the help and support we need and deserve to live alongside others in a useful, constructive, integrated way. The idea of 'reasonable accommodation' should be applied to us as much as to people who can't see, or people in wheelchairs, in that workplaces or work generally should be made accessible to us, in whatever way is suitable, such as allowing us to work from home, or to use an iPod while working, or to have time off to see a therapist, or whatever is needed to enable us to do work that we can do and make a contribution to society. Such contribution may also be by voluntary work rather than being forced into unsuitable jobs. (ENUSP discussion forum, February 2013)[2]

We fully support these rights claims. However we find ourselves asking: why should having a psychiatric diagnosis be the pre-condition for accessing these rights? Shouldn't they be available to all whose lives are disrupted by distress or madness? We believe that any person can come up against a situation which renders it difficult for them to exist and function in the world; we would rather have a society where the right to an adequate standard of living and support was not based on arbitrary medical expert assessment that reinforces 'othering'.

Given the way the societies in which we live are currently organised (around neoliberal principles of profit and individual competition), we certainly do not see acceptance or rejection of an official status of disabled as a free personal choice. But rather than sharpening divisions among users/survivors around this issue, we suggest shifting our attention to collective action. As people who *know* madness and distress, and have also experienced dominant societal responses to it, we are responsible for further exploring, advancing and sharing our knowledge to achieve a different, non-damaging and non-medical framework. Inspired and encouraged by the social model of disability, we also see no one better equipped for this task than ourselves. Our joint efforts in this direction could lead us beyond divisions based on psychiatric assessments to 'a society brave and moral enough to eschew the whole paradigm of mental health and illness, replacing it with a creation of real community, and real help' (Shimrat, 2013, 156).

The organisational level: achieving our advocacy goals

Survivors of psychiatry have long exposed the violence and degradation we endured in the name of care and treatment as *human rights abuses.* We have argued that the special laws, labels and 'treatments' devised for us alone amount to discrimination. However, these claims have lacked external recognition, being roundly ignored and dismissed by governments, psychiatrists, courts and the public. While our quest for equal rights is not new, what has shifted in recent times is the basis on which it is being pursued. Increasingly, human rights advocates, both within and outside our movement, are identifying us as beneficiaries of the UN Convention on the Rights of Persons with Disabilities. This treaty provides a solid and prominent international platform from which to launch our human rights claims.

The convention has justly been celebrated as a remarkable achievement by and for user/survivors globally. Our extraordinary influence on the negotiation and drafting process marked a moment of political participation and influence unheard of in the short history of our international movement. This was the fruit of a unique, equal partnership with international disabled people's organisations:

> Working together closely, over the course of several years, in person at the UN and by email discussions, we brought user/survivor issues into the heart of the disability

movement and found a rich common ground. (WNUSP, 2008, 4)

While our exact identity as disabled people is not clear in the convention – the language of 'persons with a psychosocial disability', suggested by some WNUSP activists, did not make it into the text – our values and our voices resound throughout.

It is this enshrining in international law of human rights *defined from a user/survivor perspective* that makes this treaty such a powerful tool for our advocacy. The users/survivors who drafted the CRPD aimed to bring an end to practices that deny our equal personhood and dignity such as forced psychiatric treatment and guardianship. They also sought to ensure access to a range of voluntary, healing community supports for people who experience emotional crisis. Stunningly, in the years since CRPD adoption, these same activists have succeeded in getting these long-term goals of our movement endorsed by the United Nations, the highest legal and moral authority on human rights abuses. Some UN treaty bodies have urged governments to dismantle their psychiatric detention, coercion and guardianship regimes and to provide a 'wide range of community-based services and supports...that respect the person's autonomy, choices, dignity and privacy, including peer support and other alternatives to the medical model' (CRPD, 2012, paragraph 38). The UN Special Rapporteur on Torture and Other Cruel, Inhuman and Degrading Treatment or Punishment (Méndez, 2013) also recently concluded from the treaty that routine psychiatric practices such as restraint, seclusion and forced drugging constitute torture. This finding profoundly validates our experiences and would not have been thinkable without the convention.

Alongside these breakthroughs, it is hard to ignore a growing debate about the impact of the convention's disability framework on our identity. At the core of this discussion is the question of whether we need to become a movement of people with disabilities in order to contest abuses and assert our human rights. Human rights lawyers and NGOs, increasingly active in post-convention lobbying, have insisted, for example, that if we want a place at the table with governments, we should abandon our outdated user/survivor identities and re-make ourselves as organisations of people with psychosocial disabilities. Moreover, they claim, we must team up with national disabled people's organisations who are stronger, better organised and have more influence.

Perhaps these ultimatums from outside are not surprising. We are, after all, used to having the terms of our participation (as 'the mentally ill', 'consumers' 'people with mental health problems' and so on) laid down by professionals without any consideration of the suitability or meaning of those titles for us. What is more concerning though is the haste of some in our own organisations to declare our transformation to people with disabilities a *fait accompli* and the only enlightened way to move forward. In contrast, the UN bodies that enforce the convention have given no sign that we must identify as disabled in order to access its full protection. They recognise that self-described user/survivor groups are treaty beneficiaries without hesitation, and do not demand that we identify as psychosocially disabled (or as having an underlying impairment). Our right to invoke the convention to end forced treatment and other human rights abuses stays sacrosanct.

Given this situation, we feel that the push within our movement to convert to a disability framework speaks to a desperation about our lack of political influence. To be sure, this is a pressing issue, calling up serious questions about resources and capacity. However, we believe that the strengthening of our organisations cannot happen by way of the strident insistence on a single approach. We also hold that any alliances with the disability movement (or any other political movement) must rest on altogether different principles. What is needed is dialogue among our respective organisations searching for common ground and shared interests. Outside our work as equal partners with disabled activists in developing the convention, we are not aware of any process like this in the history of ENUSP.

Closing thoughts

There are no easy answers to many of the questions we have raised. However, we believe that our discussion demonstrates the value of asking and exploring these tough questions together, even if we do not always arrive at new, groundbreaking answers or agree on every point. We are conscious that these kinds of explorations among us are all too rare. One ENUSP member has legitimately noted that 'there is little room to have evolving thoughts on complex issues' and stressed the difference that opening up such room could make: 'The important thing for me here is not to "win the discussion", but to come to a better understanding' (ENUSP discussion forum, March 2013).

This encourages us to come back to the personal level and share where we have both arrived in our thinking about disability at the time of submitting this chapter (end of 2013).[3]

Jasna

Many years have passed since my first encounter with the concept of disability in ENUSP. In the course of what for a while felt like a personal war, I actually never spoke about my friend Jessie. I learned to slow down my emotions as much as I can. I also learned about different realities and met people for whom the status of disabled continues to be life-saving. If I am honest, I don't know what Jessie would say herself if she was alive. Maybe she would have moved to Denmark and have happily received disability benefits (if she could have accessed them as an immigrant). I don't know. I know that moving to Germany saved me. This is where I finally stopped being a psychiatric patient. The cost of achieving permanent residence here was to never even think about any kind of state support. Maybe that is what formed me. Maybe that is how simple we all are at the end. But there are bigger things than my own little life and my strategies. To me, that is coming together as people labelled mad and establishing our place beyond the place that society and the psychiatric system have designated for us. As I am particularly interested in establishing such a place in the 'science' about us, in recent years I have kept coming across the field of disability studies and emancipatory disability research. I don't need to identify as disabled in order to see the beauty and the potential of this approach. The respect I have for both the social model of disability and the experience of madness prevents me from any attempt to simply bring them together without the due effort that such an undertaking deserves.

Debra

How has my thinking about disability shifted over the last few years? The biggest shift is that I have had the chance to do human rights advocacy with people from our world-wide movement. These activists from the global north and south are extraordinarily varied in backgrounds, experiences, self-definitions etc. Some identify proudly as people with psychosocial disabilities, while others bristle at the thought.

I have been struck by the thinking, advocacy and community work that the UN disability convention is helping these activists to do. This includes long awaited, vital progress towards the recognition of psychiatric force and guardianship as legal and moral wrongs. But it goes further to imagining communities that value and fully respect the rights of people who experience madness and distress. This work gives me hope at both a community and a personal level. I have glimpses of a world where I might be able to move forward with my life as someone who still experiences overwhelming emotional crises. Do I identify, then, as a person with disabilities? The truth is that there are times when I do and times when the phrase feels alien and politically dangerous. I worry that many understand it as a substitute for 'mentally ill'.

'*We, users and survivors of psychiatry and people with psychosocial disabilities*' is the broad, unwieldy phrase I have seen in our documents lately. Right now I am grateful for the space for diverse and shifting self-identifications it offers. I can hear more of our voices speaking in unison, but on their own terms.

There are two things we know for sure. One is that international user/survivor networks include an extraordinary range of people with different backgrounds, experiences and opinions. And the second is that if we commit to working towards common and inclusive principles and positions, this diversity could become our greatest resource. We strongly believe in the power of an ongoing dialogue among us and maintain that this is essential, especially before entering alliances.

Notes

[1] This formulation of this dilemma comes from the working title of this book.

[2] This is a private discussion forum.

[3] We regret that we were not aware at that time of criticism of the ways the user/survivor movement (re)produces disablism (see Withers, 2014) and hope to have a chance to engage with that discussion in the future.

THREE

Inconvenient complications: on the heterogeneities of madness and their relationship to disability

Nev Jones and Timothy Kelly

Our goal, in drafting early versions of the current chapter, was to ask hard questions about the potential synergies between the disability rights movement (and associated academic theory) and mad movement(s). To that end, we initially included a targeted section, centred on recent work on impairment, pain and embodiment within disability theory under the premise that this would facilitate an exploration of how work within disability studies might inform activist theory focused on madness. However, as we struggled through this analysis, we came to feel that our efforts were distinctly premature. While theoretical traction can certainly be gained from hybridisation across and between disparate domains, the complexity of movement-specific identities, social values and theoretical commitments seemed to demand that we grapple with our own problems, before too seriously looking elsewhere.

We came to this task informed and also constrained by our own complicated and often confusing personal experiences of psychosis. If there is a point in the lives of activists when they feel a relative sense of certainty and stability in the way they view the politics of their movement(s), we have not yet reached it. In this sense, our theoretical hesitations undoubtedly reflect a more personal feeling of caution and uncertainty.

Both of us grew up in the shadow of a parent with enduring and, in a very real way, 'disabling' struggles with psychosis. Unlike us, these members of our family – our mothers – live at the margins of society with no voice in either academic circles or centres of political organising. Like Spivak's (1988) subaltern, it is questionable to what extent, in an authoritative or publicly legitimated way, they can speak at all. Our own trajectories have been very different: we will soon join the ranks of the less than 1 per cent of the US population with doctorates; when we speak, at least a large portion of the time, we are able to make ourselves heard. The differences between us (Nev and

Timothy) and between both of us and our mothers, serve as a constant reminder of the often pronounced differences in the experiences of individuals diagnosed or labelled with psychotic disorders in the United States. In our work as clinicians, peer facilitators and researchers, these differences – and their human and sociopolitical costs – have only become clearer and more pressing as time has gone on.

With this personal context – these motivations and concerns – laid out, we turn to our chapter. The first section attempts to set out what we see as the key areas of diversity and variance among individuals labelled with psychiatric disorders, followed by a brief discussion of similar diversity within the disability rights movement. In the second section we include a brief discussion of broad similarities and differences between the user/survivor and disability movements, then turn to a few more concrete differences foregrounded by media perceptions of the Oscar Pistorius trial. We conclude with a discussion of the risks, and importance, of critically interrogating the identity politics internal to madness.

Heterogeneities of madness and disability

There is no single, universally accepted, term for individuals labelled with serious mental illnesses. Instead, the proliferation of terms and labels underscores the many ways in which unusual psychological or mental experiences play out in terms of identity, activist goals and sociopolitical positioning. This multiplicity of positions is further complicated by the fact that the meanings of existing labels themselves fluctuate depending on the particular contexts in which they are deployed.

Discussions of how madness or mental illnesses have come to be constituted as objects of medical discourse are numerous and beyond the scope of this chapter. It is nevertheless worth noting that many influential academic texts, including Canguilhem's *On the Normal and the Pathological* (1950) and Foucault's *History of Madness* (2006), while often illuminating, have implicitly de-emphasised many of the tensions at issue in this chapter. Indeed, in his critique of Foucault's *History*, Derrida (1978) charges the latter with the employment of 'a popular and equivocal notion of the concept of madness…as if…an assured and rigorous precomprehension of madness…were possible and acquired' (p 41). While we readily acknowledge the contributions of careful genealogies of madness as a singular category, our analysis begins from a place of discontent or dis-ease with the inattention paid to the *varieties* of madness and their implications.

Over-generalisation is, of course, not limited to scholarly texts; informal activist discourse also often adheres to parallel processes of ideological narrowing. Pronounced differences in the natural course and meaning of psychosis, ranging from a few limited (sometimes even productive) episodes to chronic, debilitating impairments of language and communication are rarely acknowledged. In activist circles, these processes often occur through the policing of identity claims. For instance, MindFreedom International, a leading activist organisation, describes its members as 'people *labelled* with psychiatric disabilities' (website). This statement emphasises the experience of labelling while distancing itself from or, at the very least, implicitly decentring impairments, limitations or experiential alterations. In terms of activist projects, MindFreedom accordingly focuses on contesting practices of psychiatrisation. Ostensibly less radical consumer activists such as members of the Occupy-affiliated Mental Health Movement in Chicago, have fought to *preserve* psychiatric clinics that primarily serve homeless and/or severely economically marginalised 'consumers' with chronic psychiatric problems.

In her ethnography of the US consumer/survivor movement, Linda Morrison (2005) captures (or inscribes) this tension as a dichotomy between radical activists – those who reject labels and identify as survivors of the psychiatric system – and reformist consumers whom she aligns with the 'biomedical brain disease model of mental illness' (p 168). She observes:

> While the c/s/x [user/survivor] movement is working hard to be inclusive, and represent a range of persons who are oppressed by psychiatry, the consumers who take the arch-conservative position...(analytically, a fully internalised deviance, medicalised deviance, fully psychiatrised position) are seen by the more radical activists to represent the most oppressed psychiatrised group. (p 169)

This characterisation illustrates how insistence on a continued need for care in the face of ongoing impairment can come to be framed as internalised deviance by more anti-psychiatric activists. Thus, in a parallel process to the scholarly work discussed above, differences across and within madness(es) can be obscured under homogenised survivor and consumer identities. In the subsections that follow, we focus on five core areas of this heterogeneity: language; severity and dimension; course or temporal trajectory and intersectionality with other domains of social marginalisation or exclusion.

Language of, and for, madness

In the United States, key identifying terms include: consumer, service user, survivor, person with lived experience, person with (or labelled with) a mental illness, person with a psychiatric disability, and mad or mad-identified. On the surface, each of these terms privileges or centres a particular aspect of psychiatric experience: use or survival of mental health services; first person experience in a general or more specific sense (for example, of mental or psychological differences or protected legal status); distancing from or centring of mad experience as a core sense of personhood (that is, person-first vs mad-first language); and legal status. In practice however, specific sociopolitical trends and geopolitical contexts have further inflected them with a range of more nuanced connotations. For example, the term 'survivor' often indicates a more explicitly political and, at least rhetorically, radical self-positioning than 'consumer', which is negatively linked to Reagan-era neoliberalism in some circles; while 'person with a psychiatric disability' may index a stronger degree of allegiance with US cross-disability organising efforts and coalitional work. These broader cultural inflections notwithstanding, self-identification as a consumer in rural Illinois may signal adherence to a far more radical sociopolitical position than self-identification as a consumer in Western Massachusetts or other centres of alternative mental health activism in the US. Finally, the same individual may use different terms depending on their immediate context. To use ourselves as examples, we typically identify as user/survivors with fellow activists, but as individuals with a psychiatric disability when meeting with university officials in charge of disability-based academic accommodations and as mad-identified in discussions with humanities theorists.

Severity and dimensions

Although explicit hierarchies of severity or suffering are often discouraged in activist discourse, experiences of madness and the severity and dimensions of such experience are in fact extremely heterogeneous. These heterogeneities, in turn, carry important implications with respect to social acceptability, degree of risk for discrimination and social exclusion, centrality to identity and access to valued social roles and norms. What is important is that intersecting sociocultural factors – including race, religion, sexual identity, socioeconomic status and co-morbid chronic illness – have an impact not only on stigma, but on all aspects of mad experience, from meaning to outcome. Thus the relative prevalence of psychiatric disorders, the form that voices or other unusual perceptual experiences take, and the effectiveness and appeal of particular interventions can vary dramatically across cultural and socioeconomic groups.

Multiple empirical studies, including systematic reviews, attest to the divergent ways in which both specific disorders and symptoms are culturally framed and placed into hierarchies (for example, Pescosolido et al, 2010; Schomerus et al, 2012). Both schizophrenia (presented as a categorical diagnosis) and psychotic symptoms typically elicit preferences for substantially greater social distance and higher reported fear than do depression or non-psychotic bipolar symptoms. These differences are mediated by social beliefs concerning diagnostically-based differences in degree of social appropriateness, dangerousness and prognosis (Norman et al, 2012). Even *within* categorical diagnostic domains, specific experiences or symptoms may carry different cultural connotations. Voice hearing, for instance, has recently been tied to a rich history of spiritual experiences and religious revelation (for example, McCarthy-Jones, 2012) while, to our knowledge, no such –genealogical work has been carried out on so-called negative or deficit symptoms or disordered thought found in psychosis, nor on the cognitive difficulties associated with severe depression.

Certain impairments also have different interpersonal consequences. For example, catatonic mutism or severely disorganised speech may have more severe consequences for the person than a preoccupation with unusual beliefs which do not alter their subjective communication to the same degree. To put this more bluntly, the struggles of a distressed individual who can nevertheless communicate with others, can and must be distinguished from an individual with thought disorder so severe that he or she can no longer be understood, even in the most basic of ways. Similarly for some individuals, madness engenders changes in personality and belief capable of driving even the most pacifistic person to acts of symbolic, interpersonal or physical violence (Jones and Shattell, 2014). For others, insight into the consequences of their actions never appears to be compromised.

Mainstream psychiatry's dependence on categorical disorders limits the usefulness of much of this work. However, psychiatric research has helped to establish the differential impact of a range of psychiatric diagnoses. Transnationally, quality of life and distress outcomes are consistently the worst in longitudinal studies of individuals with schizophrenia spectrum diagnoses, followed by bipolar disorder and depression (Goldberg and Harrow, 2004). Symptom dimensions also play out in divergent ways; for example, while voices are found across diagnostic categories, rates of frequent or chronic voices may be substantially higher among individuals diagnosed with schizophrenia versus bipolar or affective diagnoses (Goghari et al, 2012). Side effects of psychotropic medications are likewise not all equally severe; tardive dyskinesia, potentially resulting in irreversible involuntary movements or grimaces, occurs only in the context of antipsychotic use (Tarsy and Baldessarini, 2006) while low-dose antidepressants may have comparatively few serious negative side effects (Papakostas, 2007). However the addictive potential and withdrawal effects of benzodiazepines (primarily prescribed for anxiety) are notoriously severe (O'Brien, 2005).

Finally, some disorders listed in the DSM seemingly occupy a grey zone between the psychiatric and the somatic, organic or neurological. Salient examples include childhood conduct disorders (often categorised as neurodevelopmental disabilities rather than mental illness); anorexia; so-called organic psychoses stemming from traumatic brain injury, neurological conditions, or chronic alcohol abuse; and geriatric dementias (Arciniegas et al, 2001). It is often unclear how, and on what basis, certain conditions, labels or diagnoses have come to be included or excluded in broader categorisations of madness or psychiatric disability by activists, clinicians and scholars. Still other conditions, such as chronic fatigue syndrome, have sparked significant controversy precisely because of the extent to which they blur the boundaries between physical illness and psychological or psychiatric distress (Horton-Salway, 2007).

Course or temporal trajectory

By 'course' we refer not only to specific prognostic patterns (for example, improving or deteriorating symptoms) but also to the differences engendered by ongoing versus episodic experiences of madness, the relative frequency of episodes and the presence of long-term psychiatric problems (or functional disabilities) versus full recovery following a discrete period of distress. In some cases, life trajectories may also involve multiple types of mental health experiences; for example, depression during adolescence, anxiety in college, and paranoia beginning in late young adulthood. The meaning and value of experiences might also change; voices might start out as benign or helpful and only later become more menacing and distressing, or vice versa.

Clinical and activist discourse concerning recovery further colours the social significance of course. In some circles enduring symptoms may be attributed to iatrogenic harm (Whitaker, 2010), to cultural differences such as the relative degree of life stress in particular regions or societies (Myers, 2010) or to biological factors including genetic polymorphisms and inflammation (Sullivan et al, 2012). Recovery and ongoing madness may also be positively or negatively valued. For instance, narratives of recovery may in some cases be offered as examples of desirable individualistic, neoliberal self-overcoming (Myers, 2009) or as testaments to effective external (that is, clinical or pharmacological) intervention. Conversely, among other stakeholders, *on-going* experiences of madness or mental diversity may be positively formulated as sources of creative maladjustment, positive mental diversity or spiritual transformation (Farber, 2012).

Treatment

Likewise, treatment varies widely, both within and across psychiatric diagnoses, not necessarily coincidental with severity, clinical dimension or temporal course. Depending on their history, socioeconomic resources, prevailing family attitudes and social support, individuals with the same set of experiential changes and/or degree of distress might have very different contact with psychiatry. Some may be able to avoid the mental health system entirely and never come in contact with clinicians; others may be prescribed a psychotropic drug by a general practitioner with no other intervention, and still others may be hospitalised voluntarily or involuntarily for extended periods of time. Some individuals might find themselves captured by the forensic mental health system, incarcerated, subject to involuntary outpatient treatment orders, and so on. Others may have sufficient resources, or simply luck, that enables them to avoid these experiences altogether. Treatment may be long- or short-term, intensive or infrequent, harmful or helpful, and all shades in between. Current or ex-service users may come to see very similar treatments or interventions in profoundly different ways. For example, some may perceive maintenance antipsychotics (or even ECT) as life-saving, while others will view these as extremely harmful, perhaps even constituting serious human rights violations.

Intersectionality

All of the domains of heterogeneity listed above should be seen as further complicated by intersections between madness and such factors as race and ethnicity, religious affiliation, gender, class, housing and physical health status. A core tenet of intersectional theory is that confluences of social and biopolitical identity alter experience – not only in degree (that is, additively) but, what is more important, in kind (Collins, 1998). Relative to a white, middle-class college graduate who hears voices, a black, high-school drop-out from a socially deprived neighbourhood who is perceived as paranoid is likely to experience not merely more stigma, but stigma inflected by assumptions which link violence and social dysfunction to blackness, gender, class and mental illness in complex and synergistic ways (compare Metzl, 2009). Social class, including both educational background and degree of poverty or wealth, also profoundly influences access to and type of mental health services and/or community supports (Walker et al, 2012). Identity constructs such as mad pride or consumerism may also develop in ways that reflect or reinforce group-specific norms or assumptions, for instance as a product of predominantly white middle-class values. Notably, the participation of persons of colour in US user/survivor activism and research, particularly in leadership positions, is disproportionately low; a dynamic which rarely merits more than passing reference in either formal publications or informal activist forums (Jackson, 2002).

In our own work within the community mental health system, we frequently cross paths with service users from severely marginalised backgrounds; people living well below the poverty line, dependent on welfare, isolated from family or other social support systems, living in sub-standard group homes or shelters and who in many cases, never had the opportunity to finish high school or attend college. Unsurprisingly, the advocacy goals of individuals living in these circumstances often strongly diverge from those of more privileged activists. Yoga, meditation, intensive psychotherapy and other activities that the latter frequently tout, may understandably appear as frivolous or bourgeois to individuals whose priorities centre on bare essentials such as warm food, housing and basic health care.

Heterogeneities of disability

The experiences generally included in the categories of physical and developmental disability are as wide-ranging and heterogeneous as those implicated in madness. On the severity spectrum, non-psychiatric disabilities range from conditions in which mobility or language may be profoundly affected, even absent, to those in which the impairments in question are invisible and/or minimally impairing, allowing the individual in question to pursue a normal (even conventional) career and life trajectory. Onset and course may be stable, deteriorating (as is most often the case for diseases such as Parkinson's and multiple sclerosis), improving, or episodic (as in certain forms of epilepsy). Type and intensity of service use is equally variable; ranging from occasional physical, cognitive or rehabilitative therapy to institutionalisation and designation as a ward of the courts. Like individuals living under a diagnosis of a serious psychiatric disorder, disabled individuals may be placed high on the socioeconomic ladder, or be forced to live off subsistence-level disability and welfare benefits in public housing projects or group homes.

When a diverse cross-section of disability activists and advocates is considered, there is arguably no more consensus regarding preferred language and the boundaries and terms of identity than exists within the broad user/survivor movement. Some disability activists advocate for person-first language, citing a desire to distance their core sense of personhood from their disability, while others strongly defend disability-first or even explicitly diagnosis-first language (Linton, 1998). Some medical diagnoses, including autism, have been embraced by activists, while others have been strongly rejected, for example hearing impairment or loss versus Deafness (Davis, 1995; Broderick and Ne'eman, 2008).

As is true of user/survivor activism, the disability movement has tended to privilege certain sub-groups and symbols (most notably mobility-based disabilities and the iconic wheelchair) and to exclude others (for example temporary impairments such as broken limbs and in many cases, disabling terminal illnesses such as AIDS and many forms of cancer) often without any clear theoretical justification (Deal, 2003). In this vein, some disability studies scholars have drawn a distinction between so-called healthy and unhealthy disabilities. The latter includes conditions generally understood as illnesses or diseases that lead to deteriorating health, ongoing physical pain and in some cases, premature death, while the former includes more stable impairments that otherwise do not affect physical health in any extreme way (Wendell, 2001). Only members of the former group generally embrace an active disability identity. Finally, as is also the case across diverse user/survivor groups, there are disability advocates who strongly support more medical research and intervention (for example, cochlear implants to restore hearing or a cure for other disabling conditions) and others who see such interventions as oppressive and even, from a more radical perspective, veiled forms of genocide (Blume, 2009).

Across disability and madness

Differences: the cultural construction of identity

While there are thus a number of parallels between the disability and mad movements in an Anglo-American context, this overlap is often more superficial than it might initially appear. Deep culture-bound differences often underwrite diverging public conceptions of the mind, brain and body in ways that have subtly, but fundamentally, influenced the particular sets of institutions and practices that have congealed around them. The brain of autistic neurodiversity activists, for instance, clearly functions in a way that diverges from the brain invoked in critical user/survivor circles even at times when the rhetorical parallels appear strong (compare Ortega, 2009). For many autism activists, the brain appears to serve as a somatic marker of positive (ontologically stable) difference, whereas in user/survivor discourse the brain generally operates as a testament to biopsychiatric processes of biological reductionism and pathologisation.

The historical and sub-cultural trajectories of disability and mad activism have also taken very different shapes; differences mediated by an array of specific institutions and practices. In his special message to congress in 1963 for example, President Kennedy combines mental retardation and mental illness under the umbrella of mental disability, but frames each condition in fundamentally different ways. Advances in biology and pharmacology, he suggests, will eventually lead to cures for mental illness, but prevention takes centre stage vis-à-vis intellectual disability. For example, given links between intellectual disability and pre-natal nutrition, as well as child and maternal health, Kennedy proposes strengthening welfare benefits and early childhood education, while community-level psychosocial interventions are noticeably absent in his strategy for mental illness. This is despite the fact that Kennedy affirms that the majority of the mentally ill could be rehabilitated with progressive community care while retardation, once ensconced, holds no parallel promise of a potential return to normal social and community life. Contemporary medical technologies, including pre-implantation screening, pre-natal testing and elective early abortion have indeed made the prevention of certain intellectual and developmental disabilities possible, to an extent not found in psychiatric disorder, critically shaping both advocacy and the goals and means of public intervention.

It also bears remembering that, from a more global perspective, categories of impairment, disorder and illness may in fact be divided or conjoined in markedly different ways across cultures (Ginsburg and Rapp, 2013). At the most basic level, for instance, western umbrella terms such as disability and madness may simply have no cultural currency or they may be configured according to qualitatively distinct rubrics. Littlewood (1988; 2006) reports that in Trinidad the term *doltishness* includes both intellectual disability and dementias of old age, conditions indicating a relatively normal slowing down of mental functions, while *madness* more narrowly maps onto psychosis and is believed to stem from the involvement of non-human spirits. Conversely, in rural Ireland persons with intellectual disabilities, but not psychosis, are often seen as touched by God by virtue of their divine simplicity. Although the focus of our chapter is explicitly Anglo-American, we discuss these cultural variations in order to foreground the degree to which the etiologies, boundaries and identities of physically or neurologically universal conditions (for example, a broken spinal cord; epilepsy) may radically vary across cultures. Arguably these variations are not absent, but simply subtler, more naturalised or better concealed in western contexts. Conditions such as chronic fatigue syndrome/myalgic encephalitis (CFS/ME) foreground the contemporary liminality of conditions that simultaneously and ambiguously span the psychiatric and the physical, leading to enormous tensions over whether the mind or the body, but not both, is the defining site of pathology or dysfunction.

Differences: violence, vulnerability and narrative

Media coverage of the recent trial of Oscar Pistorius, a celebrated sprint runner and double amputee, underscores several further key cultural distinctions between made between physical disability versus psychiatric disorder. Accused of killing his girlfriend, Reeva Steenkamp, in a moment of either intense fear or jealous rage, Pistorius's status as disabled has been linked with issues of violence in very different ways that other public figures who have psychiatric, particularly psychotic, histories. As Liddiard (2014) describes, physically or developmentally disabled men are rarely depicted as efficaciously violent, but rather simultaneously 'weak, dependent, non-violent, and safe; and yet bitter, caustic, revengeful and angry' (*An (Extra)Ordinary Death*, para 2). While some early commentators focused on the possible benefits of a temporary insanity case, premised on extreme fear, discussion of mental instability more generally has been all but absent. De Wet (2014) reports that, in the light of the Pistorius case, disability activists have, in private, been advocating the provision of subsidised handguns for individuals with disabilities, given their increased risk and vulnerability. This suggestion is strikingly at odds with widespread popular concerns over any form of gun access for individuals with psychiatric (particularly psychotic) histories.

In our reading, a key difference is not just that madness and violence are more tightly coupled in the popular imaginary, but that fears of 'the psychiatrically insane' are uniquely grounded in perceptions of fundamental mental instability, unpredictability and acts of violence. These are seen as explicable in terms of a diagnosis, but generally not by way of a relatable psychological story-line. In place of the understandable, even pitiable fear or insecurity ascribed to a figure like Pistorius, the actions of the psychotic or mentally-ill offender are most often framed as random, coming from nowhere, distinctly non-narrative or *un*emplotted. Indeed the moral un-understandability of violent acts is a core requirement of successful insanity defence pleas according to US Law (Insanity Defense Reform Act, 1984).

But then again...

Each time we mention a specific instance of divergence or intersection between madness and disability we are reminded of the heterogeneities within madness that implicate only some diagnoses or clusters of experience and not others. The history of deinstitutionalisation described in Kennedy's (1963) special statement, for example, is of questionable relevance to individuals with so-called adjustment problems or mild forms of depression and anxiety; even though, over the past few decades, these problems have fallen under the gaze of biopsychiatry and exposed large numbers of people to psychotropic drugs. Likewise, the intersections of violence and madness in both public and legal imaginaries, particularly violence directed at others rather than the self, directly affects only a subset of mental health service users and survivors. In this sense, broad comparisons between physical, intellectual and psychiatric conditions are bound to fail, to the extent that they have not grappled with and unpacked differences within madness and disability.

Up to this point we have perhaps insufficiently stressed the identity politics and potential controversies at stake in our foregrounding of heterogeneity. On the one hand, we risk strengthening and legitimising a hierarchy of suffering or marginalisation within madness, with potentially negative implications for the possibility of coalitional user/ survivor organising. We also arguably risk contributing to the further reification of questionable categories of madness. On the other hand, to leave intra-psychiatric differences untouched would be to allow questionable practices of representational over-reach – such as the continued representation of individuals with very severe, chronic psychiatric issues by those with mild, non-disabling or fully remitted conditions – to continue unchecked. It would also fail to consider the impact of hierarchies of class, education, socially valued identity and access; all factors that so often underwrite these processes of representation and influence.

Conclusion: complications we can't ignore

> Documentation and publication…constitute interventions…
> that affect the rights of other participants…It thus behoves
> practitioners to ask themselves where their work – and not
> just their good intentions – places them in relationship to
> struggles for access to and control over public discourse.
> (Briggs, 2004, 184)

As emphasised in our introduction, we are acutely aware of the extent to which our (largely academic) privilege has enabled us to write, authoritatively (if not expertly), about issues of difference, inclusion and exclusion within the user/survivor experience. Yet it feels important to raise these issues because they rarely make their way into literature on madness or user/survivor discourse. We certainly see our intentions as good but, to borrow from Briggs, how does our 'work…place [us] in relationship to struggles for access…and control'? Our aim is definitely not to intervene in the sense of directly affecting processes of activist representation and leadership, nor, for that matter, to solve anything, even at the level of scholarship. Instead, our goal *at this stage* is to call attention to complications and absences frequently ignored in much academic and activist discourse. We insist that, whether or not more constructive directions are then taken, these complications be acknowledged and addressed.

FOUR

Unsettling impairment: mental health and the social model of disability

William J Penson

Introduction

This chapter advances an account of the social model of disability (SMD) that questions impairment and the application of the model in the areas of mental health and distress. It does so by critically examining the relationship between *impairment* and the *social,* which, in a simplistic application of the social model, is often taken as unproblematic. The concerns voiced here cannot be resolved within the chapter, nor without the involvement of a mad and disabled constituency. That said, my purpose is to advance a critique that unsettles notions of impairment in both psy science (this is the term used throughout this chapter to denote the psychiatric and clinical psychological sciences) *and* the social model of disability. Whether or not this critique suggests the necessity of a different iteration of the social model for mental health remains to be seen, and it should not be read as a criticism of the achievements made for disabled people through the application of the social model so far. Rather, this chapter aims to crystallise what I believe is a crucial tension in advancing the rights of people with mental health problems who identify as disabled. This tension is that if medical and psy sciences lack the evidence to supply a cogent account of impairment in mental health, then the social model of disability, which relies equally on notions of impairment, is destabilised. The dilemma is whether the social model can, or should, overlook this unsettled impairment.

The shifting ground of impairment and disability.

The social model of disability is ensconced in disability and equality legislation, which considers long-standing psychosocial distress to be a disability while relying upon psychiatric diagnoses and classification. The social model is, moreover, widely acknowledged as the preferred way for disabled people to have their needs met and to articulate their experience. While the social model appears to have been embraced, legislation, policy and practice remain clinical, using the language of the helping professions. Take for example the following passage from an article in the British Psychological Society's (BPS) periodical *The Psychologist*: '*Most of the time we think* about *clinical conditions*, such as autism or ADHD or schizophrenia or depression, individually. Yet *in reality* it is *extremely common* for people to show more than one condition together' (Ronald, 2014, 164, my emphasis). This article was written less than a year after the BPS published its position on the then new diagnostic manual, DSM5, stating that it would recommend psychologists not to use DSM5 in clinical practice because it lacks validity and pathologises everyday experience (BPS, 2013). Yet Ronald goes on to celebrate aspects of diagnostic changes in the new DSM5. When the quote above is read with my emphasis we see an invitation to join the author's assertion and professional positioning (we), that there are accepted entities for study and treatment (clinical conditions), and that there is both an epistemological and an ontological certainty (in reality). Furthermore, we are invited to accept that clinical diagnostics arriving at a singular diagnosis are partially correct, and those that arrive at an integrated diagnosis offer a different scale of accuracy. I suggest that Ronald's quote exemplifies the current situation in mental health and the social model of disability. That is, that despite the demands of law and policy, and the disciplinary objections to unscientific diagnostics, it remains permissible for disciplines to continue to objectify disabled people. Snyder and Mitchell (2006) point out that this can even be a problem within service user-led research.

A critical, historical account of disability highlights the intersection of ideas and practices that made possible the 'disabled person'. Ideas about impairment are crucial to this. First, the growing acceptability of pathological science late in the seventeenth century enabled natural scientists to compare organs and model functions noting those that depart from the regularity of bodily repetition (Foucault, 2010). Second, in the early 1800s, with greater urban populations, there is the advent of demographics, government figures in Europe and the study of statistics (Davis, 1995). Given the imperialist projects of the time, and the preoccupation with ancestry, primitivism and subnormality, there are the conditions necessary and amenable for a science of eugenics. If industrialisation relies on a capable and efficient workforce within a European context of white Christian, masculine superiority, it raises the question of whether the body can become increasingly perfected and efficient (Foucault, 1991). In the nineteenth century there is the somewhat arbitrary separation of 'retarded development' from 'madness' on the basis of presumed aetiology and course (Foucault, 2008). These intellectual and material conditions make it possible for a segment of the population to be designated as undesirable and unproductive. The segregation of the unproductive disabled (alongside the idle and criminal), became a lesson to those that do not work. The potential for removing them, both from the factory and from the gene pool, became more apparent in post-Darwinian discourse. With economic activity and productivity linked increasingly to upstanding morality, aspiration and material conditions, a self-serving rationale is developed for both identifying non-normative forms of being and the necessity of the disciplines that survey and ameliorate their expression.

Conceptions and contestations of 'impairment' within the disability field.

Given this history, impairment is usually defined as a deficit, lack, dysfunction or abnormality that negatively reduces or changes function. The assessment of impairment is usually arrived at through clinical judgement on the basis of statistical infrequency or professional consensus, or both together. The first notes that a given difference or phenomena is infrequent when measured, and so it is abnormal by dint of its relative rarity. Such measurement is presumed to be reliable and valid. The second (professional consensus), can be operated in a variety of ways and merely requires enough agreement by those people exercising sufficient power to decide whether what is being measured or assessed is impaired. For instance, depending on where the assessment is made, HIV status could be either statistically common or rare but, either way, it is viewed as a sufficient health state to be impairment. In contrast, sexual minorities have, in professional and political terms, historically been viewed as ill and pathological. This was simply a (prejudiced) consensus view and did not require a coherent account of illness or impairment.

There is an implied, and often accepted, constancy to impairment, based on the assumption that impairment is medically describable and relatively stable. Impairment is often seen as an *acultural* and *atheoretical* classification that merely describes a *true* physical or psychological state. This *neutral* notion of impairment has been questioned and challenged (Tremain, 2006; Penson, 2011). If medicine and psy science represent their knowledge as neutral, then what they point out during diagnosis is merely the 'fact' of the abnormality. However, as Foucault suggests, the belief 'that the body obeys the exclusive laws of physiology and that it escapes the influence of history...is false' (Foucault, 1971, 87). Thus, what appears initially to be an unproblematic assessment of physical or psychological difference is actually embedded in social experience. Moreover, it becomes subject to disciplinary discourses and practices. The perceived stability of impairment is also in question given that only 15 per cent of disabled people are born with their impairment (Davis, 1995). Among the rest there is great variation in how impairment is acquired, to what extent, under what circumstances and to what effect. This notion of impairment (assumed, distinguishable and constant) is seen as underpinning the variable social experience that follows. According to the social model of disability, it is the combination of impairment and social response that demarcates 'disability'.

The current application of the social model could be accused of failing to re-integrate the impairment and the social after making the initial separation. In actuality, impairment is always in an environment, is socially described in clinical knowledge in advance of its expression, and impairment is always socially located.

If impairment is contested there are two implications. First, the presumed stability, clinical neutrality and fixity of impairment as something knowable and describable that sits anterior to the disabled experience, is removed. Second, and by extension, a *double-social model of disability* is implied. By this I mean that, if the neutrality of impairment is placed back within discourse, there is no component of the social model that is not social, and so impairment and disability both become subject to social, disciplinary and cultural forces. In the initial separation of impairment and the social in the social model, construction and meaning was seen as only located in the social response. In a *double-social model of disability* both the impairment and the social response are constructed. Impairment is equally as socially constituted as is the social response; it is not a natural, essential category outside of human designation.

Impairment in mental health and psy science

The state or identity of *disabled* relies on the assessment of an underpinning impairment, of sufficient presence to disrupt a range of normative expectations. Psy science holds the view that states of madness, mental illness and pathological distress carry with them an underlying set of deficits that constitutes impairment.

Yet there are two main problems with this. First, that there remains little clear evidence of underlying pathology in any of the functional mental health diagnoses; and second, it is not clear what constitutes a deficit rather than a variation, and a presumed deficit may not be the impairment but rather a sign of a further underlying difference. This is not to doubt the existence of a biology of distress, but to question whether distress and unusual experiences are illnesses and diseases. As we have seen, the concept of impairment is open to question – even in physical disability where it is arguably more amenable to description. If this challenge is accepted then the categorisation of psychiatric 'impairments' must be even more contestable. This offers a conundrum for the social model of disability in mental health and distress. If it is essential to the social model for the split between impairment and disability to be made, what is the impairment that we can reliably call upon in mental health and distress? The following section identifies the problem with other ways of defining impairment which might be proposed to try and get around this difficulty.

Problems with others ways of defining impairment.

One might propose that being prevented from full participation in society, or not being able to respond to life's normative demands, because of social exclusion and oppression, is sufficient for a disabled identity. However, this would include other people, such as asylum seekers, who are excluded and living on fractions of a survivable income, but without impairment. Similarly, we might suggest that certain bodies are excluded and disabled because they differ from those in mainstream, normative society. However, physical difference alone is insufficient to be judged as impairment even where that difference is characterised as inferior. People from ethnic minority groups are excluded on the basis of such physical differences when white, European benchmarks of skin colour are used (Davis, 1995) against a historical backdrop of eugenics, racist ideology and colonialism. What is the threshold for differences to become impairments? What about health differences? Or risk of ill-health? Health differentials can be seen in multifactorial risk models of aetiology. These include familial histories of heart disease and cancer. Could we see negative health potentialities as impairments? This is unlikely to be popular as a means of assessing disability because it would include all poor people in a population, since poverty is a determinant of poor physical and mental health. Yet, while some ill-health potentialities have no disability status (poverty), others do. For instance, dietary-controlled diabetes, multiple sclerosis and cancer in remission, and a non-symptomatic HIV positive status, can all constitute a disabled status even with no evident impairment. In these cases, it is the social responses and psychological adjustment to the health status that are problematic.

These examples show that while the social model of disability differentiates impairment from the social response, in practice, impairment is socially inscribed; impairment *is* a social response. Difference and variety are natural occurrences, but how we then note them and classify them is not. To arrive at the knowledge of being impaired, either by one's own or another's definition, is to have judged the social response as viable – you come to know your own difference. An exemplar of this is found in *The Reason I Jump* (Higashida, 2013) which is an autobiographical account of autism. Higashida writes in his preface,

> When I was small, I didn't even know that I was a kid with special needs. How did I find out? By other people telling me that I was different from everyone else, and that this was a problem. True enough. It was hard for me to act like a normal person... (Higashida, 2013, 15)

Higashida confirms that, for him, impairment was not an originary moment but rather it is the social response towards him which in turn confirms his presumed impairment. This begins his knowledge of difference.

Distress, norms and the social model of disability

The notion of impairment is only plausible on the grounds that there is a normal body and mind, visible, measurable and desirable, against which non-normative bodies and minds can be benchmarked. While some people do have bodies and minds at variance with others, this remains a somewhat arbitrary matter of degree. How far does one need to deviate from a culturally formulated norm to be constituted disabled? Currently, this problem is resolved primarily through diagnosis.

In mental health, this brings particular complexities. The World Health Organization (WHO) predicts that by 2030 depression will rank as 'the leading cause of disease burden globally' (WHO, 2011a, 1). Remove the clinical language and this evokes a picture of many, if not most, people being persistently miserable by 2030, with psychiatry as our main response to this 'pandemic' (critiqued by Mills (2014). If we accept this proposition, we might ask a further question: if mental health is a disability, and disability is a state that is beyond the norm, what are the implications for practice when the persistent states of misery (depression) and fear (anxiety), are so prevalent they become the new norm? What is the useful separation that can be sustained in the social model of disability or medicine when the disabled population is so expanded. How do we understand stigma and exclusion on the basis of attitudes to impairment if so many people are impaired? Perhaps this demands a shift in focus, to that of interrogating normality, not difference.

If my argument, that impairment and disability are fluid, that *both* are socially construed, is accepted, we then entertain the idea that there are fundamental flaws in the way that the 'activities of helping' are organised, not least of which is the problem of classification on which all else is predicated. In this scenario, the helping role is not redundant,

There are three implications for impairment that arise from the World Health Organisation prediction. The first is a system of classification that by its own assessment of scale seems over inclusive and without the means to corroborate a diagnosis (no blood test, scan or urinalysis). Those that seem to have the most to gain from this are disciplines that extend their influence and place more people under their 'necessary' purview, and increase 'market demand', for example, for the products of Big Pharma (Mills, 2014). Second, given World Health Organisation predictions, services would need to be so nuanced and responsive that the costs, burdens and adjustments would be of far too great a scale. The third implication relates to the cause of this increase. If, as predicted, the global south is to bear the brunt of the rise in depression by 2030, why is this happening? Is it a biological predisposition thus far unexpressed but which is accelerating? If so, how far is this from racist and eugenic propositions of the early twentieth century?

Linking the social model of disability, policy and practice

The social model of disability has become influential in health and social care policy and this can be critiqued on two levels. First, adopting it for mental health to inform legislation unintentionally imports unquestioned assumptions about impairment (such as the ones outlined thus far in this chapter). Second, there is an acceptance that systems of classification already in operation (here, psychiatry) are relevant, reliable and valid as the basis for assessing such impairment. Altered states associated with bipolarity and psychosis, and problematic mood states such as anxiety and depression, make the transition from psychiatric categories to legal categories of disability. This implies that, while anxiety and depression are disabling (in clinical and policy terms), grief and anger are lagging behind. I think that this has two effects: the first is to suggest that some mood states rather than others have credibility as disabilities, and so should be privileged in their induction into the order of disability. The second is that psychiatric classification must be worthwhile because the mood states that it describes are disabilities; a self-perpetuating circularity. Thus, it appears, disciplines can 'sift' impairments.

Arguably, the social model of disability has colluded in the induction of people both into psychiatry (through deploying diagnostic labels) and into our legal/administrative systems (through employee assistance and welfare benefits). Medicine, through its own activity and that of other health professionals, is still the gatekeeper to assistance and adaptation; self-definition only gets one to the first gate. The limitations of the social model and some shrewd manoeuvring on the part of disciplinary interests (see Trueman, 2013, for an account of how the Royal College of Psychiatry used its position to skew its level of involvement in the amendment of the Mental Health Act), have resulted, I would argue, in this unacceptable status quo. This is not least because a model of activism has been co-opted and assimilated, rendering the disabled/mad dissident voice impotent. How does one find a voice, and talk back to the people who advocate one's own model of dissent (but who may then practice through the objectionable medical model)? Disciplines are trading on their status as helping professions that are scientifically validated and ethically rigorous, but the life outcomes for the disabled generally, and for people with mental health problems specifically, remain poor (Schizophrenia Commission, 2012) found people with this diagnosis lose on average 15 to 20 years of life compared to a non-clinical population). This is despite dominant narratives of recovery and optimism.

The social model of disability is driven by the intention to gain protections for the people concerned. However, there is a cost to accepting medicalised definitions of impairment and there appears to be no acceptable alternative way of defining impairment which is so loose that it would include substantial sections of the population. This is not a plea for greater exclusivity in who is (or isn't) awarded disabled status, but rather it raises the question of what psy science and medicine gain by their participation in the lives of people with mental health problems.

Conclusion

The absence of a discernible disease-based impairment – despite biological psychiatry's own claims of a biological basis for mental ill health – has not stopped distress and misery from being inducted in to the pantheon of disability. This cements the psy sciences as the 'impairment certifiers' and confirms the 'mad' and miserable in their status as disabled. Furthermore, the possibility that misery and madness are consequences of urbanisation, poverty and capitalism is denied; political responses are nullified, and dissent is typified as resulting from lack of insight or the marginal ramblings of academic malcontents. By engaging with normative, medical and psychological models, humans remove the possibility of viewing madness as a human variation and misery as a natural response to circumstance. Perhaps *the Mad* would prefer a position analogous to that adopted by Deaf communities, of being a linguistic minority and not disabled (Davis, 1995). Rather than being pathologised, segregated, subject to inhumane treatment and rehabilitation, through theories of sub-normality, *the* mad would then become a natural variation, a sub-culture with a changing membership, with degrees of participation.

It is not new for subjugated populations to be benchmarked unfavourably against a supposed neutral, racialised, gendered, able norm. All civil rights movements have had to contend with their members being construed as physically, psychologically or spiritually inferior. Perhaps mental health problems would be better articulated as neurodiversity, or post-traumatic growth, allowing for the arguments of social justice to be mounted without a commensurate acceptance of an underlying pathology or deficit; difference, without capitulation to inferiority or the abnormal. This would remove the concept of impairment from the social model of disability and replace it with one of difference that is variably maltreated and unaccepted. We could therefore alleviate distress through social and political means, without recourse to disease models that result in stigma and damaging treatments (this is part of what the social model aimed to achieve).

This critique of impairment is not easily resolvable through a new term or idea. Arguably, continuing to use a wrong notion because it is what we have, and has a certain tradition, is even more problematic. It is what Feyerabend (1975) refers to as the 'material force', the political power of traditional thinking which limits what it is permissible to say and do within a given field. Rather than seeking to fit mental health and distress into the SMD, issues raised in this chapter might result in its transformation. If impairment itself is mutable perhaps, as

I have argued, a *double-social model* has explanatory power. In the first instance this double-social model might require a renewed vigour in questioning how disciplines operate models of impairment in practice. It might also question the implied normativity that seems to be a fiction for most people. Lastly, it might build bridges between groups of disability activists dissatisfied with the ways in which their difference and variation is only ever referred to in normative terms (such as 'function').

Despite these problems, the social model of disability has a productive history in the campaign for disabled civil rights. So, while the working out is done – and for so long as psychiatry is practiced (even in the absence of robust evidence), the social model retains an important place. The social model of disability does explain why disabled people have certain social experiences past the point of diagnosis. However, on-going scholarship and activism should be cognisant of the possible concession that advocates of the social model of disability in mental health might be making on the notion of impairment. The range of experiences falling within the reach of psychiatry continues to extend; whether that is advantageous to people in distress is questionable. However, there remains a paradox for activists and people with mental health problems alike. Currently, to forgo psychiatric diagnosis is to forgo the social recognition of impairment, and subsequently the conferment of a legitimised disability, along with the help that follows. This paradox has far-reaching implications for people who are struggling with mental health issues but do not accept notions of impairment and the psychiatrisation of their distress.

Part Two
Theorising distress and disablement

FIVE

Towards a socially situated model of mental distress

Jerry Tew

Mental health and mental distress, like sex and gender, and impairment and disability, sit uncomfortably at the intersection between biology, personality and social experience. They represent a site at which power relations operate and a politics of difference may be enacted – ruthless processes of 'othering' which have the potential to permeate both one's social relationships and the entirety of one's being. But these are processes that may be resisted and transcended through individual and collective struggle – not only can the inter-personal be made political, so too can the intra-personal. Developing a conceptual vocabulary to make sense of mental distress is important to these struggles – both theoretically and politically – if we are to move beyond the limiting perspectives provided by biomedicine.

The social model of disability has been remarkably successful in shifting thinking and practice in relation to the situations faced by people with impairments, challenging the implicit tragedy/deficit model that was underpinned by a medicalised form of understanding. Its validity and impact has stemmed from being rooted in the situated knowledge of those with direct experience of impairments. However, as has been discussed in the other chapters, this model – although useful in many respects – has not proved quite able to address some of the key issues that have been seen as important by people with mental distress who have sought to make sense of their experience.

Mental health has had its own history of activism and, although willing to consider alliances with the wider disability movement, there have been concerns about the specific priorities of mental health users becoming lost if mental distress were to become subsumed as just another instance of impairment. Furthermore, the notion of impairment has never quite seemed to capture the actuality of mental distress – although disabling societal and (medicalised) professional responses to mental distress can be just as discriminatory and debilitating as those towards physical and mental impairments.

Within the field of mental health a number of alternative perspectives have emerged – both challenging the reduction of experience to medical diagnosis and recasting the idea of 'recovery' in social/ existential terms, rather than equating it with remission of 'symptoms'. However, these ideas have yet to coalesce into a way of thinking that has had the impact of the social model of disability – and the agenda can be in danger of being appropriated by professional interests.

The social model of disability and the politics of stigma

In its original simplicity, the social model of disability was transformational: it constructed a new way of seeing which challenged the way in which mainstream society and medicine had colluded to define impairment as a shameful tragedy for the individual and those close to them. Instead it problematised the exclusionary attitudes, practices and environments that constituted the everyday assumptive world of the 'normal'. Using a civil rights based discourse, it offered disabled people an opportunity to take power for themselves in demanding inclusion, and it set the terms of a very different agenda for professionals in assisting and enabling this. In its original conception, it did not quite capture the entirety of disabled people's experience, leaving a need to further interrogate the notion of impairment itself (Shakespeare and Watson, 2002), and to acknowledge the psycho-emotional dimension of living with impairments and experiencing social disablement (Reeve, 2004). Nevertheless, it has largely stood the test of time in providing a core framing for disabled people's experiences and for collective action to address oppression.

Politically and theoretically, it opened up two interrelated perspectives. One was a more practical concern with the material barriers faced by people with impairments in terms of accessing physical, economic and social spaces – issues that could be remedied, to a significant extent, by awareness campaigns, assertive action and anti-discriminatory legislation. The other was more complex and related to the politics of identity (Corker and French, 1999) – and the subtle (or not so subtle) ways in which people are situated within discourses of inferiorisation and marginalisation, fixed within a sometimes unrelenting gaze of stereotyping and misrecognition. As Jenny Morris describes it, disabled people can be 'faced with the knowledge that each entry into the public world will be dominated by stares, by condescension, by pity and by hostility' (1991, 25).

As with women and Black and Minority Ethnic groups, people with impairments are faced with invidious choices within dominant discursive structures – accepting a pre-given identity that is signified on the basis of a supposedly inferior biology, or trying to pass as 'normal' by denying something that is actually an important part of their identity. Either strategy may be experienced as damaging, at a psycho-emotional level, to a person's self-esteem or sense of self (Reeve, 2004). In response to this, particularly in the United States, some people with physical impairments chose to self-define as 'cripples' or 'crips', emulating the appropriation of the term 'queer' by lesbian and gay groups in asserting a political identity on their own terms (McRuer, 2006).

Both of these perspectives have relevance for people with mental distress. Whether experiencing longer term mental health difficulties or recovering from more acute forms of breakdown, people may benefit from disability legislation that requires employers to make 'reasonable adjustments' to work environments. However, this may often not address the key barriers that people face. It may often not be practical arrangements that are the crucial issue; instead it may be attitudes and perceptions. In common with people with physical or sensory impairments, people with mental health difficulties may face being patronised or excluded, or being defined as a 'problem'. However, over and above this, people with mental health difficulties may face a particularly extreme form of vilification or demonisation (Laurance, 2003). They may be situated in identities that not only construct them as devalued, but also as constituting a threat to the 'normal' populace. As Foucault (1967) has suggested, this phenomenon is not mere coincidence. Whereas the social order in traditional societies depended on deference to the unquestioned authority of religion, monarchy and aristocracy, the institutional and discursive structures of modernity are legitimated on the basis of rationality – and hence any expressions of irrationality may be seen as potentially subversive to the very fabric of social relations (Tew, 2005a).

Whereas the concept of stigma has had relatively little traction within the wider disability movement, it has been embraced more strongly within the field of mental health (Thornicroft, 2006a; Corrigan et al, 2011). The notion of stigma starts to capture this social repudiation of those identified as suffering from mental distress, something that goes beyond what is usually denoted by terms such as discrimination or injustice. Through visible markers such as talking to one's voices or walking with an unusual gait, or through becoming the object of whispering and gossip, a person may find that their whole being becomes socially discredited. Labels such as 'psycho' and 'schizo' can construct identities that are inseparable from 'mad axeman' stereotypes. The further concept of 'stigma by association' is helpful in making sense of how carers and family members may also find themselves tainted with identities that are stigmatising – that they may somehow also be 'carriers' of infectious irrationality, or that they have failed in their public duty to contain or suppress irrationality within their household.

Although social interactionist theories of stigma and labelling tended to neglect inequalities of power – and hence who was in a position to impose a stigmatised identity on whom – more recent applications of this approach have taken this dimension more seriously (Link and Phelan, 2001). This has helped shift the focus from a concern with how people with mental distress should learn social skills in order to assimilate into the mainstream, to addressing social attitudes within the wider community through anti-stigma activity (Pinfold et al, 2005; Thornicroft, 2006a) – and exploring individual and collective strategies whereby people may resist the internalisation of such stigma (Sibitz et al, 2009).

Due to their emotional vulnerability and to the disruption of their 'pre-illness' identities associated with their breakdown, people with mental distress may be particularly prone to taking on and internalising within their sense of self, many aspects of the stigmatised identities that are attributed to them (Rusch et al, 2006). Interestingly, lacking 'insight' into one's illness (that is, not accepting one's diagnosis) can also work as a strategy for resisting any acceptance of the social stigma attached to the label (Lysaker et al, 2006). Whether or not one is able to resist such internalisation, being subject to ongoing stigmatising social interactions may constitute a significant additional source of stress and potentially exacerbate one's levels of distress – a process that is very similar to that denoted by the idea of psycho-emotional disablism.

Challenging stigma has not been a straightforward process. Some people with mental distress have worked in alliance with professional groups and other bodies on national campaigns to change public attitudes, such as See Me in Scotland and Time to Change in England. However, such strategies have brought up their own contradictions, particularly in terms of how mental distress is discursively constructed (and by whom). Psychiatry has been keen to promote, as a normalising idea, the notion that mental distress is 'an illness like any other'. However, rather than creating a discursive space in which people could construct an ordinary identity as a person first (who happens to have an illness), this foregrounding of 'illness' served to reify inter-personal differences as biological, thereby rendering the identities of people with mental distress as irrevocably 'other' and reinforcing 'us' and 'them' thinking within the general population (Dietrich et al, 2006; Read et al, 2006a). An alternative strategy that eschews professional colonisation has been the more overtly political Mad Pride movement which has modelled itself on similar movements by Black and gay people. 'Mad' becomes a political term – a positive assertion of alternative identity that distances itself from any biological signifier and which celebrates irrationality rather than seeking to erase it from public view.

The social meaning of mental distress

As with physical and sensory impairments, many people have found dominant medical discourses to be at best insufficient, and at worst positively destructive, as explanatory frameworks with which to make sense of their experience (although the mental health user/survivor community has been quite divided on this issue). For some, accepting a diagnosis and taking medication has enabled them to resume worthwhile and satisfying lives. For others, this has not worked so successfully. For many, irrespective of whether they have found medical treatment useful in managing certain experiences, there has been a desire to make sense of their mental distress in their own terms and within the context of their lives (Wallcraft and Michaelson, 2001; Geekie, 2004).

Although being acutely aware of issues of discrimination and exclusion, mental health activists have tended to give even greater focus to problematising the notion of 'mental illness' and the somewhat limited vision of 'treatment' that stemmed from this. For them, in order to reclaim power over their lives, the first step needed to be reclaiming authorship over their experiences. Viewed within the terms of the social model of disability, the political and intellectual focus was at least as much on challenging dominant constructions of their 'impairment' as it was on challenging disabling social attitudes and practices. However, many found the term 'impairment' itself to be unhelpful as it tended to conjure up the very notions of 'chronic mental illness' against which they were struggling.

In relation to experiences such as hearing voices and behaviours such as self-harm, service users and survivors started to articulate their own frames of understanding – supported by peer support organisations such as the Hearing Voices Network and the Bristol Crisis Service for Women. Building on the perspectives of the 1960s anti-psychiatry movement, and the work of Laing and Szasz, their starting point was to see distress experiences, not as symptoms of an underlying 'mental illness', but as meaningful responses to 'problems of living'. Whereas the idea of psycho-emotional disablism helps us to focus on how people may turn inwards aspects of the oppression they experience in relation to their impairment, the experiences of many mental health survivors pointed to associations between prior exposure to social trauma, humiliation and subsequent incidence of mental distress (Plumb, 2005) – although other issues such as neglect and non-recognition may also have their own impact. Such associations between adverse life experiences and 'mental illness' have become increasingly supported by research evidence (Bentall and Fernyhough, 2008).

Mental health survivors have been careful not to situate themselves as passive victims of external circumstances (however extreme these may have been) and they have started to reinterpret distress experiences, such as self-harming or hearing voices, as their best available coping mechanisms to deal with challenging life experiences such as sexual abuse or racial harassment (Spandler, 1996; Dillon, 2010). Thus, instead of seeing distress experiences as something simply to be eradicated (by medication or cognitive reprogramming), people suggested that these were to be respected as creative (but desperate) ways of surviving in almost unliveable circumstances. If they were symptoms at all, they were symptoms of unresolved personal and social issues – a direction of understanding that was profoundly social, but took people beyond the social model of disability as a frame of reference.

Unlike notions of impairment or illness, these perspectives started to re-situate people as having some sense of agency in relation to their distress experiences, despite the fact that these experiences may seem to have taken on a disturbing momentum of their own (Tew, 2011). However painful the realisation, people could begin to explore how they might, consciously or unconsciously, be deploying coping mechanisms that had purpose and meaning – albeit ones that usually came at a price in terms of subjective distress and ability to function.

Such seemingly out-of-control coping mechanisms may also be seen as representing a way of expressing experiences and embodied memories that cannot easily be expressed in any other way. Sharon Lefevre, a self-harmer, described the unbearable existential isolation of feeling disconnected from, and unable to communicate the inner reality of her experiences of sexual abuse with those around her. In such situations, 'language is survival', but everyday language was inadequate (1996, 28). The only way out of this impasse may be for self-harm, voice hearing or other forms of mental distress to provide an 'intermediary language' that gives voice (often somewhat obliquely) to the jarring and extreme elements of inner experience that cannot be expressed in any other way (Lefevre, 1996, 30). The content and identity of voices ('auditory hallucinations'), the nature of fixed and unusual beliefs ('delusions') and the apparently meaningless sequences of word-salads may all provide metaphoric clues as to underlying issues that cannot be spoken of directly.

Such understandings have led to a new form of praxis which may be seen as complementary to the social model of disability. It represents a very different form of taking power – one which focuses much more on the personal but viewed through a lens that is profoundly social. As with the social model of disability, it involves renegotiating one's relationships with one's impairment or distress experiences – but the journey is somewhat different. For a person with a physical or sensory impairment, the impairment usually remains a given; what alters is its social signification – and the journey may involve negotiating an identity that takes account of, but is not dominated by, biology. For a person with mental distress, the journey may be rather more complex. It may involve developing a relationship with their distress experiences that is respectful and even collaborative – working with their experiences to discover what may be their underlying social meaning – while at the same time, finding ways of developing a more assertive and equal power relationship with their distress experiences, no longer allowing them to dominate or take over their lives to the same extent.

Such shifts in relationships with one's distress experiences are hard to accomplish alone – and opportunities to share and try out ideas within peer networks such as the Hearing Voices Network have proved crucial in developing this new praxis. Voice hearers have shared insights and strategies for talking to and negotiating with their voices. Out of this have been developed workbooks and techniques such as 'voice dialogue' in order to develop ways of exploring what may underlie the content of the voices and what they may be trying to communicate both to the voice hearer and to the wider world (Coleman and Smith, 1997; Corstens et al, nd). Alongside this, people have developed simple but effective strategies for being more assertive with their voices – for example, talking back to an intrusive voice and saying, 'I'm busy now, but I will talk to you in half an hour.'

Similarly, a self-harmer may learn to respect their impulse to cut, but may negotiate a 'breathing space' in which they will try an alternative coping strategy, while reserving the option still to cut if the other strategy proves insufficient in this instance (Inckle, 2010). Alongside this they may start to explore, with the emotional support of peers or others, what they may be trying to communicate through the intermediary language of self-harm. Although perhaps harder to make sense of at the time, people coming through experiences such as depression, where there may be less overt 'content' with which to engage, may nevertheless find that, through the depression, they have learned something valuable about themselves and their social relationships (Ridge and Ziebland, 2006). It is heartening to note that such approaches are now achieving recognition within some mental health services.

Whereas the notion of impairment suggests something that is relatively stable and predictable, the coping mechanisms of mental distress – and the urgency to have recourse to an intermediary language – are inherently more fluid. They are likely to be triggered (or not) by particular aspects of a person's current context of social interactions. Conversely, certain sorts of social relationships – and, in particular, those characterised by commitment and mutuality – may act as an effective buffer against such triggers having any lasting impact. This provides a further social and contextual dimension to the analysis and praxis: managing distress experiences through actively changing one's social environment or the ways in which one interacts with it.

Making some sort of sense of distress experiences may be a pre-requisite for re-establishing agency – and the agency that one establishes may need to take account of the context, content and meaning of one's impulses and experiences. Ultimately the goal may be to transform both one's relationship to one's distress and what it may signify, and one's current social relationships, identities and ways of being in the world.

Recovery

Emerging somewhat separately from the debates about the social meaning of mental distress, the idea that has made the greatest impact, in terms of how we may think about mental health services, has been that of *recovery*. Originating particularly through the work of survivor activists in the United States, a movement developed in which people with mental health difficulties demanded an alternative to the assumptions and worldview of traditional medically dominated mental health services. While some activists, such as Pat Deegan (1992) drew inspiration from the Independent Living Movement, they tended not to engage specifically with the conceptual structure of the social model of disability (which has tended to be less influential in American disability politics).

Central to this new conception of recovery were ideas of personal and collective empowerment, linking to the work of Judi Chamberlin (1997) and others within the mental health survivor movement. This involved people taking the initiative in reclaiming control over their lives and becoming agents of their own recovery, rather than passively waiting for professionals to 'make them better'. It also involved inviting others to see them in this way.

Although its subsequent relationship with psychiatry has been somewhat ambiguous, the movement initially coalesced around the idea that people could reclaim the term recovery from its association with medicine. No longer was recovery to be seen as a successful response to therapeutic interventions to be measured in terms of remission of medically defined symptoms. Instead, it was re-conceived in social capability terms as achieving whatever people defined for themselves as 'a life worth living' (Hopper, 2007; Wallcraft, 2010) – irrespective of whether they continued to hear voices, experience mood swings or hold on to unusual beliefs. An analysis of the (now quite substantial) conceptual literature suggests that the core processes of recovery are seen to comprise:

- empowerment and reclaiming control over one's life – negotiating more equal relationships with professionals, family and friends, and developing strategies for managing, rather than being dominated by, distress experiences;
- rebuilding positive personal and social identities (including challenging stigma and discrimination and dealing with its impact);
- connectedness (including both personal and family relationships and wider aspects of social inclusion);
- hope and optimism about the future; and
- finding meaning and purpose in life (Leamy et al, 2011).

Despite the pessimism that has dominated mental health services over the last century, there is overwhelming evidence that, for the majority of people with serious mental distress, a substantial degree of recovery is possible in the longer term – whether this is defined in social *or* medical terms (Warner, 2004). Furthermore, rather than medical treatment and remission of symptoms being the necessary precursor of social recovery (as suggested by the biomedical approach), the reverse would seem to be the more typical route to recovery. At a population level, it would seem to be social opportunity that can provide the most effective key to long-term symptom remission. Throughout the twentieth century, in developed countries, both social and medical recovery rates were shown, not to correlate with any advances in medical treatment, but with reductions in national unemployment rates (Warner, 2004). This forms part of a wider theoretical and evidence base which links a range of social factors to successful recovery outcomes (Tew, 2012; Tew et al, 2012).

This approach to recovery also opened out a consideration of what people might need to recover from. This could comprise, not just distress experiences themselves, but also the traumatic dislocation to people's identities and relationships that resulted from others' responses to their distress, including the potential damage done by oppressive or insensitive service interventions which could be experienced as 'spirit breaking' (Deegan, 1990). In this way, the starting point for recovery thinking was very similar to that of the social model of disability – highlighting the degree to which social and professional responses to distress/impairment could be profoundly disabling. However, underlying this apparent similarity was a more fundamental difference of inflection. Whereas the social model of disability proposed that the focus of action fell fairly and squarely within the field of social and political activity, recovery implies an equal focus on intra-personal experience as a key site for awareness raising and change.

Taking charge of one's therapeutic journey takes one into a very different discursive space in which an interrogation of the personal meaning of one's distress may become as important as challenging social stigma or social and economic discrimination. If mental distress comes to be viewed, not as a (biological) impairment, but as a desperate 'coping strategy' or an 'intermediary language', recovery may also involve acknowledging and coming to terms with a legacy of stressful or abusive life circumstances that may have contributed to one's initial breakdown. This intertwining of social and personal experiences is thus not easily reducible to any simple dualism of impairment and disability – with no part that is fixed or 'given' in any sense.

Despite its cautious acceptance by more progressive elements within professional groups, and its espousal within certain government policy documents (Care Services Improvement Partnership et al, 2007), recovery has not yet had the sort of decisive impact upon the dominant ways in which mental distress is understood in Britain that has been achieved by the social model of disability. This is probably a reflection of two factors. First, in mental health, the medical model is structurally and institutionally more entrenched than in relation to physical or learning impairments. Second, the recovery model is conceptually more complex – which may be necessary in encompassing what is important in people's experience, but has also led to a certain slipperiness and lack of conceptual clarity (Pilgrim, 2008), which has allowed for subtle (and not so subtle) colonisation of the idea of recovery by professional interests.

While the idea of recovery provides a framework which opens up both disability *and* impairment as potential sites for struggle and transformation, there is a danger that mental health services tend to neglect the former and latch on to the latter. In particular, they may try to reassert the claim that they have the expertise to 'treat' the impairment/'illness' and thereby bracket out the social meanings that may be represented in people's distress. What has been most troubling for mental health service users and survivors has been instances where their radical conception of recovery has become appropriated and used against them – sometimes as a new label for old style professional-led interventions, or as a legitimation for wholesale removal of services, or as a way of blaming people if they did not manage to 'get better' within an externally prescribed time period. In this sense, it has shown itself to be less politically robust than the social model of disability.

Despite these concerns, however, the recovery model has still proved influential in opening up the prospect of people with mental health difficulties reclaiming power and agency for themselves. In common with the social model of disability, it has achieved a switch of meaning which has challenged prevailing models of signification – and there are signs that this has destabilised some of the dominance of biomedical reductionism within some (parts of) mental health services. For example, we are now witnessing the emergence of Recovery Colleges in the United Kingdom which, as the name implies, aim to provide a discursive space that is framed within an educational rather than a medical ethos, and where those with lived experience of mental distress may take a lead role in setting the terms of the conversations and activities that take place within such spaces (Perkins et al, 2012). Similarly, across a number of states in Europe and North America, there is a growing interest in implementing the principles of Open Dialogue within services – creating a therapeutic space for people experiencing mental distress and their wider family and social networks to make sense of their experiences in their own language, rather than viewing it through the prism of illness and diagnosis (Seikkula and Olson, 2003).

Towards a socially situated model of mental distress

Neither the recovery model nor the social model of disability may be seen to provide a clear or sufficient basis for (re)conceptualising people's experiences of mental distress. However, they may both be potentially useful in offering political frameworks that are rooted in lived experience – and within whose parameters we may be able to develop key elements of a socially situated model. Both frameworks foreground the idea that societal and (some) professional responses to mental distress can be profoundly disabling. However, we may need to go beyond this and argue that both mental distress *and* social responses need to be seen as (at least in part) socially constructed and infused with a continuing legacy of oppressive and exclusionary power relations. As suggested by both the recovery model and psycho-emotional disablism, this requires a both/and approach to seeing the importance of the personal and the social.

Whatever may be its biomedical correlates in terms of brain functioning, and whatever part may be played genetically derived sensitivities, we start with the foundational position that mental distress may be understood as a meaningful response to life circumstances. Specific distress experiences ('symptoms') may be understood as coping mechanisms – but ones that seem to have taken on a momentum of their own and which may come at a price in terms of levels of subjective distress, confusion and impaired functioning. They may also be seen as 'intermediary languages' that are seeking to express some of the pent-up reality of social experiences that have become intolerable. While we must be careful not to make assumptions as to what may be the sorts of life circumstances that may drive people over the edge, we know from survivor narratives and wider research that social issues such as sexual abuse or racial discrimination are often implicated.

Equally important is the social environment within which a person experiences their mental distress. Within modern societies, expressions of irrationality can be seen as particularly threatening, triggering responses from families, communities and professionals that are defensive and destructive. Such stigmatisation can go beyond discrimination or disablement and can violate or invalidate a person's personal and social identities. Research around stigma and stigma resistance has highlighted how constructing mental distress as a medical 'illness' can have unintended consequences in terms of reinforcing perceptions of otherness within the wider population and increasing the likelihood that people will internalise stigmatising attitudes and beliefs towards themselves.

Drawing upon the insights of the various perspectives discussed above, we may see mental distress as a situated and potentially fluid response to a particular confluence of personal and social circumstances. As the recovery movement has argued, whatever their ongoing vulnerabilities or experiences, people may be able to reclaim valued and meaningful lives through some combination of personal struggle and social opportunity – processes that may be actively disabled by services that are exclusively oriented towards the treatment of 'illness'. It is important to recognise that people may need to recover from some combination of the socially situated impacts of oppressive and abusive life experiences, how these may have become internalised as mental distress, and how this may have become exacerbated by insensitive and discriminatory societal responses to their distress. At a theoretical level, while conceptualising disability as social remains a core part of this understanding, making sense of mental distress requires a move beyond both the social model of disability and psycho-emotional disablism in taking apart the notion of impairment – and seeing this also as an encapsulation of oppressive social constructions.

SIX

The Capabilities Approach and the social model of mental health

Jan Wallcraft and Kim Hopper

A recent national study in the UK canvassed a diverse range of mental health service users/survivors opinions about the relevance of the social model of disability (Beresford et al, 2010). In conclusion, the authors pointed to the need for a social model of madness and distress. One approach, they suggested, would be for proponents of the social model of disability to consider how it might be made more accessible to mental health service users, enabling them to explore its relevance to their own lives. They also called for mental health survivor leaders and activists 'particularly those concerned with the movement's value base and philosophy' (Beresford et al, 2010, 31) to engage with the social model of disability in more depth.

This chapter takes up this challenge. We contend that the Capabilities Approach provides a way forward in this ongoing debate about the social model in disability and mental health. Although the Capabilities approach was developed in economics to analyse issues related to standards of living and the underlying axioms guiding international aid and poverty abatement, we believe that the framework may be deployed to address critical issues in social response to mental distress, support and recovery.

We think the Capabilities Approach offers a solid underpinning which service users, survivors and allies need to mount a serious challenge to the dominance of the medical model. This is because it supplies what is usually missing in even expanded medical models (like the biopsychosocial model) – a profound understanding of *structural* constraints and enablements. It provides a clear, practical and rights-based answer to the call for a social model of mental health which could offer a real alternative to the medical model in terms of policy and planning; engagement of service users in creating new services to meet their expressed needs; and research and evaluation of service outcomes. Therefore, this chapter will outline what the Capabilities

Approach offers our understanding of disability and how it can be applied to mental health to prevent long-term 'psychiatric disability'.

Before we explain this in more detail, we need to understand how the Capabilities Approach differs from other approaches to disability.

Theoretical models of disability

While to the layperson, disability usually means 'the inability to do something', there are actually no commonly accepted ways to define or measure disability, which has been subject to many definitions in different disciplines and for different purposes. We start by reviewing some of these (drawing on Mitra, 2006).

The medical model

The medical (or biomedical) model considers disability to be a problem of the individual that is directly caused by a disease, an injury, or some other health condition and requires medical care in the form of treatment and rehabilitation. In contrast to the social model, impairment is thus synonymous with disability. This model attributes the problem to the individual, who has a condition that is unwanted and that places him or her in the 'sick role' (Parsons and Fox, 1952). This model is 'normative' – that is, it is the duty of the sick person to try to get well, and compliance with this expectation is part of the social bargain struck in exchange for dispensation from ordinary responsibilities. When the 'sick role' is prolonged, and it becomes clear that a full return to one's former capacities is unlikely, the sick role can be formally recognised as 'disability', that is, the person cannot function as a 'normal' person does. The medical model works at the political level to ensure the provision of healthcare and rehabilitation services and to manage the expectation that the recipient of the services is 'responsibly sick' (Susser et al, 1985; Mitra, 2006).

The social model

The social model of disability draws an important distinction between impairment and disability, stating that 'impairment' exists in the real physical world, while 'disability' is a social invention, defined through language and practice within a complex system of shared meanings, discourses and limitations imposed by the environment at a particular time and place. It thus has its philosophical foundations in social constructionism.

The social model recognises that some individuals have physical or psychological *differences* which can affect their ability to function in society, but suggests that it is the organisation of society that leads to *disability*. People are not disabled by their impairments but by the barriers that exist in society which fail to take their needs into account. These barriers are of three kinds: environmental, economic and cultural (BCODP, 1981). Persons with disabilities face discrimination and segregation through sensory, attitudinal, cognitive, physical and economic barriers. Their experiences can therefore be perceived to be similar to those of any other oppressed minority group. In important ways, *failure to recognise* (the needs of people with impairments) can be disabling (Fraser and Honneth, 2003; Hopper, 2006).

However, even in the disability movement there are disagreements about this strong version of the social model, which asserts that disability is caused not by impairment but by the social barriers (structural and attitudinal) which people with impairments face. Leading theorists (Shakespeare, 2007; Thomas, 2008) have critiqued the extent to which the social model of disability allows for the subtleties and complexities of the relationship between factors intrinsic to the individual person and those arising from the wider cultural and social environment. The nature and severity of the actual impairment and the attitudes of others are compounded by economic and social issues and together make up the extent to which a person with impairments finds them*selves* disabled.

Other models of disability have tried to combine the social and the medical, in a formulation of functional limitations.

The disablement model: functional limitations

The disablement model (Nagi, 1965) sets out how pathology and functional limitations lead to disability. 'Pathology' refers to an interruption of normal body processes which can lead to 'impairments', defined as anatomical or physiological abnormalities or losses. 'Functional limitations' are the restrictions that impairments impose on an individual's ability to perform normal daily activities and fulfil expected social roles, for example in relation to work, childcare, community membership and self-care (Nagi, 1991). According to the disablement model, impairment is at the source of a causal chain leading to disability, which eventually becomes a social construct. For example, a 12-year-old girl with learning disabilities who stays home with her parents helping with household chores may not be seen as 'disabled' if she lives in a society where young girls are not expected to go to school but may be 'disabled' if her culture expects school attendance. The disablement model therefore promotes a social and cultural relativist view of disability.

International Classification of Functioning, Disability and Health (ICF)

The World Health Organisation developed the International Classification of Impairments, Disabilities and Handicaps (ICIDH) in the early 1980s. It was recently revised and renamed the International Classification of Functioning, Disability and Health (ICF) (WHO, 2001a). According to Hemmingson and Jonsson (2005) this revision was in response to critiques from the disability movement and the emergence of the social model of disability. Conceptually, the ICF is presented as an integration of the medical and the social models and is sometimes termed the biopsychosocial model of disability. Similar to the disablement model, it sets out the view that disability is the result of a health condition that leads to impairments, which then result in limitations in activity and participation within specific contexts. Impairments are defined as 'problems in body function or structure causing a significant deviation or loss'. The World Health Organization calls ICF 'a synthesis, in order to provide a coherent view of different perspectives of health from a biological, individual and social perspective' (WHO, 2001, 20).

It also states that ICF emphasises a shift in focus, from disease to health: 'ICF has moved away from being a "consequences of disease" classification (1980 version) to become a "components of health" classification' (WHO, 2001, 4).

Hemmingson and Jonsson, however, refer to ongoing critiques from the disability movement in relation to ICF's continued reliance on labelling and classification which has 'historically contributed to the stigmatisation and oppression of persons with disabilities' (2005, 571). Such critiques also note the lack of a focus on subjective dimensions of 'functioning' such as role satisfaction and happiness, or the importance of environmental factors such as local culture.

An alternative model: the Capabilities Approach

Beginning in the 1970s, Amartya Sen developed the Capabilities Approach, which radically rethought the conventional framework of welfare economics, bringing together ideas that had been excluded or not properly described in this area (Sen, 1979; 1985a; 1989; 1999;

Sen and Nussbaum, 1993). Sen's work was revolutionary because he did not think income and goods-oriented measures were enough to capture individual wellbeing. Along with political philosopher Martha Nussbaum, Sen has been able to make the Capabilities Approach the leading paradigm for policy debate in human development. It has led to the creation of the UN's Human Development Index (HDI) which has supported discussion of equality of opportunity especially in relation to gender equity.

The Capabilities Approach emphasises locally valued functional capabilities, termed 'substantive freedoms', such as the ability to live to old age, engage in economic transactions, or participate in political activities. Poverty is seen as capability-deprivation. Resources or assets are prized, not in themselves, but by virtue of the valued things people are able to do or be as a result of having them – the capabilities they command. In other words, genuine welfare depends less on what I own or have access to, than the real opportunities open to me as a result. Central to this approach is the distinction between capabilities and functionings.

Capabilities and functionings

Under Sen's approach, capability does not constitute the presence of a physical or a mental ability; rather, it is understood as a practical opportunity. Disadvantage (for example, poverty, impairment or 'mental illness') and the social devaluation and 'degradation' that so often accompany it, can harm in ways that are both lasting and tricky to discuss and address: by restricting a person's opportunities. This means its effects are ultimately moral as well as material – they go to the heart of whether we recognise and value a person, and how we assess their worth.

The Capabilities Approach distinguishes between what a person *actually* achieves and what he or she could *possibly* achieve. Functioning is the actual achievement of the individual, what he or she actually achieves, through being or doing, in the course their life. By contrast, a person's 'capability set' includes all the various combinations of functionings that he or she *could* achieve. Again, capabilities are 'substantive freedoms' – the potential to do or be something that is socially valued. Capabilities take in the full set of possibilities, or realms of life engagement actually available to each person.

Because they have to do with possibility, rather than how freedoms are actually exercised, capabilities are difficult to measure and functionings are often used instead to assess situations and progress towards personal goals. This puts the importance less on what a person chooses than on the range of valued options which are available to them. In assessing whether capability has expanded, what is needed is evidence that a person can realistically engage in informed and competent consideration of locally valued alternatives.

Disability can be understood as a deprivation, in terms of capabilities or functionings, that result from the interaction of (a) an individual's personal characteristics (for example, age and impairment); (b) the basket of available goods (assets and income); and (c) their environment (social, economic, political and cultural). What people can actually achieve with the resources at their disposal varies with socially recognised diversity, including disability. For example, ridicule from colleagues can poison a workplace so that a visibly disabled person, however capable, may prefer to stay at home on benefits. Custom complicates matters further. For example, a woman may be literate and live in an area with libraries available, but be confined to her home by custom.

The Capabilities Approach has been widely debated by political theorists, philosophers and social scientists in the area of health (for example, Venkatapuram, 2011; Ruger, 2012). However, although it has been used in international development to analyse the links between disability, gender discrimination and poverty (Welch, 2002), its usefulness in relation to disability and mental health policy has not yet been widely considered. The following section explores the value of his approach to disability, arguing that it is an improvement on other disability models.

The value of the Capabilities Approach to disability

Scholars such as Mitra (2003; 2006) have extended the Capabilities Approach, from its original use in poverty, to people with disabilities. Disability, like poverty, can be re-described as deprivation of capabilities, because it interferes with a person's ability to make valued choices and participate fully in society. Intervention can occur at the level of the original impairment (or, 'psychiatric disorder') or at the level of 'disability' – the social reception and consequences of impairment.

This approach helps to explain the importance of the economic causes and consequences of disability and is closely related to the ICF (WHO, 2001). In the disablement model and the medical model, there is no concern for the lived experience of the individual, nor for her achievements or aspirations. Asking a person if she can work (in the disablement model), or lift 10 pounds with one hand (in the medical model), regardless of whether she wants to or needs to, whether there is any job for her in the economy, or whether she has anything that heavy to carry, becomes irrelevant if the concern is about the activities the person values.

While the social, medical and the disablement models have a fixed and limited set of criteria for disability, the strength of the Capabilities Approach is to make the selection of relevant evaluative dimensions for disability an explicit exercise in social choice. For example, under the capability rubric, the 12-year-old girl with learning difficulties (described earlier) who stays home with her parents helping with household chores would still be seen as capability-deprived, whether she lives in a society where young girls are not expected to go to school or if her culture expects school attendance in either case. This is because, in both scenarios she would be deprived of choices.

In line with the Capabilities Approach, the ICF is concerned with the lived experience of the individual. That is, it takes into account what matters to people (Sayer, 2011). However, the term 'functioning' has different meanings in the ICF and in Sen's Capabilities Approach. In the ICF, it includes functionings that are directly related to health (body functions and structures) as well as activities and participation in a wide range of life domains (for example, education, self-care, work). Sen's concept of functionings is broader in that it includes activities (for example, playing soccer) as well as desirable states of persons (for example, being fit), and it can be general (for example, being free of thirst) or specific (for example, drinking wine).

Mitra (2006) argues that the range of functionings under consideration in the ICF includes those that are relevant to disability, and is broad enough to reflect the lived experience of the person. As such, the ICF can be understood as a specification of the Capabilities Approach to disability. An additional similarity between the two approaches is that disability in the ICF has the same meaning as 'actual disability' in the Capabilities Approach: both refer to functioning deprivation. However, in order for the ICF to be a faithful specification of the Capabilities Approach to disability, it would need to be modified to take account of economic constraints, as well as the personal characteristics (for example, gender) that may exacerbate the capability deprivation that results from impairment. This is particularly important for the ICF since it is being implemented worldwide, in a lot of countries where disability often goes hand in hand with poverty. In addition, the ICF is intended as a universal classification of health, functionings and disability applicable across cultures. By contrast, the Capabilities Approach promotes a relativist view of disability, recognising that selecting the dimensions whereby disability is determined is a social/cultural exercise and will therefore vary from society to society (Mitra, 2006).

Tools for implementing a Capabilities Approach

These tools have been devised as ways of conceptualising the Capabilities Approach; they set out the rights perspectives, for example, the basis of substantive freedoms to which all human beings should have a right, and the sets of beliefs and concerns that underpin the approach. Using these tools it is possible to devise practical strategies to address endemic social injustice for people with disabilities.

Ten conceptual tools of the Capabilities Approach

1. A substantive freedoms approach to human flourishing that places a huge emphasis on *agency* (the exercise of self-determination) and, in consequence, casts a critical eye on developmental or assistance programs that target wellbeing but ignore or impair agency
2. A sustained concern with *context*: the social machinery that enables people to *convert* resources and rules into real opportunities
3. A working hypothesis that among the lasting effects of deprivation is the toll it takes on one's 'moral self' or soul
4. A belief held by people with difficulties that their limitations are fated, if not just, and that adjustment of aspirations downward is the safest way to go
5. A conviction that social wrongs and harms – and thus the local ledger of injustice – must include both material and symbolic forms of deprivation and devaluation
6. The idea that assisted development schemes should be judged by how well they enlarge the actual field of valued options in an ordinary life, and by the process through which they accomplish this
7. The belief that planning a life and social participation – including the 'social bases of self-respect' that underwrite one's commitment to both of these – are two core capabilities
8. Concern with the tension between an assured but other-defined wellbeing and the riskier road to fulfilment that one maps oneself, often haltingly, through mishaps and instructive failures
9. Concern with the distinction between a weak sense of agency (intentional action) and a strong sense that includes a *reflective* component – or what might be called 'critical agency'

10. The idea that two frameworks are possible: a) an applied/modified social model of disability, interpreted from a capabilities perspective; b) and a more thoroughly reconfigured, if still work-in-progress, interpretation; one that subjects the category of impairment itself to close scrutiny.

How the Capabilities Approach can strengthen a social model of mental health

In this section we will draw on some recent work which has begun to apply the Capabilities Approach to mental health (Hopper, 2007; 2012; Ware et al, 2007) to rethink how to prevent or minimise 'psychiatric disability'. We will use two examples to illustrate this. First, we will use the example of recovery from 'schizophrenia'.[1] Second, we will go back to first principles for successful early intervention in psychosis, or what has been called 'first break'.[2]

The Capabilities Approach and recovery from 'schizophrenia'

The focus on securing the resources and opportunities needed to craft a life worth living represents a promising framework to improve the quality of life for people coping with long term mental illness such as 'schizophrenia'. The Capabilities Approach's focus on the *meaning* of a good life – a life of one's own authorship, aimed toward flourishing, not merely coping – is compatible with seeing 'recovery' as an ongoing process that takes place within social contexts. Recovery is not only about overcoming or 'managing' illness, symptoms, or presumed deficiencies; rather, it is about reclaiming the possibility of a real life, the kind of life that people (with choices) want to live. 'Recovery asks not what such people should be content with but what they should be capable of, and how that might be best achieved and sustained' (Hopper, 2007, 875).

If we reconceptualise living with schizophrenia in terms of the viable identities and real prospects available to people, then 'recovery' becomes a social project, not just a treatment regimen. There may be treatments and technologies, including medicines and 'illness management' skills to manage voices, which can reduce the 'impairment' of schizophrenia and increase capacity. However, the Capabilities Approach also insists that 'enablements' be in place to ensure 'enhanced capacity' can be converted to valued social roles and activities. Here, then, it anticipates the need for wider social technologies such as supported employment, job coaching and social enterprises which can provide the right environment to enable a person to make choices. Further, recovery must be about shared 'meaning-making' as well as material provision of things like housing and work. So a capabilities-informed social recovery is about citizenship as well as health, and about what enables people to thrive and flourish, not merely to survive. This can put it at odds with convention: 'Eying custom critically [the Capabilities Approach] seeks out suppressed discontent and invites people to question received roles and life courses. It prizes choice but makes unexamined commitments problematic. Taking capabilities seriously means creating imaginative space where other-than-conventionally prescribed possibilities might be glimpsed' (Hopper, 2007, 874).

This, in turn, draws attention to the link between disability studies – concerned with how impairment is transformed into socially relevant limitations and restrictions – and the Capabilities Approach – concerned as well about the suppressed assumptions regarding moral worth and limited capacity. Each approach seeks to interrogate the taken-for-granted ways in which injuries of body and mind are transformed into locally defined distinctions with practical consequences (such as discrimination) and emotional impacts (such as shame). But the Capabilities Approach explicitly examines past experiences and unexamined assumptions which have set invisible standards for the subjective and objective measurement of quality of life – standards that are in wide currency and easily internalised by individual disabled people.

Quality of life studies of people with schizophrenia repeatedly show that people tend to be more positive about their lives than would appear objectively justified, which seems to be because they have adapted to their circumstances and lowered their expectations (Pinikahana et al, 2002). Disturbingly, these studies are too often accepted uncritically, without examining or questioning this apparent satisfaction with limited life choices (Wallcraft, 2011). A Capabilities Approach questions whether people's current expressions of 'satisfaction' are representative of what they *might have chosen* if real opportunities presented themselves. Perhaps they are survival strategies patched together to navigate a world that consistently counsels cramped hopes and small futures. The Capabilities Approach teaches us that when schooled by deprivation to self-contain and repress, disappointment can be pre-empted if one trims one's hopes to what's possible.

Therefore, we must re-emphasise that it is not just about how people actually function, but their having real options, genuine opportunities – the practical *choice* – to function in important ways *if they so wish*.

Examples might include: basic education, freedom to form a family, to pursue a career, become an artist, etc. People can be deprived of such capabilities in many ways, for example, by ignorance, government regulation, political oppression, lack of financial resources, or their own (conditioned) unawareness or 'misrecognition' of their real situation (sometimes called 'false consciousness'). See Tang's (2013) study of the recovery journeys of Chinese mental health service users living in the UK for an in-depth exploration of such factors.

The Capabilities Approach is also about ensuring that the 'social bases of self-respect' are seen as essential capabilities (Rawls, 1971; Nussbaum, 2000).

> The social bases of self-respect are features of institutions that are needed to enable people to have the confidence that their position in society is respected and their conception of the good is worth pursuing. These features depend upon history and culture. Primary among these social bases in a democratic society are the conditions needed for equal citizenship, including equality of political rights and fair equal opportunity, as well as personal independence and adequate material means for achieving it (Freeman, 2014).

Institutionalised disrespect compounds the suffering of those already struggling with the experience of psychosis. Forging a life plan of one's own making, and having it command the regard of respected others, is how the social bases of self-respect translate into practice.

Therefore, taking action based on the Capabilities Approach could include making an inventory of what valued 'beings and doings' are currently available to people living with schizophrenia, and documenting the day to day realities of disadvantage, and assessing the capabilities-enhancing potential of existing interventions. This is a starting point for an exercise to find out what the deficiencies are in access to information, mobility, engagement with others and debate, and the problems that people might have in planning their lives in a situation of poverty and isolation. If people with schizophrenia are to participate in public debate and in the transformative exercise of reworking cultural templates of disability, many will need specific support to develop the relevant skills and confidence, coping skills and ability to manage their mental health problems.

Finally, the recovery literature shows that people are not simply asking for social recognition in the 'identity politics' sense. People are actually calling for redress of past injuries and neglect (from the cumulative impact of confinement, unwelcome regimens of surveillance, discrimination and exclusion, all of which can cripple imagination and weaken moral agency). People are also seeking reparation (for homes, better health, companionship, decent work and respect from others). All of this requires the development of an active user/survivor movement and alternative communities of practice able to make recovery a collective and contested project (Hopper, 2007).

The adoption of the Capabilities Approach as a rights-based social model of disability, and as a form of analysis of which aspects of a valued life people with diagnoses of severe mental illness have been deprived of, could help the movement to unite with allies and to argue for programmes of reparation which take into account the wide variety of forms which capabilities-deprivation can take and the variety of solutions needed. The struggle for reparation should link with international human rights legislation, in particular the UN Convention on the Rights of Persons with Disabilities (CRPD).

The Capabilities Approach and early intervention

A first experience of a psychotic breakdown is often a threshold event in a young person's life. Young people can be vulnerable to breakdown at transition points such as leaving home, starting work or college and loss of family or relationship; as well as where issues of sexuality are concerned. Breakdown can be the culmination of a vexed sequence of confusion, non-communication, fear and desperation. If undeflected, psychiatric hospitalisation can mark an irreversible initial step on the road to long-term patient-hood (Wallcraft, 2002). Expectations are cut back, routines changed, old social networks fade and more limited ones take their place. Hopes for a once bright future are dashed and plans reconfigured. Family members and friends can become uneasy and tentative in their interactions with the troubled young person. At risk of being 'written off' (Russo, 2009), a young life is socially redefined and tacitly sidelined from normal developmental trajectories. Young people in crisis risk being diverted from gaining basic core competencies they need for their stage of life, skills which can only be gained by taking risks and learning by trial and error.

These early experiences, coupled with ongoing real and perceived constraints – pre-set assumptions and discrimination – can instil in people a sense of limited prospects and opportunities. People can become convinced of their own inferiority, which can damage their ability to hope and see beyond what is given them to what might be possible (for example, ways in which women are prevented from achieving their aspirations, especially in some societies). In poverty studies, one may read about dreams that never reach formulation or aspirations blocked before they can be entertained. Mental health system survivors experience something similar. Sen called this 'adaptive preferences' (Sen, 1985b) – a self-initiated tamping down of what one wants or allows oneself to hope for.

So, how can a Capabilities Approach assist us in preventing this situation? A Capabilities Approach to transitional crises could support young people to plan their lives, providing an alternative to the negative social definition of mental patient-hood (albeit now mainly community-based since long-term hospitalisation has become rare). This approach would seem to favour non-medical crisis alternatives (such as crisis respites, Soteria houses, or early intervention services) which minimise the physical and social disruptiveness of institutionalisation and long-term medication. It could offer opportunities for:

- personal crisis to be reframed as an unwelcome but potentially productive ordeal – an opportunity to re-assess one's values and goals;
- incorporating 'peers' who have been there themselves and can reassure the person in trouble that they've come to right place and will find security, guidance and welcome here;
- interrupting the disablement process at the point of initial reception so that the disruptive impact and negative social consequences of using mental health services are muted;
- minimising biographical disruption by appropriately timed alternatives (that is, not only in the wake of the *failure* of conventional treatments) to help prevent social exclusion in the first place.

In this way, a Capabilities Approach can inform preventive approaches to help ensure that people experiencing a first episode of psychosis do not also have to experience long-term psychiatric disability. In other words, alternatives informed by a Capabilities Approach would de-medicalise 'first break', seeing it as a transition (albeit severe and painful) and provide experienced 'guides' who are confident that the person can make it through and who are able to provide support and reassurance.

Conclusions

The social model of disability has been a powerful lever for legislation and adaptations to make the world more accessible for the physically disabled. This is relatively straightforward compared to what is needed in mental health, which calls for a transformation in how we view madness and mental/emotional problems, and adaptations to make the world accessible for us. Although the social model of disability can be applied to mental health in theory, in practice what is needed is so much more complex and goes against the grain of current assumptions about 'severe mental illness'.

We have argued that the Capabilities Approach could provide the 'social model of mental health' if it can be specified as valued *locally embedded practices* which are open to debate and discussion. On-going opportunities, such as focus groups and workshops, could be created to debate the Capabilities Approach and to encourage service users and allies to draw out the real life meanings of the term and how these could be practically applied in their locality or with reference to particular sets of needs and issues. At present the arguments may seem over-complicated set against the simplicity of the social model of disability. However, oversimplifying it might lose the subtle and complex adjustments it leads us to make – and miss out on the potentially clarifying effects of further debate.

We have begun to explore how the Capabilities Approach can be extended to make 'recovery' and 'prevention' really work in mental health. This would reconfigure the social model by subjecting the categories of impairment, functioning or mental illness itself to close scrutiny, and analysing the power of diagnosis and treatment to create capability deprivation. It would build on progress the service user/survivor movement has been making towards self-management and peer support, but make this part of a broader, shared understanding that people need mainstream funded support, while being given space to make decisions based on their own values and enabling them to work towards their chosen goals.

In the UK today, given the retraction of public services, this seems a distant dream. However, the elaboration of the Capabilities Approach could lead towards an international movement to enable people who have been labelled and treated as 'mentally ill' to develop their capabilities and exert their freedom to choose from a range of personally and socially valued forms of help and support, claiming and exercising their rights alongside other disabled people. This approach helps us to support the extension of people's substantive freedom of choice in mental health. It also enables us to recognise and compensate for the damage done to service users and survivors by denial of those freedoms in the past.

Notes

[1] 'Schizophrenia' is a highly contested diagnosis (see Thomas, 2013; Coles at al, 2013).

[2] We draw on the proceedings of a working conference, co-sponsored by the Center to Study Recovery in Social Contexts and INTAR, held in New York in November 2009, especially the working papers by Jasna Russo 'Reclaiming of a life written off: Survivor perspectives on first breakdown' and Kim Hopper's 'Reframing early psychiatric crises' (Hopper, 2012).

SEVEN

Psycho-emotional disablism in the lives of people experiencing mental distress

Donna Reeve

Introduction

The social model of disability has been criticised for adopting a medicalised view of mental distress and for failing to take account of people's lived experience of mental health problems (Plumb, 1994). In addition, insights from the mental health survivor movement have largely been overlooked by academic writing in the field of disability studies (Beresford, 2000). This omission may result from the fact that structural disablism – with its emphasis on barriers to activity – is perceived to have limited relevance for those experiencing mental distress or 'mental illness' (I will use the term 'mental distress' throughout this chapter). It will be argued that psycho-emotional disablism (Thomas, 2007), by contrast, is a much more common form of disablism in the lives of people who experience mental distress, often in the form of negative attitudes, prejudice and internalised oppression. One consequence of psycho-emotional disablism is that it can lead to increased levels of anxiety and stress which, in turn, increase the level of mental distress the person is experiencing.

This chapter will discuss psycho-emotional disablism and consider its applicability to people experiencing mental distress, arguing that this concept has particular relevance here, because of the focus on barriers to being rather than restrictions on activity (Thomas, 2007). In particular, this chapter will explore the ramifications of framing mental distress as arising from an interaction between the psyche and society rather than from a pre-existing impairment, distinct from the experience of disablism. If disablism *'constitutes the very thing that is deemed the illness itself'* (Spandler, 2012, 15, emphasis in original), then the experience of mental distress has important implications for ongoing theoretical debates within disability studies about the complex, blurred relationship(s) between disablism and impairment. In short, this chapter teases out the connections between the concepts of mental distress, disablism and impairment and considers how they are mediated by structural disablism, psycho-emotional disablism, and the psycho-emotional effects of impairment.

The extended social relational definition of disablism

The social model of disability has done much to improve the lives of disabled people through identifying and challenging the economic, cultural, social and environmental barriers which exclude people with impairments from mainstream society. Drawing on the same UPIAS statement which underpinned the social model of disability (UPIAS/ Disability Alliance, 1976), Thomas (2007) has proposed an extended social relational definition of disablism: 'Disablism is a form of social oppression involving the social imposition of restrictions of activity on people with impairments and the *socially engendered undermining of their psycho-emotional wellbeing*' (Thomas, 2007, 73, my emphasis).

This means that the social oppression experienced by people with impairments is placed in the same domain as racism, sexism and ageism. This chapter will largely use the term 'disablism' when referring to the processes that marginalise disabled people in society, particularly those that operate at the psycho-emotional level. 'Disability' is associated with the disabling barriers approach of the social model of disability and its prevalence within the literature means that this term will also be used in this chapter where appropriate (see Thomas, 2007, 13).

Disablism can be broken down into two strands: structural disablism and psycho-emotional disablism. Structural disablism has a direct impact on what people can do and refers to the disabling barriers which operate at the public level, such as exclusion from the built environment, discrimination in the work place or information in inaccessible formats. Structural disablism refers, in other words, to the disabling barriers typically associated with the social model of disability. Psycho-emotional disablism, on the other hand, operates at the private level, restricting who people can be. Examples of psycho-emotional disablism include having to deal with the hurtful comments or stigmatising actions of others, along with internalised oppression which can all undermine someone's psycho-emotional wellbeing and sense of self (Reeve, 2008). It is important to note that the experience of psycho-emotional disablism is not inevitable; it can vary with time and place, and may be influenced by personal history, other aspects of identity such as ethnicity or gender, as well as by experiences of impairment and structural disablism (Reeve, 2008).

While the social model does not deny the reality of psycho-emotional disablism, structural disablism has dominated discussions within academia, policy and grassroots activism. This has resulted in psycho-emotional disablism, and its long-term consequences, being overlooked. Having to deal with the stares and comments of strangers can exclude someone from the built environment as effectively as a flight of stairs, showing how barriers to being can also result in barriers to doing. In addition, the impact of psycho-emotional disablism can be likened to that of emotional abuse because of its long-term and cumulative effects (Reeve, 2006). Consequently, how someone deals with current psycho-emotional disablism can be affected by their past experiences of psycho-emotional disablism or abuse. The failure to take account of psycho-emotional disablism may arise, in part, from a reluctance to engage with psychology, due to its preoccupation with individual tragedy models of disability and association of disability with loss. Whatever the reasons, the impact of psycho-emotional disablism on the lives of disabled people has been neglected.

Psycho-emotional disablism and mental distress

People who are given a psychiatric diagnosis by the mental health system are identified, in terms of legislation, as disabled people – whether or not they self-identify as such (Beresford, 2000). This brings a measure of protection against discrimination in the workplace although prejudice against this group of people often remains because of the prevalence of associations between 'mental illness' and dangerousness (Beresford et al, 2010). In line with the finding that people are more prejudiced towards people with mental health conditions than those with physical or sensory impairments (Staniland, 2011), people with mental health conditions experience disproportionate rates of disablist hate crime compared to most other impairment groups (Sin et al, 2009).

Disablist hate crime is an extreme form of psycho-emotional disablism carried out by a perpetrator whose actions are based, at least in part, on their assumptions about the invalidity and less-than-human identity of someone they perceive to be disabled. For example, leaving the house can make someone vulnerable to name calling by neighbours, based on prejudices such as 'psycho', 'nutter', 'freak' and 'schizo' (Mind, 2007, 6). It is not difficult to see the negative impact that this form of psycho-emotional disablism can have on emotional wellbeing. Stigma, verbal abuse or harassment, particularly if experienced on a daily basis, might be expected to exacerbate the experience of mental distress. This point will be returned to later in this chapter.

I can see how the conventional social model of disability with its focus on removing *structural barriers* appears to have little to offer people experiencing mental distress. A social relational definition of disablism, by contrast, highlights disabling barriers that operate at both the public and private levels and is better fitted to this group of people, for whom psycho-emotional disablism is likely to be the most disabling. The harassments and prejudice that people with (perceived) 'mental illness' experience need to be labelled, not as prejudice, but as forms of *disablism*; this renaming highlights the role played by cultural and ideological beliefs that position 'normal' people as being superior to those perceived to be impaired. In addition, it can be argued that the medical profession operates a form of institutional psycho-emotional disablism where 'mental illness' is diagnosed and associated with incurability and hopelessness.

Internalised oppression is another form of psycho-emotional disablism which happens when someone internalises the devalued and stigmatising messages about madness and mental distress. 'We are generally seen (even by ourselves?) as being at fault – "not coping", "not fitting in" of "holding strange views" or "behaving oddly"' (participant in Beresford et al, 2010, 18).

Internalised oppression is insidious and difficult to counter because it largely acts at an unconscious level. As well as having a potentially damaging impact on someone's self-esteem and sense of self, internalised oppression is likely to exacerbate their level of mental distress by increasing fear and anxiety levels. Beresford et al (2010) call for more attention to be paid to helping people challenge their own internalised oppression through support from survivor-led organisations. Developing a positive sense of identity goes a long way towards helping people resist the negative messages and attitudes of others; for example, organisations such as Survivors Speak Out (Plumb, 1994) or the Hearing Voices Network (Hornstein, 2009) have directly challenged negative, dehumanising and medicalised identities that circulate in society.

Finally, because psycho-emotional disablism arises from relationships that a disabled person has with others, positive relationships with a single person can have a healing effect on the disabled individual, and may mitigate the negative effects of psycho-emotional disablism (Reeve, 2008). For example, Tew (2011) points out that many 'recovery' narratives feature a single individual who continued to offer acceptance, respect and recognition of a person experiencing mental distress, at a time when other social support had faded away. This *humanising* response counters the *dehumanising* impact of stigma and verbal abuse which can exacerbate the experience of mental distress. It may come in the form of a professional who goes the 'extra mile' or a peer supporter based in a user-led organisation providing support to those recovering from/learning to live with mental distress.

Mental distress as a different way of being

Plumb (1994) argues that what is termed 'mental illness' is often the result of culture and adverse social experiences rather than being down to a chemical imbalance in the brain or faulty genes. The idea of impairment is obviously inappropriate for those people who see themselves as *being* different as opposed to *having* a deficit or chronic illness. So, if mental distress has its roots in relationships that the individual has with society and others (past/present), then there is also a need to recognise diversity of 'being'. Unfortunately our society is not very accepting of difference: 'We all identify with each other, but we don't live in a society, despite the facts that we speak about individuality, we really don't like difference, do we? Anybody who's slightly different, reacts differently, get 'em out as quickly as possible, or try and change them' (participant in Beresford et al, 2010, 26).

This is one of the points of departure from the social model of disability. Disabled people tend to be fighting for inclusion into mainstream society. However, for others, it may be the experience of being a 'round peg in a square hole' which causes the mental distress in the first place, which then gets labelled as 'mental illness' (Plumb, 1994). Therefore, for some psychiatric survivors, rather than being shaved down to fit the allotted hole, the fight is for a changed society which recognises diversity and allows for new and creative ways of being.

Psycho-emotional disablism stifles these diverse ways of being and invalidates and rejects the person experiencing them. Combating these effects is one of the important functions of survivor-run mental health organisations. For example, an important contribution of the Hearing Voices Network has been to advocate *listening* to what people's inner voices are saying, and making sense of the role they play in the context of someone's life, rather than simply silencing these inner voices with drugs (Hornstein, 2009). Ontological validation is important to people experiencing mental distress, particularly when they may have experienced years of having their fears and experiences labelled by 'experts' as unreal fantasies, delusions or symptoms (Kristiansen, 2004).

In many ways, the ontological questions being asked here are similar to some of the debates going on in the neurodiversity movement. Here 'neurodiverse' ways of being are valued alongside the conventional neurotypically-informed 'norms' of being (for more exploration of this, see Chapter 16 by Steve Graby in this book). In both cases disablism emerges when the behaviour and actions of those who are neurodiverse or are experiencing mental distress 'clash' with societal norms of *behaviour*, which of course varies with culture, time and place. This is substantially different from the case of other groups of disabled people where the disjuncture is more connected with societal norms of moving, comprehension and perception and where the removal of disabling barriers – such as installing a lift, making information accessible or the provision of tactile pavement edges at street crossings – is 'common sense' (Plumb, 1994, 14).

Disabled *and* experiencing mental distress: an invisible group of people?

While increasing attention has been paid to how service providers can meet the needs of people with mental health difficulties or those with physical impairments, the needs of people who fall into both categories have been largely overlooked (Morris, 2004a). Adverse social experiences can happen to anyone, so people with physical impairments are at least as likely to experience mental distress as non-disabled people. Research located in the medical and psychological sciences generally reports that disabled people experience *higher* rates of mental distress than their non-disabled counterparts (see for example Okoro et al, 2009).

Most research about people who have both physical impairment and mental distress assumes, however, that mental distress is caused by the experience of impairment itself (Morris, 2004b). Thus the 'psycho-emotional effect of impairment' (Thomas, 1999, 47) is usually assumed to take the form of depression, despite limited evidence of any firm correlation between the degree of depression and the severity of impairment (Morris, 2004b). Other forms of mental distress are also attributed to impairment; for example, one woman discovered that her medical notes stated that she had an 'understandable personality disorder because of her disability [sic]' (Begum, 1999 cited in Morris, 2004b, 8).

Thus the impact of living with the experience of *disablism* is usually overlooked, not helped by the continual elision of impairment/ disability in everyday language (as seen in the short quote above).

For example, disabled people with congenital impairments might be predicted to have higher rates of mental distress, given the increased likelihood of their having been abused as children (Westcott and Cross, 1996). Disability is also associated with increased poverty, lower socio-economic status and unemployment and these factors are recognised as increasing the likelihood of mental health difficulties developing from existing adverse life experiences such as trauma or abuse (Tew, 2011). This would suggest that the experience of disablism itself (social oppression and associated poverty, exclusion, stigma etc) could contribute to rates of mental distress among disabled people. This would include those with pre-existing impairments, as well as those who develop impairments as consequences of mental distress; for example as a result of accidental and self-inflicted injuries or as a direct result of psychiatric intervention, for example through the side-effects of medication (Morris, 2004b).

I would argue that the experience of psycho-emotional disablism, along with other adverse life experiences such as childhood abuse, is likely to contribute more to mental distress than the experience of any impairment per se. It should be noted that many research studies into mental distress explicitly exclude participants who have other medical conditions, despite the fact that such participants make up the bulk of the population experiencing forms of mental distress such as schizophrenia (Jeste et al, 1996 cited in Morris, 2004b). This erases the voices of disabled people who are also experiencing mental distress (other than depression 'caused' by impairment).

The relative absence of impaired bodies from the literature about mental distress, in turn, has implications for disabled people experiencing mental distress who require accessible inpatient care and community-based support. In a survey carried out in 2004, ward managers reported that 87% of wards were accessible to those with mobility impairments, but only 64% of wards were fully/partially accessible for those with sensory impairments (Garcia et al, 2005). In contrast, research carried out in the same year with people with physical impairments, rather than ward managers, found that six out of ten people rated their experience of in-patient care as poor or very poor (Morris, 2004a); these figures are similar to inpatient satisfaction rates generally (Mind, 2004). Difficulties were reported with physical environments which were not fully accessible, a situation which was made worse by staff attitudes and responses. Some participants felt that the failure to meet their physical needs while in hospital caused considerable stress and in some cases had actually made their physical impairment worse.

Deaf people face disproportionate rates of social exclusion and unemployment, because the language needs of those who rely on British Sign Language for communication are poorly met within education and work environments. While the exact numbers are unknown, because the psychiatric system (and research) is based on the experiences of a hearing population, a clear causal link between mental distress and the experience, for deaf people, of living in a hearing world, has been drawn: '…pressure all though my life with people not accepting my Deafness, being under pressure to conform, to be normal, to be a normal person. Sometimes I just feel like I have no strength, no energy, nothing. That's why I became ill' (respondent in Prendergast, 2003, cited in Tuohy and Cooper, 2007, 28).

Indeed the disproportionately high rates of mental distress in the Deaf community have been officially recognised as a *'consequence of being Deaf in a hearing world*, rather than an innate predisposition' (Department of Health, 2002, 11, my emphasis). In addition, it has also been suggested that internalised oppression (psycho-emotional disablism) is very common among Deaf people, leading to very low self-esteem (Tuohy and Cooper, 2007).

The stickiness of 'impairment' within accounts of mental distress

Plumb (1994, 4–5) argues that mental distress is actually analogous to disablism rather than impairment, because the roots of mental distress are to be found within an individual's relationship with society rather than in a chemical imbalance or other impairment. The 'causes' of mental distress are complex, multifaceted and rarely follow a tidy causal chain. Mental distress can develop as a consequence of traumatic childhood experiences, chaotic lifestyles and tensions within personal relationships along with current stresses, oppression and humiliation. Difficulties in the here-and-now may be exacerbated by unresolved issues from the past. In the absence of access to social support and social capital, and where resilience may be compromised, unease in someone's life can develop into mental distress (see Tew, 2011, 88–98).

Research carried out by Beresford et al (2010) suggests that people experiencing mental distress do not generally consider themselves to have an impairment. They often express ambivalence about the term, although they do articulate the need for something closely related to it: 'Well, I've always felt a bit uncomfortable about this, but it's there isn't it…I mean there's an impairment that's imposed on people in some kind of way, I suppose it is the equivalent, it's not a very good word, but it is the equivalent' (participant in Beresford et al, 2010, 28).

For those who do see mental distress as an impairment, the latter is seen as socially constructed and fluctuating, not as 'objective' and 'measureable' as are the physical, sensory and intellectual impairments typically associated with a social model of disability. Many participants in this research saw their mental distress as a temporary phase from which they would recover, rather than a situation which was permanent.

The ambivalence noted above may be due to confusion about what 'counts' as disability or impairment. Kristiansen (2004) challenges the construction of impairment as purely social, arguing that this denies aspects of the experience of mental distress in itself – such as discomfort, terror or physical pain caused by hearing loud voices – which do not originate from society or relationships. Recognising that 'impairment' may refer to something less straightforward than a paralysed limb or poor vision, Kristiansen suggests that it may be more helpful to see disability and impairment as blurred, rather than in terms of the dichotomy suggested by traditional social model approaches. For example, one participant in her research with women experiencing mental distress in Norway described how: '[p]eople I know avoid me on the streets, look the other way...my doctor says I'm paranoid, oversensitive...I don't feel I am, but I just don't know...I don't think the medicine helps, but what else can I do?' (participant in Kristiansen, 2004, 379).

In reality, what is seen as being caused by 'impairment' and what is down to 'disability' is unclear as the two threads are tightly interwoven. Certainly traces of 'impairment' persist in many of the accounts of those experiencing mental distress; for those who 'see themselves as somehow "crazy"..."something" feels very real, and whatever "it" is, it sometimes feels physical and "inside the head"' (Kristiansen, 2004, 378).

Therefore, theoretical analyses of mental distress need to include reference to impairment in some form or another. How then, based on the discussion so far, might impairment, disablism/disability and mental distress interplay and have an impact on each other?

Interactions of mental distress with disablism and impairment

Throughout this chapter I have considered the different ways that mental distress is considered (or not) to interconnect with disablism and impairment. While this has largely revealed the part played by psycho-emotional disablism in the experience of mental distress, I have also explored the role played by impairment. I now want to build on these arguments to consider the *interaction* between these three very different terms: disablism caused by society and social relations; impairment linked to medical conditions (usually of the body); and mental distress (linked to being).

In my view, it is necessary to look at mental distress in this interlinked way in order to appreciate the complexity of the experience. Below I have identified factors which contribute to each of the pairs of interactions between disablism, mental distress and impairment:

Interactions between disablism and mental distress:

- People experiencing mental distress have to deal with the prejudices and attitudes of other people in society; in other words, they can experience psycho-emotional disablism due to the hurtful reactions of others.
- Internalised oppression (a form of psycho-emotional disablism) is possible if someone absorbs and starts to own the negative messages about mental distress circulating in society.
- The negative impact of psycho-emotional disablism on self-esteem and self-confidence, can cause additional stress/anxiety which, in turn, exacerbates mental distress. This is more significant than the impact of psycho-emotional disablism on impairment described below.
- Structural disablism has less of an impact than psycho-emotional disablism, but can still exist in areas such as discrimination in employment and housing. The experience of discrimination, like psycho-emotional disablism, can cause additional stress which in turn exacerbates mental distress.

Interactions between impairment and disablism:

- People with impairments face structural disablism such as discrimination and inaccessible environments which prevent them from participating fully in society.
- Structural disablism is likely to be more significant for those living with impairments than for those living with mental distress because of environmental barriers such as inaccessible buildings.
- People with impairments can experience psycho-emotional disablism arising from the prejudices and attitudes of other people in society.

- Internalised oppression can result if someone absorbs and starts to own the negative messages and images about disability circulating in society.
- Structural and psycho-emotional disablism can have an adverse impact on impairment; for example pushing a wheelchair up a ramp which is too steep can cause shoulder problems; dealing with the thoughtless comments of others can cause stress which can make pain and muscular problems worse. However, the experience of disablism exacerbates impairment less than it does mental distress.

Interactions between mental distress and impairment:

- Medical treatments for 'mental illness', such as drugs, often come with side effects which can cause physical impairment (Breggin, 2008). This has often been called 'iatrogenic harm', in other words, the negative effects of medical intervention.
- People experiencing mental distress are at higher risk of acquiring physical impairments as a result of accidental and self-inflicted injuries (Morris, 2004b).
- There are some aspects of the experience of mental distress which feel very 'real' to the individual, such as discomfort or physical pain associated with hearing loud voices (Kristiansen, 2004). These could be considered as forms of 'impairment'.
- Psycho-emotional effects of impairment (Thomas, 1999, 47) refers to the emotional difficulties that are 'side-effects' of living with some impairments. For example, chronic pain is often associated with depression and anxiety which could contribute to (the likelihood of) mental distress.

These three pairs of interaction can be represented in Figure 7.1 showing the complex interplay between mental distress, disablism and impairment for someone experiencing mental distress. It is also important to note that for each person who experiences mental distress, the interconnections will weigh differently; each interaction will vary with time, place and personal experience, as well as in relation to any existing impairment.

Figure 7.1 is an attempt to represent the complex interplay between mental distress, disablism and impairment for people experiencing mental distress. However, it should be noted that in reality these interactions are far more intertwined, interdependent and blurred than simple arrows can imply. Figure 7.1 builds on these four guiding principles:

- It considers mental distress as disablism: and it replaces 'society disables us' with 'society distresses us' (Plumb, 2012a, 21).
- It recognises mental distress as a valid way of being.
- It differentiates so-called 'mental illness' from impairment, but still takes account of 'something' that feels 'real' and 'inside the head', that can cause confusion and pain such as discomfort associated with hearing distressing voices (Kristiansen, 2004, 378).
- It includes experiences of disabled people (with impairments) who also experience mental distress.

Figure 7.1: Interactions of mental distress, disablism and impairment for people experiencing mental distress

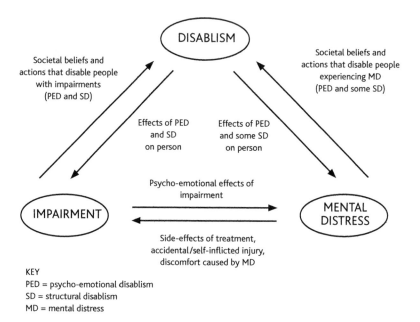

KEY
PED = psycho-emotional disablism
SD = structural disablism
MD = mental distress

In particular, I have separated out aspects of oppression (largely psycho-emotional disablism) which can and must be challenged within society. However, I acknowledge that I have continued to use the terms structural and psycho-emotional disablism which, in their definition, refers to 'impairment'. While I acknowledge that this is problematic for some writers (Plumb, 1994), it does continue to stress the related social oppression experienced by both disabled people and those experiencing mental distress, and it is difficult to formulate an alternative strategy at this time.

Conclusions

This chapter has explored the relevance of psycho-emotional disablism for people living with mental distress. Leaving aside the discussion about whether this group of people self-identify as disabled or not, they are seen as 'different' by other people in society and experience psycho-emotional disablism in the guise of derogatory comments, name calling and prejudicial attitudes. Psycho-emotional disablism also includes the pathologisation of ways of *being* that fail to fit narrow definitions of 'normal'. Thus psycho-emotional disablism is a reality in the lives of many people living with mental distress and, moreover, often exacerbates mental distress because of the stress and anxiety that psycho-emotional disablism can cause.

Mental distress reflects diverse ways of *being* rather than different ways of doing, sensing or learning. As such, mental distress has more in common with neurodiversity than with other impairment groups relating to physical, sensory or intellectual impairments. Society is becoming much better at including people with physical and sensory impairments, largely because the accommodations required are perceived as 'common sense', such as a ramp for a wheelchair user or lift buttons labelled with Braille. The journey for those experiencing so-called 'mental illness' is much harder because the changes needed at a societal, cultural and institutional level are much more 'challenging'. The need to accommodate a wheelchair user is easy to comprehend; the need to accommodate a person who behaves differently to the 'norm', who breaks social etiquette about appropriate behaviour, is seen as much more difficult and controversial.

For those who reject a biomedical explanation of mental distress, in favour of a social model understanding, directly equating mental distress with impairment makes little sense. Nonetheless there are some that argue that the experience of mental distress in itself – such as discomfort, terror or physical pain caused by hearing voices – cannot be explained with reference to society or disablism alone (Kristiansen, 2004). Therefore the question of whether mental distress is impairment or disablism or both is slippery, precisely because of the particular characteristics of the experience of mental distress. In addition, as I have shown, this becomes more complicated when taking into account the experiences of people who both have impairments and experience mental distress.

A consequence of these discussions is that any attempt to theorise the experience of mental distress needs to take into account disablism and impairment, as well as mental distress. The concept of psycho-emotional disablism is a vital part of this analysis because it provides clear recognition of the damage done by forms of social oppression that adversely affect emotional wellbeing and restrict diverse ways of being. Although the diagram I have used to illustrate this necessarily over-simplifies the messiness and complexities of real life, it does show the complex interplay between mental distress, disablism and impairment. As such, it contributes to arguments I have made elsewhere about the need to take impairment into account when understanding experiences of disablism (Reeve, 2012b).

Part Three
Applying social models of disability

EIGHT

Psycho-emotional disablism, complex trauma and women's mental distress

Shelley Briggs and Fiona Cameron

Introduction

This chapter will explore the complex and intergenerational trauma that many women with psychiatric diagnoses such as borderline personality disorder experience. We propose that labelling responses to trauma as mental illness often results in further trauma, in stigma and psycho-emotional disablism. Practice responses and the reactions of other people can then contribute further to the distress experienced. However, if individuals' responses to trauma are understood as psycho-emotional adjustments that open up possibilities for alternative reactions on the part of services and communities, that are empowering, build strengths, reduce further risk-taking and boost resilience. The work of Thomas (1999) and Reeve (2004) on expanding the concept of the social model of disability, provides a useful starting point for unpacking this complex interaction.

The social model of disability challenges the medical model as 'an artificial and exclusionary social construction that penalises those... who do not conform to mainstream expectations of appearance, behaviour and/or economic performance' (Tregaskis, 2002, 457). Those who experience mental distress may be seen as transgressing all of these expectations, as a result both of the impact of their perceived impairment (for example, depression, anxiety or psychosis) and the behaviour often associated with it (such as withdrawal, lack of self-care, self-harming or talking to voices). While the social model challenges exclusionary social structures, Thomas (1999) called for its extension through a social relational model to take into account impairment effects and the psycho-emotional effects of disablism.

Carol Thomas defines disability as a 'form of social oppression involving the social imposition of restrictions of activity on people with impairments and the socially engendered undermining of their psycho-emotional well-being' (Thomas, 1999, 60). For her, psycho-emotional disablism involves 'the intended and unintended "hurtful" words and social actions of non-disabled people (parents, professionals, complete strangers, others) in inter-personal engagement with people with impairments' (Thomas, 2007, 72). Donna Reeve's chapter in this book (Chapter Seven) uses this notion to analyse the complex interplay between impairment, mental distress and disablism. In this chapter we build on her work by exploring complex trauma as a form of psycho-emotional disablism, particularly for women. The concept of psycho-emotional disablism is useful here because of its emphasis on forms of disablism and distress that are often unrecognised. We argue that women's experience of abuse is often compounded by the hurtful negative reactions of others, especially to the ways they have found to cope with their abuse.

Drawing on our practice experience, we present the story of a woman's experiences of, and responses to, trauma. To illustrate the effects of psycho-emotional disablism we specifically highlight the negative impact of her family, community and services in effectively re-traumatising her, and relate this to our wider experience of working with women experiencing complex trauma.

Complex trauma

People's reactions to trauma are varied and complex, and for many women who have had a series of abusive and traumatic experiences throughout their lives, the trauma is intergenerational. There is increasing awareness of the links between abuse and mental ill-health, especially psychosis and schizophrenia. For example, there is now some evidence to support the view that psychosis can be caused by trauma; that experience of psychosis can contribute to post-traumatic stress disorder (PTSD) and that psychosis and PTSD are on a spectrum of responses to traumatic events (Morrison et al, 2003). The controversial criterion for a diagnosis of PTSD has been successively broadened to include a wide range of subjective symptoms in individuals who have experienced 'toxic events' (Bowman, 1997); varying from one-off events, for example, an incidence of bullying or a minor car crash, to long-term and multiple trauma experiences either in childhood or in adulthood (Herman, 1992).

Intergenerational trauma has been defined as a 'secondary form of trauma that results from the transfer of traumatic experiences from parents to their children' (Doucet and Rovers, 2010, 94). Doucet and Rovers utilise attachment theory to understand the ways in which intergenerational trauma is transferred. They identify two pathways: direct transmission of trauma via unconscious channels of intra-psychic influences and styles of communication, and indirect transmission via parenting styles or suboptimal patterns of family interaction. Intergenerational transmission of trauma, whether direct or indirect, can lead to parents being unable to parent, the child absorbing the unresolved emotional burdens of the parent and themselves taking on a parenting role. Absorbing the parental experience of, or response to, trauma may leave the child feeling unsafe, anxious, depressed or unworthy. We use the term complex trauma to try to capture the dynamics of multiple and intergenerational trauma experienced across the lifespan and the constellation of symptoms that may result.

Background to Sally's story

We have developed Sally's story from our combined practice experience: Shelley Briggs, working with survivors of sexual abuse in the rural Scottish highlands and First Nations communities in remote northern Canada; and Fiona Cameron, working with women with forensic histories in secure and community mental health services in urban English settings. Despite these very different practice settings, we observed some striking similarities in women's experience of complex trauma. Many of the women with whom we worked had experienced traumatic events throughout their lifetime, presenting with changing symptoms, leading to different mental health diagnoses ranging from depression and anxiety to schizophrenia or borderline personality disorder. We particularly noted a similar interplay between individuals, their families and communities, and their diagnosis and treatment in mental health services.

Canadian First Nations communities have the highest level of deprivation in Canada and when women leave their reserves, often in remote and isolated locations, they tend to experience exclusion and discrimination (MacDonald and Wilson, 2013; McCaskill, 2012). The communities in which we worked in Scotland and England had suffered multiple levels of deprivation, with high unemployment, low income and low levels of cultural and social capital, often leading to a reliance on drugs, alcohol, welfare or crime (Savage et al, 2013). In both UK and Canadian contexts, the communities were on the margins of society and had developed their own cultural norms and values. While these communities experienced exclusion from wider society, their cultural norms were often very patriarchal with women often being marginalised, oppressed and abused. Paradoxically, while women experienced violence and trauma, the community also offered them some form of protection from wider societal disapproval and negative reactions, precisely because of its marginalisation and location outside the gaze of mainstream society. However, staying in the community had a significant impact on the level of disablement women experienced, leading many to leave and seek help outside the community. In the British context, we worked with women from a range of different racial and cultural backgrounds and, in the Canadian context, aboriginal people experienced specific historical oppression and trauma which contributed to intergenerational trauma. We have not explored these additional historical and racial complexities, but have chosen to focus on the commonality of women's experiences across these contexts. While Sally could have been located in any of these geographies, we decided to locate her in rural working-class Scotland.

The process of writing Sally's story has been a long and difficult one. We started by sharing our specific practice experiences of women who were given the diagnoses of borderline personality disorder and post-traumatic stress disorder. This work had a powerful impact on us, through our awareness of the devastating outcomes of their experiences for the women themselves (such as suicide), transference of the feelings involved and our intense frustration with inadequate service responses. Sally's story has developed over time, and we use it as a teaching aid on an Approved Mental Health Professional course, where students have been able to identify with the story and share their feelings about it.

Sally's story

Sally is a 38-year-old woman who lives with her husband and young son and close to other family in the community in which she was raised. Sally hears voices that tell her she is a waste of space and would be better off dead, and she is scared and suspicious of people. She has been diagnosed with a variety of mental health conditions over the years, such as behavioural problems, depression, PTSD, psychosis and schizophrenia. She is now under the care of the local mental health services and a psychiatrist who treats her paranoid delusions with medication that makes her feel groggy and flat.

In Sally's family there is an extensive history of trauma with a series of alcohol and drug related deaths and suicides. Sally witnessed and experienced domestic violence by her father and brothers, and was sexually abused at an early age by her uncles, grandfather and later her brother. Sally's mother, who had similar experiences in childhood, was depressed and anxious and unable to protect or support her. Indeed, in a reversal of roles, Sally took on a caring role for her mother. Incidents of domestic violence and problematic alcohol and drug use in the community are high, leading to a number of diagnosed and undiagnosed mental health issues.

Sally witnessed her mother's on-going abuse, as well as her responses to it (for example, becoming numb, withdrawn and depressed). This led to Sally having insecure/disorganised attachments with others. Her attempts to trigger care-giving, by being alternately distressed and then angry, sadly resulted in further rejection from her mother as she was unable to respond to Sally's needs.

When Sally was younger she enjoyed school, but her attendance was intermittent. When her frustration and anger in response to what was happening at home led to her being aggressive, she was expelled. With no escape from the abuse at home, Sally left at 14, moving to a larger city where she lived on the street before being taken in by an older man who introduced her to drugs, prostitution and further violence. She then started to hear voices and experience flashbacks of her childhood abuse.

After a few years, Sally managed to leave her boyfriend/pimp when she was offered help from a women's refuge centre. A gender sensitive approach was adopted, which acknowledged the role of oppression and abuse in her life, and tried to help her develop the skills to recognise potentially harmful situations. As a result of this extension to her repertoire of coping strategies, Sally managed to move into her own flat. However, due to funding cuts, the women's centre was no longer able to provide on-going outreach support at this important transition time. Without this specialist support, and in the face of continued exposure to potentially threatening situations in the community, Sally returned to less helpful coping strategies.

Sally gradually isolated herself in response to acute feelings of anxiety and insomnia and she returned to using drugs to cope with her situation. After a drugs overdose, she was admitted to a psychiatric ward and had her first contact with mental health services, which unfortunately focused on symptom management with limited attention to the abuse she had suffered. She was diagnosed with drug induced psychosis and treated with indifference, sometimes with hostility, by the overworked hospital staff who viewed her mental distress as the result of her wilful drug use (and, by implication, her own fault).

When she was discharged, Sally returned to her home community where, despite her experience of abuse, she felt some sense of belonging. Sally had some connection with her mother and sister but was unable to discuss the abuse she had experienced as a child. It had always been made clear to her that you do not 'snitch' on anyone in the community, especially your own family. She met her husband who, like many of the men in the community, was controlling and violent. Sally's husband reinforced her low self-worth by taunting and bullying her and telling her she was useless and stupid. After a difficult pregnancy, and the birth of her son, the violence in her relationship decreased though she increased contact with male family members which rekindled traumatic memories.

Sally continued to cope by using alcohol, painkillers and a variety of other substances as well as self-harming. While some of these coping mechanisms are similar to those used by other women in her family, when Sally talked to her voices and was suspicious of those around her she was either ignored or teased as the 'mad stupid bitch'. As the incidents of self-harm increased, her family and people in the community reacted with further bullying and taunting, stating that she was worthless and should have 'completed the job'. Sally's levels of self-harm increased and, after a number of suicide attempts, she was admitted to another psychiatric ward and re-diagnosed as having borderline personality disorder. She encountered negative attitudes from staff on the ward where she was viewed as difficult and attention seeking. As the voices became more persistent her suspicions of others increased, leading to further isolation. Over the next few years Sally was in and out of hospital and became a 'revolving door' patient, diagnosed as having a severe and enduring mental illness.

Complex trauma and psycho-emotional disablism

Sally has experienced complex trauma which has occurred throughout her life. This has included sexual abuse in childhood and, in adulthood, abuse from partners, family, community and mental health services. It has also included indirect intergenerational trauma because her mother required parenting as a result of her own psycho-emotional adjustments to the abuse she had experienced before and following Sally's birth; and direct intergenerational trauma because of her mother's inability to provide a safe base for Sally to develop a secure attachment. This contributed to Sally's belief that the world around her was unsafe and untrustworthy. The dissociation she experienced meant that was unable to keep herself safe in adulthood. It is worth noting that mothers with high levels of betrayal trauma in childhood, and interpersonal re-victimisation in adulthood, have been found to have higher levels of dissociation (Hulette et al, 2011). In addition, their re-victimisation has been associated with a higher likelihood that their children would have a history of betrayal trauma, suggesting a persistent unawareness of threat to self and child (Hulette et al, 2011).

There is a complex interplay between Sally's experience and the way in which she has internalised and interpreted these experiences, compounding her feelings of guilt and worthlessness. Sally experienced direct and indirect trauma, and the behaviours she used to cope with this were negatively responded to by her family, community, services and society. These reactions can be understood as psycho-emotional disablism (Thomas, 2007) that causes further distress and trauma. Thus Sally becomes stuck in a spiral of re-traumatisation.

Jokes, taunts and suggestions that she 'might as well top herself' from within the family and the community played a significant role in Sally's experiences of social isolation. The malevolent voices she hears reinforce these external reactions and compound the abuse she suffered. This demonstrates the complex interaction between psycho-emotional disablism and her distress. Sally responds to this with behaviour that elicits further negative community reactions, leading to further mental distress and impairment. This becomes a vicious cycle out of which it is difficult to break. To explore this complex interplay between Sally's experience of, and reactions to, trauma and psycho-emotional disablism, the next section will discuss, in turn, responses to trauma at the individual, family, community and service level.

Individual responses to trauma

The behaviours that resulted in Sally being diagnosed as mentally ill can be seen as psycho-emotional adjustments to long-term and multiple trauma experiences which can include acute anxiety and wariness of social interaction, self-medicating with substances and self-harm (Herman, 1992). Sally's responses varied from hyper-vigilance, which reinforced her paranoid thinking, to repeated self-exposure to high risk situations and relationships. A chronic lack of self-esteem and confidence made it very difficult for her to escape from abusive relationships.

It is now well established that self-harm is often a way for people to manage painful memories, thoughts and feelings (Spandler and Warner, 2007). However, these strategies have often been misunderstood as maladaptive behaviours or symptoms of a mental illness. It is important to understand and appreciate how women develop coping strategies to deal with abuse. For example, Warner (2009) states that women learn to cope with repeated sexual abuse in a variety of ways; initially by denial, then by distraction and dissociation. When dissociation is extended beyond the initial abuse, or is retriggered by further abuse, it may result in hearing voices or seeing visions related to the original fear. The meaningfulness of these experiences is lost when they are perceived as symptoms of mental illness rather than 'historically-located coping strategies' (Warner, 2009, 17).

How people make sense of traumatic experiences is vital in determining outcomes. The extent of trauma-induced impairment depends on the degree to which an individual internalises both their oppression and abuse and the reactions and beliefs of others. Individual responses will also depend on age of onset and severity of abuse; length of exposure; level of hostility and violence involved; responses to disclosure; and whether the victim blames the perpetrator or themselves (Morrison et al, 2003). Plumb identifies a variety of responses to trauma which she describes as 'logical, rational and necessary for the person to achieve their 'prime directive' (survival)' (Plumb, 2005, 113). These can include guilt or shame, self-hate, anger, low self-esteem and confidence, negative self-image and fear of weakness. However, she is keen to emphasise that the nature and degree of these responses is influenced by a wide range of factors such as the person's personal qualities, support structures, relationship with the abuser and cultural, gender and class contexts. Given all these variables, our understanding needs to go beyond the individual and consider the interplay between the individual's response, their family network, community and wider society.

Family responses

Intimate relationships, friendships and families can provide much needed support or, alternatively, can further stigmatise and reject a person experiencing abuse or emotional distress (Thornicroft, 2006b). Unfortunately, in Sally's case, her family had a negative impact on her mental distress and level of impairment. Sally's oppression as a woman was perpetuated by her family culture where women were not valued, but subjugated to sexual and physical abuse by men. The traumatic experiences of abuse that triggered Sally's psycho–emotional adjustment took place within a family where violence towards women had become normalised. Sally was affected by her own experiences of trauma as well as intergenerational trauma manifesting in her mother being unable to care for and protect her, which left Sally in the caring role for her mother. Sally also internalised her mother's sense of low self-worth.

While she did have a relationship with her sister and mother, who provided some support, this also resulted in contact with her abusers.

As Sally felt pressure to maintain the cloak of silence in the family about the abuse, she felt trapped in an impossible situation. Not only did the contact with her abusers cause her further trauma, she also experienced the negative response of her family to the ways she had found to cope with the situation, her psycho-emotional adjustments.

Community responses

Communities play an important part in the establishment and regulation of cultural norms. In Sally's community there were cultural norms around the patriarchal family, engagement with wider society, and what can or cannot be disclosed. Like families, communities can alleviate mental distress through supportive social connections (Kawachi and Berkman, 2001). Equally, however, communities can have a negative impact on individuals by responding in hurtful ways, which can be seen as a form of psycho-emotional disablism.

Cultural norms within Sally's community dictated that experiences of violence and abuse should not be disclosed and therefore, by default, not challenged. Just as the abuse and trauma in Sally's family was intergenerational, so too were the coping strategies that Sally, her mother and other women in the community adopted. Moreover, some of Sally's own ways of coping, such as using substances, were, sanctioned within her community; and this served to reinforce the silence around the abuse and violence that women experience. Disclosing her abuse would have violated cultural norms and moving away risked her becoming isolated and rejected both by her own community and mainstream society. For example, when Sally talked about leaving her abusive relationship, she received little support in the community. However, as we have seen, Sally also received little help from health and welfare services.

Service responses

Unfortunately, Sally experienced further exclusion and oppression through psychiatric assessment, diagnosis and pharmacological interventions. When she sought help from mental health services, Sally was understood, not as making psycho-emotional adjustments to complex trauma, but as mentally ill. Too often women find themselves in a 'catch 22' situation where medically based practices further oppress and traumatise them, exacerbating their oppression. In particular, the diagnosis of borderline personality disorder has historically been associated with manipulative or attention seeking behaviour (NIMHE,

2003; Commons Treloar and Lewis, 2008) and has a very negative stigma. Also, despite findings that link childhood trauma and psychosis (Read et al, 2005), most psychiatrists still prioritise biochemical and genetic factors. In this way, diagnosis can be experienced as a form of psycho-emotional disablism in that it effectively misrecognises women's experiences of trauma and misinterprets their psycho-emotional adjustments as symptoms of mental illness (Reeve, 2004).

Not only did the intervention from mental health services lead to further exclusion, Sally's 'impairment' was compounded by the side effects of antipsychotic medication. The medication made Sally feel tired, groggy, flat and unable to engage. Sally became further impaired as she was unable to care for herself or develop positive and meaningful relationships.

We contend that mainstream psychiatric interventions continue to pathologise, oppress and re-traumatise women. Mental health practitioners can be seen as contributing to psycho-emotional disablism. Mental health services could shift their understanding of women's emotional distress by making the links between disabling social arrangements, structures and attitudes and inter-generational and complex trauma. Women-only mental health crisis services have developed that embrace this way of understanding women's mental distress, providing a safe haven for women. For example, Drayton Park Women's Crisis House and Resource Centre in London has an all women staff team. Women can self-refer and are enabled to talk about past experiences of abuse in a contained way alongside things like massage, support with accessing other services and healthy eating. There is also some capacity for children to stay, preventing their being placed separately (Killaspy et al, 2000).

Conclusion

We believe the concept of psycho-emotional disablism is useful in highlighting the complex interplay between the individual, the family, the community and wider societal responses. For women who experience complex trauma there is a vicious cycle between their experience of trauma, their psycho-emotional adjustments to trauma and societal reactions; which leads to further trauma, impairment and mental distress. Psycho-emotional disablism may help us understand this cycle for, as Reeve (2004) points out, negative responses by others can be as disabling as structural barriers.

Unpacking the link between impairment, distress and disablism is, however, not easy. For those experiencing emotional distress, it can be difficult to separate out impairment effects from the effects of psycho-emotional disablism. For example, to what extent are Sally's responses a normal reaction to her abuse rather than a symptom of an underlying illness? In addition, to what extent is Sally experiencing impairment effects arising from the negative voices she hears, and to what degree are these being triggered by psycho-emotional disablism in terms of negative reactions from others?

While it is difficult to untangle the causal relationships between mental distress, disability and impairment, psycho-emotional disablism does offer a way of understanding the interplay between individuals and society in relation to mental distress and complex trauma. If, as research has suggested, prevailing beliefs that mental distress is located in individual pathology or brain abnormality are correlated with increased fear and prejudice (Read et al, 2006b), then moving away from this may start to shift people's responses and reactions to mental distress. Therefore, we suggest that utilising the idea of psycho-emotional disablism, and reframing symptoms as psycho-emotional adjustments to trauma, could help to nurture more positive social reactions and responses to complex trauma (Kawachi and Berkman, 2001). This, in turn, this could address the vicious cycle of mental distress, disablism and impairment.

NINE

Linking 'race', mental health and a social model of disability: what are the possibilities?

Frank Keating

Introduction

Individuals from Black and Minority Ethic (BME) groups who experience mental health problems, already face what some have termed 'double jeopardy'. Therefore, to situate their experience within a social model of disability (or other models of disability) as well may add another layer of unnecessary complexity. However, I will argue that insights from a social model of disability can offer a way of theorising and addressing mental health inequalities and disparities for BME communities. To do this, however, it needs to integrate insights from Critical Race Theory, and ideas around intersectionality, embodiment and 'othering'.

The struggle to achieve racial justice and equality for BME people with mental health problems has mostly occurred in isolation from, or on the margins of, other social movements, partly as a result of 'silo thinking'. This chapter starts from the premise that a single frame of analysis is unhelpful in understanding the linkages, connections and contradictions pertaining to mental distress, 'race', racism and disability. Focusing on a single aspect of identity cannot fully explain other dimensions and experiences of individuals and groups because we cannot disentangle 'race' and ethnicity from other social categories, divisions or status such as gender, class, disability or sexuality. Focusing on single identities can lock groups into hierarchies of oppression and can lead to binary thinking such as black vs white, woman vs man, or gay vs straight. People actually experience multiple oppressions simultaneously (Stuart, 1992).

The chapter will be sequenced as follows. First, I will set the context for understanding mental distress and the experience of racialised minority groups in the UK. Second, I will discuss the advantages and disadvantages of using a social model of disability as a frame of analysis for BME service users. Then I will present some theoretical insights which I argue help us understand the experience of BME communities. Finally, I will use these insights to suggest some ways forward to help bridge the gap between theory and practice.

The context: mental distress and racism/racialisation

The longstanding disparities for black and minority ethnic (BME) or racialised[1] (minority) groups in relation to mental health and mental health care in the UK have been well documented, but not always adequately understood or explained. Differences between groups or categories of people are a natural, if not an essential, dimension of human experience and the driving force for a diverse and evolving society. However, when these differences are evaluated negatively or become disproportionate they should be construed as disparities. Such a conceptualisation should aid an analysis of inequality and how this is sustained and maintained in contemporary society. In order to fully appreciate and understand the contexts for racialised groups in relation to mental health it is necessary to first consider their general status in society and then their particular position in terms of mental health. BME communities constitute 12% of the population in England and Wales, yet fare worse across all indicators of economic, health and social well-being. For example, the initial findings from the 2011 census (ONS, 2012) indicate that they have considerably higher rates of unemployment, are more likely to report poorer health and that racial harassment is still a common experience for these communities.

Turning to mental health, there is well-documented evidence of the disparities for BME groups. They are three times more likely to be admitted to psychiatric care, 44% more likely to be compulsory detained, have elevated rates of schizophrenia, are more likely to have police involvement in admissions to psychiatric care, and to be on the receiving end of excessive use of control and restraint once there (Care Quality Commission and National Mental Health Development Unit, 2011). Explanations for these disparities have been sought from a range of perspectives, but primarily from a bio-medical perspective to the exclusion of more social explanations.

The medicalisation of mental illness means that containment, control and compliance become essential features of mental health practices. The experiences of racialised groups seem to be dominated by practices that resemble some BME communities' experiences in everyday life – that is, exclusion from school, stop and search practices, and over-representation in the criminal justice system. This is particularly pertinent for African and Caribbean communities. It has been argued elsewhere (Robinson et al, 2011) that a solely medicalised approach locks people into a stalled cycle of recovery. For example, people avoid mental health services at all costs; thus they come to the attention of services in a more severe state of distress; receive more coercive treatment; and, when they are 'better', they disengage from services and the cycle repeats itself.

Cultural approaches have attempted to shift this medicalised discourse by advocating a deeper understanding of the role of culture in mental illness and proposing cultural competence as a solution (often called 'culturalist' approaches). Cultural explanations for health inequalities suggest that individual behaviour and the social norms of minority groups (such as immigrants) are influenced by a person's culture and, in turn, this has a negative impact on health outcomes (Viruell-Fuentes et al, 2012). However, culturalist approaches have their own difficulties as they tend to locate the issue(s) at individual, cultural and community levels and ignore the deleterious consequences of racism, racial inequality and structural disadvantage. In addition, experiences of BME communities are homogenised and 'the problem' is situated within the 'cultures' of these communities, thus blaming the victim or pathologising their experiences of distress. While stress is an everyday experience which can derive from family life, peer relationships, work, and so on, there is little or no acknowledgement of the stress that can be derived from belonging to a marginalised or racialised minority group.

Brown (2003) argued that psychiatry disregards narratives about how racism hurts and how it can cause mental distress despite the fact that racialised experiences have been linked with mental illness (Fanon, 1967; Karlsen et al, 2005). Distress that derives from these experiences can be construed as racialised stress and Xanthos (2012) has categorised this as racism–induced stress and racial minority status stress. The latter has been defined as the stress that minority groups experience due to their in/visibility and identifying with a minority group. Racism-induced stress, refers to racial discrimination and harassment. I prefer to refer to this as 'race trauma' because of the disturbing, distressing and traumatic impact of racial discrimination and harassment. Nazroo (2003) suggests that social and economic inequalities are chief explanations for inequalities in health and mental health and found that experiences of racial harassment and discrimination have been consistently linked to poorer self-reported health and outcomes. An online survey to explore popular views on the links between racism and mental illness found overwhelming agreement that racism can cause mental illness (Beresford et al, 2010).

Distress, 'race' and the social model of disability

The social model of disability locates disability in physical, social, attitudinal, economic and political barriers that disabled people face (Oliver, 2013). Disability is viewed as a social construct and proposes that focusing on society and its disabling institutions can facilitate access to resources, empowerment and social justice (Morris, 1993). It is clear from many of the other chapters in this book that mental health service users are divided about the desirability of identifying as disabled (Anderson et al, 2012). Plumb (1994) has cogently highlighted some of the difficulties with integrating mental distress within broader disability politics.

Activism in mental health has tended to be focused on three areas. The first is that of challenging the dominance of the medical model and its narrow focus on diagnosis and medication. However, because this challenge has been framed in the context of the fear of being further 'discounted' by psychiatry, activism has also focused on challenging the absence of 'the user voice' in the discourse about mental distress. Therefore, the second area has been a focus on re-conceptualising the experience of mental illness and mental distress itself (Anderson et al, 2012). Third, social activism has focused on transforming the relationship between people who experience mental distress and mental health services. The goal here has been to achieve greater levels of partnership and involvement in developing and providing mental health services, rather than a focus on how society disables mental health service users (Beresford, 2004).

An added layer of complexity is the fact that BME service users were largely absent from this drive for involvement and partnership in mental health services. Their struggles for racial equality have been fought on two levels. They have challenged both the Eurocentric psychiatric discourse on mental distress *and* the white hegemonic nature of the mental health service user movement.

Before we consider whether the social model of disability might be helpful to BME mental health service users, we need to examine how the issue of 'race' has been addressed (or not) in the disability movement. At best, issues of 'race' and racism have been at the margins of the disability movement (Stuart, 2012). I therefore view the social model as a single frame of analysis because, historically, it has advocated for the rights of disabled people over other forms of struggle, such as 'race' and gender (Morris, 1993; Stuart, 1992). Some concern has been raised about the lack of engagement between the disability movement and BME communities (Barnes et al, 1999; Oliver, 2013), but there is little evidence that this has been taken seriously. There seems to be an ongoing lack of critical race analysis within disability studies (Gorman, 2013) and material from the margins is rarely included (Meekosha, 2011). Stuart (2012, 142) argued that 'patriarchal and Eurocentric assumptions underpins the social model of disability, which makes it difficult to consider ways in which BME communities imagine and construct disability'.

BME service users have not been involved in either the drive for involvement in mental health services nor development of the social model of disability. They may have been understandably mistrustful and reluctant to engage in discourses that are perceived as exclusionary and discriminatory. A complicating factor is the fact that within BME communities disabled people and those who experience mental distress have advocated separately and in isolation from each other. This has made it difficult for their voices to be heard.

BME service users who experience mental health issues *and* physical disabilities also face considerable challenges in terms of having their needs met. Dewan (2001), for example, writes about her struggles to persuade mental health practitioners to acknowledge her disability. Adding disability to the equation means that we can think of 'triple jeopardy'. While mental distress and disability are rarely considered jointly, discussion of the links between distress and disability within BME communities is even rarer.

It is against this backdrop that I now turn to the possible advantages and disadvantages of utilising a social model of disability for BME service users. Despite the above criticisms, an analysis informed by a social model of disability can offer a sound theoretical foundation or platform that can assist BME service users to take forward a political agenda (Barnes and Mercer, 2004). It can, for example, aid an understanding of how social policy and legislation serve to marginalise BME service users, and that in turn, can be used to advocate for their rights and responsibilities as service users.

The focus on their struggles can be redirected from individualistic analyses of mental illness to the processes of social oppression, discrimination and exclusion – everyday features of their lives (Mulvany, 2000). This shift from an individualistic and often blaming construction of 'illness' can be less pathologising. Goodley (2012) further suggests that such theorising gives a different way of accounting for mental distress beyond symptoms and diagnoses showing how distress is framed in different social contexts.

A social model of disability can offer a way of understanding how BME service users are located at the interstices of 'race' and mental distress (Erevelles and Minear, 2010). A focus on oppressive structures requires an extension of our view beyond medicalised services. We need to include broader spheres such as housing, education, leisure and employment. I have argued elsewhere that the issues for BME service users are not purely medical, that is, biological – they are social, economic and political. Therefore, psychiatry cannot 'go it alone' (Keating, 2007).

The social model emphasises rights, needs and entitlements rather than impairment (or what I have called the embodiment of distress). Essentially this means that the subjective experiences of disability at a very personal and individual level and how people make sense of their physicality is overlooked or deemed less significant (Mulvany, 2000). In other words, the social model of disability has failed to address embodiment and the lived experiences of distress (Tomasini, 2012). As we shall see, the embodiment of distress is very pertinent for BME service users. Therefore, the social model would need to incorporate a focus on how distress is embodied in racialised contexts. The biggest challenge for applying a social model of disability to the distress of BME service users, is the need for a fuller recognition of the ways in which 'race' has been marginalised in both the discourses of distress *and* disability. A further challenge is that to overcome the Eurocentric assumptions of the social model would necessitate an integration of critical race theory with critical disability studies and not just adding 'race' as another issue to consider. Therefore, in the following sections I explain some theoretical insights that I have found helpful in understanding racism, mental health and disability. These ideas can help to support and strengthen the social model.

Critical race theory (CRT) originated in the US to challenge traditional and liberalist approaches to understanding 'race' and racism. It has been defined as a theory that, describes and explains iterative ways in which race is socially constructed across micro- and macro-levels and how it determines life chances implicating the mundane and extraordinary in the continuance of racial stratification (Brown, 2003, 292).

There are five key tenets to CRT (Delgado and Stefancic, 2003, 7). It proposes that: racism is endemic and ubiquitous and is a 'normal' or everyday experience for BME people; 'race' is a social construction; liberalism makes racism invisible and obscures self-interest, privilege and power of dominant (that is, white) groups; experiential knowledge is legitimate and appropriate because subordinate groups are able to explain their experiences of racial stratification, and, finally, it advocates social justice.

An understanding informed by CRT helps us to conceptualise the relationship between 'race', racism and power, but also how we can change or even transform these experiences at both micro and macro levels. At a micro level, it gives credence to the experience and realities of racism and accepts it as a causal factor in some of the difficulties racialised groups face. In relation to mental health, CRT can aid an analysis of the emotional and psychological effects of 'race' and racism (Brown, 2003).

Intersectionality is a term/theory that is closely linked to CRT. It is a way of analysing the intersections and interactions between multiple forms or systems of oppression. It aims to understand how these all work together to produce, sustain and reinforce inequality. There are various conceptualisations of intersectionality (see for example Crenshaw, 1991), but its central tenets are that:

- human lives and experience cannot be reduced to single characteristics (such as race or disability);
- social categories are socially constructed, fluid and intertwined;
- it is not an additive approach whereby one category is merely added to the next;
- it rejects the hierarchical ordering of oppression.

Tam (2013) argues that when we examine social divisions as single issues or systems, there is a danger that categories can become objectified and translated into entities and attributes that are fixed. She suggests that these systems of oppression are linked together in their formation of structures of power and inequality. Therefore, we should explore how various forms of social stratification and discrimination relate to and co-constitute one another (Hanivsky, 2002).

Applying an intersectional analysis to mental distress can aid a critique of the dominant constructions of madness, normality and sanity. It can help us explore and acknowledge the pitfalls of simplistic theorising that involves dichotomous or binary thinking that leads to oppositional constructions such as good/bad; ill/healthy; or sane/insane.

Otherness is a process that is central to how people are categorised and has been defined as, a dualistic process of differentiation and demarcation by which a line is drawn between 'us' and 'them' and through which social distance is established and maintained; 'a process that serves to mark and name those thought to be different from oneself' (Lister, 2008, 7). According to Lister, 'othering' secures and defines one's identity and notions of normality and difference (Lister, 2008, 7). 'Othering' involves the assumptions we hold about ourselves and about others, the worth we assign to ourselves and others and the comparisons we make between ourselves and others (Rosenfield, 2012). An important dimension of this process is how differences between people are translated: often negatively. Once we have cast someone as 'other' this becomes a basis for inclusion or exclusion, which in the former can lead to a sense of belonging and in the latter to a sense of marginalisation.

Otherness is a multi-faceted process. When I categorise someone as 'white', I have categorised her or him as other and different to me. It means that I may construe this difference as hostile, friendly, superior or aggressive. Simultaneously, I have categorised myself as other to them – I could perceive or construe myself as inferior, not worthy or, conversely, proud of who I am. Unfortunately, people (and society) find these processes of othering uncomfortable and often apply or invoke strategies to ignore or deny their existence. 'Otherness' often becomes obscured under the mantra of 'we are all equal' and 'I treat everyone the same'. Ultimately, however, this invalidates the experiences of people or groups whose 'differences' *are* evaluated negatively.

So how are people construed as mentally ill othered? They are measured against a hegemonic norm of wellbeing or what it means to be normal. The language that is then applied to them contains pejorative connotations: failure, dropout, weak, dangerous, risky, attention seeking etc. Disabled people are similarly othered, but in different ways. For example, they are perceived as less competent, as people with limited agency and reduced scope for participation in civic life.

The othering process for people with mental health problems from racialised groups is complex and has led to stereotypical views such as 'big, black and dangerous'. Singh and Burns (2006) in attempting to refute that racism can play a role in mental distress, suggested that we should accept that there is an epidemic of schizophrenia in the black community. The question this raises is: are black people therefore madder than other groups? Keating et al (2002) have demonstrated that stereotypical views of black people, racism, cultural ignorance, stigma and anxiety associated with mental illness often combine to undermine the way in which mental health services assess and respond to the needs of BME communities. These perceptions structure the interactions between BME people with mental health problems and professionals. These interactions are often characterised by fear, control and silencing.

'Othering' is a process from which racialised groups are not immune. I premise this on the assumption that membership of an oppressed group does not imply that one lacks agency or does not have access to power: *we all have the ability to oppress*. 'Othering' in relation to mental health within racialised groups often occurs in the domains of religion and spirituality, the family and their broader communities. Spirituality and religion are important facets in the lives of some racialised groups and help with issues of mental distress is often sought from spiritual or religious leaders. However, in some communities mental illness is often construed as spirit or demon possession and therefore something to be exorcised from the body with disastrous consequences.

Embodiment relates to how people make sense of their bodily and corporeal presence and how this has an impact on their identity or subjectivity (Mulvany, 2000). It can be seen as both a biological phenomenon and a social production (Seymour cited in Mulvany, 2000).

Our sense of ourselves is influenced by society and factors such as 'race' and ethnicity play a significant role in how people experience the world. A sense of one's own body is significant for racialised groups because their physiology and skin tones are evaluated negatively, which affects how they experience the world in relation to their physicality and corporeality. These negative evaluations can be internalised or externalised. Racialised trauma can affect self-esteem and lead to emotional distress. When trauma is discharged inwardly it may manifest itself in the form of self-destructive behaviours and when it is discharged outwardly it may become what Nelson (2006, 126) calls 'other directed destruction'. Metaphor plays an important role in the ways in which BME groups describe distress. Phrases such as 'tears were dropping in my head' or 'my spirit was low' are commonly used to portray distress (Keating et al, 2002).

Towards a social model informed by intersectionality, Critical Race Theory and 'othering'

A narrow medicalised approach does not help us to understand how racialised groups, people with mental health problems, and BME disabled people are all 'othered'. Neither does it help us understand how distress is embodied in racialised contexts; or how racism intersects with other forms of oppression. To do this, we need a social model of distress which is informed by these ideas.

Following Gorman (2013) I define a social model of mental distress as a social, relational, identity based and anti-oppressive approach to studying and responding to mental distress. So what would a social model of mental distress entail?

1. First we need to understand the *unique experiences and identities of BME service users*. This means appreciating people's experience of mental distress will be affected by processes of oppression (othering). Anti-oppressive practice should locate the experience of racialised groups within their multi-layered experiences of power and take into account other dimensions of oppression too (intersectionality). How we express distress will be informed by our bodily and corporeal experiences and evidence shows that BME communities utilise different metaphors to describe distress (embodiment). Therefore, we need to examine and appreciate the unique manifestations of mental distress for racialised groups.

2. We have to acknowledge that *values* are at the heart of a social model of mental distress. This is the essential distinction between social models and more medicalised approaches to mental distress. Medicalised approaches are premised on objectivity, rationality and neutrality whereas value based practice embraces subjectivities. Some of the values that we need to espouse are social justice, respect for diversity and empowerment.

3. A social model will not only require a shift in the value base, but should be supported by *reframing the discourse(s) of distress*. Bentall (2006) for example, suggests that we should use the term 'complaints' to refer to what is troubling people. The aim in working with individuals can then be to ascertain what areas of life and experience they are struggling with and target those. Tew (2011, 28) suggests another way of constructing madness: a shift from *disease* to *unease* to *distress*. Conceptualised in this way, distress arises out of unease with ourselves and/or our social situation. Racial induced stress can thus be considered as unease with a social situation and racial minority distress can be considered as unease with the self at an individual level.

4. We need to consider the *social impact* of the co-constructed categories of racialisation and mental distress on the social status and position of individuals. We know for example that these groups experience significant disadvantage, high levels of victimisation and harassment and are among the most socially excluded groups in society. Patel and Fatimilehin (1999) suggest that the impact of racism is psychological, social and material. The effects of this are likely to be detrimental to

mental health; for some they may be minimal, but for others they have great significance for their emotional well-being. The impact of racism has to be analysed in the context of histories of migration, alienation, subordination and the way in which these groups have been and continue to be stigmatised in society today. Practitioners should focus on the environmental and relationship factors that cause mental distress by linking it to 'problems' of living.

5. We need to explore the nature of *relationships* in which individuals are engaged, acknowledging that these will have a racialised dimension. Relationships for individuals who experience mental distress are often fractured at various levels that can include family, peers and society in general.

6. Finally, *narratives of voice and action* can help to counter or challenge hegemonic narratives of normality (Krumer-Nevo and Benjamin, 2010). Structure/policy narratives can help to unravel the specific public and policy contexts in which racialisation and racism takes place and how mental distress is conceptualised. Agency/resistance narratives can assist us to analyse the ways in which people take action with limited resources. Here we can particularly think of the limited access that racialised groups, people with mental health problems and disabled people have to valued societal resources such as employment or housing. This last point is of particular pertinence for racialised groups who have traditionally been marginalised in both, mental health and disability movements, as well as services.

So how do we apply this to practice? I suggest that the above activities should be informed by reflexive practice in which practitioners develop an understanding of how the processes of racialisation, othering, embodiment and intersectionality inform their interactions with racialised minorities.

Conclusion

This chapter has argued that narrow interpretations and approaches to understanding how mental distress affects racialised groups are not only inadequate and unhelpful but also reinforce the oppression they experience. It has highlighted that BME users have been involved in neither the drive for involvement in mental health services nor in developing the social model of disability. Integrating a social model of disability for BME communities poses significant challenges. However, a social model of distress/disability informed by theoretical insights gained from CRT, intersectionality, othering and embodiment offers a framework for addressing the disparities that racialised groups experience in relation to mental distress. The 'problems' of everyday living should be our focus and I believe it is only then that we can make our practice safe and bring about the much needed change for racialised groups in our quest for equality.

Note

[1] The term BME service users or racialised groups will be used interchangeably to refer to minority groups, acknowledging the diversity within and across these groups.

TEN

Social models of disability and sexual distress

Meg John Barker and Alex Iantaffi

Introduction

In this chapter we suggest that there is much to be gained from bringing social models of disability into dialogue with current understandings of sexual distress. First, sexologists and sexual health practitioners could benefit hugely from applying the shift from medical to social thinking about disability to the arenas of sexual 'disorders' or 'dysfunctions'. Second, it is fruitful for those studying and working with disability to extend social models to include considerations of sex and sexuality, as in some of the more recent, intersectional revisions of these models.

In order to explore the potential of such a dialogue we devote the first half of this chapter to examining how prevailing norms of sex and sexuality position many of us as mentally disordered or dysfunctional, and could therefore be said to actively disorder or disable people in a manner akin to the way in which certain material features and social norms disable certain bodies and sensory and cognitive experiences. We consider how features of the shift from medical to social models of disability can be applied in this area, to the benefit of those who are struggling with sexual distress and in ways which enhance understandings of sex and sexuality more widely. By 'sexual distress' we mean mental distress which occurs specifically around sex, for example feeling anxious about sexual situations or ashamed of sexual desires.

Following this, in the second half of the chapter, we examine the ways in which medicalised understandings of both sex and disability constrain and restrict the sexual experience and expression of disabled people. We draw out the potential benefits of applying social models of disability to this area, building particularly on recent intersectional work to enable a fuller understanding of the ways in which sexuality, disability and other aspects of identity and experience combine.

In the concluding section of the chapter we weave these strands together to suggest how social, critical and intersectional understandings of sexuality and disability could inform thinking and practice around both these areas.

Before embarking upon this dialogue we will briefly present our own understanding of social models of disability in order to locate ourselves within the broader themes of this book. We regard these models as an explicit critique of – and move away from – conventional medical models of disability which have predominated in professional and popular understandings of disability. These medical models regarded disability as a lack or impairment which limits and constrains everyday life, and is located within the specific individual (for example, in an area of their body, in their senses, or in their cognitions) (Iantaffi and Mize, 2015).

Social models of disability, on the other hand, locate disability in society rather than in the individual. For example, stairs are viewed as disabling, rather than disability residing in the body of a person who uses a wheelchair. Limits on people's capacities to conduct activities that are essential to everyday life are regarded as imposed by structural and systemic barriers. These barriers are part of a social system that constructs some bodies as normal and some as other rather than considering a broad range of bodies and possibilities. This relegates disabled people to the status of lesser citizens due to lack of access (Barton, 1997; Barnes, 2000).

Disability is therefore viewed as a by-product of a society which is organised around only certain bodies which are defined as normative, in legislation, education, institutions and popular culture (Oliver, 2004). This means that solutions are focused around societal rather than medical interventions (Oliver, 2009). For example, the provision of audio or captions would be seen as providing access to a wider community, rather than addressing a specific individual need (Iantaffi and Mize, 2015).

Finally, social models of disability regard everybody as interdependent, rather than locating disabled people as dependent in order to shore up a neoliberal myth of everybody else as independent. Being reliant on a carer, for example, is part of a wider system of interdependency which includes the reliance that everybody has on those who produce food, remove refuse and run public transport. Feminist models in particular, have suggested that cultural emphases on health and normativity place bodies with disabilities at the margins because people do not want to be reminded of their interdependency, limitations, pain and mortality.

They have also challenged and broadened social models of disability to include embodied experiences (Morris, 1992; 1996; Wendell, 1996).

To summarise, social models:

- are critical of normative thinking which creates binaries of people without/with disabilities (normal vs. other);
- shift understanding of disability from a lack/impairment of specific bodies, to an understanding that a diverse range of bodies exist;
- shift from locating disabilities within individuals to within society (structural, material and cultural aspects);
- regard everyone as interdependent – rather than dividing dependent disabled people from independent non-disabled people.

Please note that we recognise that we have not drawn clear distinctions here between social models and postmodern models of disability, but rather we have considered what all of the more critical/social theories have to offer in combination. Towards the end of the chapter we will turn to crip theory and other approaches which are specifically grounded on an intersectional understanding.

Disordering sex

In this section of the chapter we begin by considering how sexual distress – and sex more broadly – is currently conceptualised. Returning to the features of social models of disability (outlined above) we then explore how these apply to supposed sexual disorders and dysfunctions, outlining how an understanding informed by social models of disability would not only benefit those struggling with sexual distress, but has potential value for all of us.

As with disability, the prevailing model of sexual distress has been a medical one, enshrined within the Diagnostic and Statistical Manual (DSM-5) (American Psychiatric Association, 2013) and the International Classification of Diseases (ICD-10) (WHO, 1994). In this chapter we focus on the DSM given that this is the more recently updated of the two, and that the ICD generally follows the DSM in its categorisations. Sexual distress is conceptualised in the DSM as a 'sexual and gender disorder', either under the category of 'sexual dysfunction' or 'paraphilic disorder'.

Broadly speaking the 'sexual dysfunctions' delineate dysfunctional from functional sex, and the 'paraphilic disorders' delineate abnormal from normal sex. Anything which risks disrupting the functional, sexual response cycle of desire, arousal and orgasm is deemed a dysfunction.

Thus we have categories for lack of desire: 'erectile disorder', 'female orgasmic disorder' and 'delayed ejaculation'. There are also categories of 'premature ejaculation' and 'penetration disorder' which suggest that penis-in-vagina penetration is considered necessary for functional sex to have occurred (Barker, 2011a). Paraphilic disorders are defined as 'intense and persistent sexual interest other than…in genital stimulation or preparatory fondling with phenotypically normal, physically mature, consenting human partners', demonstrating that preparatory fondling followed by genital stimulation is regarded as normal sex, and that sexual interest in anything other than this is regarded as paraphilic (unusual or abnormal) sex. This category includes interest in certain sensations and materials, in being watched or watching others, and in mixing sex with pain, physical restraint or power (for more on the history of how such categories developed, see Irvine, 2005; Berry and Barker, 2015).

These conceptualisations of sex are not restricted to psychiatric texts and practices, but rather they form the basis of much wider cultural understandings and norms. So, for example, the same divisions of functional/dysfunctional and normal/abnormal sex are replicated in the most popular 'bibles' of sexology used in the training of health practitioners and sex therapists (Barker and Richards, 2013). They are also echoed in mainstream sex advice across self-help books, magazine and newspaper problem pages and TV documentaries. For example, most bestselling sex manuals present a model of sex as: foreplay, followed by penis-in-vagina intercourse, ending in orgasm. Such books consider difficulties with erections, penetrations or orgasm as requiring of correction, while 'alternative' sex is relegated to a final chapter of the book with many notes of caution around not straying into anything that the authors regard as abnormal or dangerous (often including 'real' BDSM and fetishes as opposed to light bondage or blindfolding, and also cybersex, or group sex of any kind) (Barker et al, in press).

People are clearly disordered by these prevailing binary understandings of sexual function/dysfunction and normality/abnormality. The most recent UK survey of sexual attitudes and lifestyles (Natsal-3) for example, found that 42% of men and 51% of women reported having a sexual problem: so around half see themselves as sexually dysfunctional (Mitchell et al, 2013). Similarly, statistics on the number of people who entertain fantasies of bondage or spanking are usually well over 50% of people (Richards and Barker, 2013) as evidenced by the huge popularity of the *Fifty Shades* series (Barker, 2013a) and yet, sexual sadism and masochism remain on the list of paraphilias. Advocates of such categories point out that under DSM-5, paraphilias are only categorised as disorders if they cause distress or impairment to self or others. However, as with homosexuality – which was only removed from the DSM in 1973 and the ICD in 1992 – the stigma involved with being regarded as potentially disordered is, in itself, a cause of distress. It can easily be argued that the sexual categories of mental disorder are making us crazy (Kutchins and Kirk, 1997).

As with medical models of disability, we can see here that binaries are created of people with and without sexual disorders. 'Normal people' have functional, normal sex, and others have sexual dysfunctions or paraphilic disorders. Interestingly though, in this case, the evidence around dysfunctions and paraphilias make this hard to sustain given that – statistically at least – it is probably far more 'normal' to have a sexual dysfunction and/or paraphilia than it is to not have one.

As with disability, sexual disorders are considered to be a lack or impairment of certain bodies and/or psychologies and are therefore located within the individual, rather than within broader systems, such as heteronormativity. Most treatment involves some form of medical, behavioural or psychological intervention (for example, PDE-5 inhibitors for erectile dysfunction, masturbatory techniques for premature ejaculation or challenging negative thoughts for orgasmic disorder) (Barker, 2011a; Kleinplatz, 2012).

So what could be gained, in this area, from applying the social model of disability? We will now return to each of the main features of social models in turn.

Rejecting binaries

First, we could reject binary models of people with or without dysfunctions and disorders for a model of sexual diversity. Many critical, queer and feminist sexologists have argued for such a shift to what Rubin (1984) terms benign variation, rather than a hierarchical model that keeps attempting to redraw the lines between what is considered good, normal, functional sex, and bad, abnormal, dysfunctional sex. For example, authors such as Irvine (2005) have pointed out how people are pathologised for wanting/having both too little sex and too much sex. On the one hand, categories relating to low sexual desire risk pathologising both asexual people and those – very many – who experience fluctuating levels of desire throughout their lives. On the other hand, while thankfully not included in the DSM, the popular but deeply problematic category of 'sex addiction' risks pathologising both those who have a high level of desire and those who enjoy certain kinds of sex such as solo sex, casual sex and cybersex (Richards and Barker, 2013).

Diversity

A model of sexual diversity could much more comfortably contain those with no, low and high levels of sexual desire, as well as attraction to more than one gender, which is currently often erased by binary models (Barker et al, 2012) and diverse sexual practices. It is also in keeping with feminist and queer approaches which have pointed out the phallocentric and heteronormative assumptions of the current model (Tiefer, 1995; Barker and Langdridge, 2013). Such an understanding of sexual diversity could encompass, for example, solo sex, partnered sex and group sex; manual, oral, vaginal and anal sex, as well as other parts of bodies rubbing together for pleasure; sexual fantasy, sex talk, cybersex, erotic fiction and visual stimulation; and enjoyment of a diversity of roles, bodies, materials, sensations and dynamics. Under such a model, few – if any – people would be regarded as disordered or dysfunctional given that erections, penetration and orgasm are not necessary, albeit they may well be enjoyed by some people some of the time. And, as authors such as Rubin (1984), Denman (2004), Kleinplatz (2012) and Barker (2013b) have suggested, attention could turn from functionality and normality to the – arguably more important – considerations such as the extent of pleasure or fulfilment experienced, whether or not sex is consensual, a focus on enjoying the process rather than aiming towards a specific goal, expansion of erotic imaginations, and ethical treatment of self and/or other/s involved.

Location of issues within society rather than individuals

The social model shift from locating disabilities within individuals to within society is also a useful shift when it comes to sexual distress. The turn to more social understandings of bodies and health (Fox, 2012) enables us to locate the body and psychological experience within social norms, societal systems and structures.

For example, vaginal tension and pain on penetration is a common experience for many heterosexual women. It is often treated with the insertion of increasingly large dilators, and/or cognitive-behavioural therapy for sexual anxiety. Applying a more social model approach, one of us (Meg John) worked with a young, white, working-class woman – Helen – who was experiencing 'vaginismus'. The work involved considering the psychological meanings that Helen had around femininity and sex, and how these were embedded within wider sociocultural understandings, as well as how they operated through her body during sex. For example, Helen placed great importance on being desirable to others, particularly to her boyfriend, in order to feel valuable. Part of this involved ensuring that her body always looked attractive, so she attempted to adopt certain positions during sex to ensure a flat belly and to avoid potential attention to the parts of her body she regarded as unattractive such as her 'muffin-tops' (a newly created bodily flaw that was currently the focus of many of the images in the magazines that Helen read and an advertising campaign for a local gym).

Like many women, Helen also controlled her bodily functions such that she waited to urinate and defecate when nobody was in earshot, she prevented herself from passing wind, and she was fearful that others would be able to tell when she had her period. All of this contributed to tension, discomfort and pain in her body, particularly in her genital region (Iantaffi, 2013). This was further exacerbated by her anxieties about not being able to provide 'proper' sex to her boyfriend, the fear that she would lose him if she did not, and the underlying belief that it would be terrible to be single (Barker, 2011b; Mize and Iantaffi, 2013). Exploring the social norms in which her distress was located helped Helen to explore different ways of relating to her body, her partner, and to others. Her 'vaginismus' ceased to be an issue when she stopped trying to force herself to have the kind of sex she thought she should be having. Kleinplatz (2012) gives other examples of sexual difficulties being created by medicalised norms about 'proper' sex, and explains how shifting these is a vital part of therapy, alongside helping people to tune in to the meaning of their particular experience.

Interdependence

As touched on previously, utilising a social model could also focus on interdependence around sex, moving away from the current model of dividing dependent disordered people from independent non-disordered people. Current mainstream sex advice books present a very individualistic, neoliberal view of sex, with themes of individuals meeting their needs, making clear autonomous choices, and engaging in self-improvement to acquire sexual capital through techniques and skills (Barker et al, in press). In contrast, a model of interdependence could re-focus upon sex as relational and socially situated. For example, it would consider the social power dynamics in play which may enable or constrain agency around practices, communication and consent (Barker, 2013a). It could also include recognition of the material things that are involved in disordering people, as with the example of stairs and physical disability. For example, long working hours, certain living situations, issues of time and space, money and energy and gender roles may all restrict the potential of people to perform the kind of great, normal or functional sex advocated by sex manuals and psychiatric nosologies.

Sex and disability

In this second half of the chapter we consider how medicalised understandings of both sex and disability constrain and restrict the sexual experiences and expressions of disabled people. This requires a turn towards social models which are informed by the concept of intersectionality (Crenshaw, 1989) and an awareness of the ways in which sexuality, disability and other aspects of identity and experience combine.

Much of the literature on disability and sexuality has focused on common assumptions that disabled people are either malignantly sexual or, more likely, asexual (Kim, 2011). We have both come across this in our work within mainstream sex therapy. For example, Meg John remembers working with a couple who both had diagnoses of multiple sclerosis and who had been told by multiple health practitioners that sex simply wouldn't be part of their lives anymore and that they should stop thinking about it, despite the vital role it had played in their lives. Alex has met several disabled individuals and couples whose doctors had never mentioned sex and sexuality. They had not been given any resources on how to use props or to consider what they *could* do sexually. Instead they were faced with the silent assumption that sex was not an option for them. Alex also has experienced living with a chronic illness (fibromyalgia) for over 15 years and has not yet met a health professional who has discussed sex with him in the context of his disability.

Medical models of disability are perpetuated and reinforced when disability is mentioned in mainstream sex advice. For example, only around half of the bestselling sex manuals mention disability at all. While the ones that do mention it challenge the myth that disabled people are not sexual, they still distinguish disabled people from everybody else in a binary manner. All of the books that consider disability include it in a separate section on 'disability and illness' or 'sex for special populations' rather than integrating the topic, or considering sex with diverse bodies, throughout the book. This further reinforces the idea that disabled people are 'other', rather than acknowledging the reality that most people will experience some level of illness or disability through their lifespan. None of the mainstream books analysed depict any disabled people among the many images of sexual bodies within the manuals (Barker et al, in press). Disability is presented as an ailment or impairment that individuals have rather than residing in society. They also perpetuate damaging myths such as the idea that the absence of one sense makes other senses grow stronger.

Most sex manuals do not suggest that an active sex life is impossible for disabled people. However, the imperatives of maintaining a varied sex life in order to be a healthy human being, and to maintain a relationship, are reproduced in specific sections for disabled people. The means of achieving this are located in messages like 'committing to making sex a priority' and having a 'willing mind' (for example, Berman, 2011, 270–1). It is worth remembering that a disproportionate number of women experience divorce following the development of a chronic illness or impairment. Given this, the heteronormative advice to be willing to have sex in order to maintain a relationship is concerning as it is likely to create pressures that remove or restrict the possibilities for consensual sex. There is no awareness of such structures and systems of gender, sexuality and disability in these texts, despite their relevance for both the kinds of sex people have and their experience of it. It is telling that the sex advice book *The Ultimate Guide to Sex and Disability* (Kaufman et al, 2007) was written precisely because of the lack of useful advice in mainstream publications.

Even when disabled people are seen as sexual beings, the range of acceptable sexual expression is narrow, and straying outside its purview can easily locate people further from societal norms. For example, queer disabled people are often seen as having chosen their sexuality because a healthy, heteronormative companion or relationship(s) are regarded as less available to them. Kinky disabled people are also seen in a similar light while also conjuring media-fed images of disabled people as either villains or hapless victims (Iantaffi, 2009). It is rare for disabled people to be viewed not only as sexual but also as sexy, as highlighted by the *American Able* campaign images, which placed bodies with visible disabilities in similar poses to bodies without visible disabilities in a popular US fashion ad campaign (Olsson, 2012).

Disabled people are not expected to have sexual capital or agency and, even when they might be regarded as sexual beings they are rarely, if ever, depicted as such in mainstream images. A recent exception was the popularity of the Oscar-nominated movie *The Sessions*. However, even in this, the aspect highlighted was that of disabled people as consumers of sex work. While this may be part of the experiences of some disabled people, it seems to be the only part that Hollywood sees worthy of representation, perhaps precisely because such depictions do not upset the status quo of disabled people being seen as lacking sexual capital.

The lack of agency for disabled people within the medical model can most clearly be seen in the enforced sterilisation of young women with learning disabilities (Brady, 2001; Human Rights Watch, 2011; Tilley et al, 2012; Stefánsdóttir and Hreinsdóttir, 2013; West, 2013). This practice is not uncommon and highlights what happens within a medical model at the intersection of femininity, youth, disability and class. Many of the young disabled women sterilised around the world had no choice about this decision, which was made either by more educated middle-class parents with the resources to pursue this, or by professionals in charge of poorer young women with little independent access to a health provider of their choice. In these cases, the denial of disabled people's sexuality becomes marked on the body, designating these young women as incapable of making their own decisions, and as potential victims of heteronormative, unbridled male libido. At the same time, systems continue to contribute to the high rates of sexual abuse among young disabled people, such as residential education, group homes and home settings in which young people are not adequately protected (Nosek et al, 2001). A social model of disability approach would attempt to tackle these social systems rather than resort to inappropriate, non-consensual medical treatment of individuals.

It is around the issues of sexual agency and consent that the lines between people with physical, sensory and learning disabilities and those with mental health issues begin to blur (if those lines are believed to be present in the first place, of course). What all the above categories have in common is that they are seen as affecting people's ability to consent or have sexual agency in their lives. For example, disabled people who are trans*[1]-identified might encounter several obstacles when trying to access transition-related healthcare services. Their identities are often questioned by professionals, and sometimes family members, who want to ensure their trans identities are not a manifestation (or symptom of) their disability. For example, Alex has seen several young people with autism who identified as trans* having to fight for their right to access healthcare services with a provider of their choice, because of their parents' lack of belief in their identity as legitimate, rather than 'another obsessive phase'. These issues are even more salient for trans* people with significant learning difficulties who are under guardianship orders. This situation is even more difficult if they express queer sexualities. Alex has seen some of these clients disappear from therapy after the initial diagnostic assessment, despite their desire to receive gender-specialist services.

People with mental health issues and users of psychiatric services often experience a similar stripping away of their agency and capacity to consent. For example, Alex often sees clients who have received no information on how prescribed drugs might affect their sexual desire, nor how medication side-effects (such as interference with menstrual cycle, increased fatigue or drowsiness) might affect their sexual lives. Further, people with mental health issues are too often depicted as undesirable sexual and/or romantic partners in mainstream media, and instead as unstable villains or figures of fun. These depictions are part of the stigma surrounding mental health issues which has a negative impact on the self-esteem and perceived sexual capital of people with mental health issues.

As mentioned earlier, the ability to be viewed as people with agency, capable of consenting to sex, is also dependent on other factors, such as class, race/ethnicity, gender and education. A white, cis,[2] middle-class, educated, heterosexual man is likely to be seen as a more viable sexual agent, than someone with disabilities and different identities. It is worth noting that when disabled characters are depicted as sexual (as in *The Sessions*) they generally adhere to all the other identities listed here.

Underlining this disparity are heteronormative foundations that also assume whiteness, class and education (Warner, 1993). Those foundations are seen as central to normative discourses of citizenship, where the ideal unit is the happy, white, heterosexual, middle-class nuclear family. To stray from these foundations is itself deviant (Rubin, 1984), and to do so while having a disability is often still regarded as pathological. Within these normative discourses, pervasive assumptions abound. For example, loss of sexual function, usually seen as the ability to have penis-in-vagina penetrative sex, is perceived to be a worse loss for men than women. In contrast, loss of one's reproductive abilities is seen as the ultimate blow for a woman and far greater than any loss of the ability to experience sexual pleasure. Similarly, the importance of creating a sexy appearance is highlighted for women with disabilities, which can include disguising one's disabilities or highlighting other characteristics to compensate, in order to participate in the enactment of acceptable sexual capital. Often men are discouraged from considering a woman with a disability as a potential partner (Shakespeare et al, 1996) especially if those men are not disabled themselves. For disabled men, a woman without disabilities is seen as more desirable as she is perceived to be better able to nurture and care-take according to traditional, heteronormative gender roles.

Disabled people, and especially people of colour and/or with trans* and queer identities have increasingly challenged these normative discourses in many ways, including contribution to theory development, such as social models of disability and, more recently, crip theory. The latter is based in intersectional understanding and draws on a range of critical theories around gender, race, ethnicity and sexuality to directly challenge normative discourses that limit bodies and pleasure to a simple binary of normative vs deviant (Sandahl, 2003; McRuer, 2006; 2011). Such intersectional perspectives are also often present in the work of disabled artists. One of the groups that has sought to challenge our understanding of bodies and sexuality through performance is *Sins Invalid* (Berne, 2008), a performing art group of disabled people, who place people of colour, queer and trans★ identities at the centre of their explorations of sexuality, embodiment and disability. Through theorising, educating and performing, disabled people are reclaiming their agency and visibility, while also challenging normative discourses of embodiment and sexuality.

Conclusions

Drawing together the two strands of this chapter it seems that the expansions of understanding suggested by social models would be valuable for everybody, not only those currently disordered by categories of sexual disorder and those currently disabled by societal understandings.

For example, critical engagement with the narrow binary versions of sex perpetuated in the DSM categories and mainstream sex manuals would enable the kind of expansion of people's erotic imaginations, and move from goal-focused to process-focused sex, which would likely improve everyone's sexual experiences (Kleinplatz, 2012).

Also, it would be a profound – and valuable – shift if people were encouraged to approach each new sexual encounter with the assumption that bodies and minds are diverse, and so they would need to explore this new body/mind and how it works. This would be a radical departure from the current popular belief that a set of sexual techniques can be learnt that will make a person 'good in bed' with everybody (and the implicit caveat that, of course, nobody would want to have sex with anybody who was disabled or sexually disordered/dysfunctional).

The approach taken by the sexual surrogate in *The Sessions* actually makes a pretty good model for all sexual encounters. This is because it involves finding out what turns the other person on through verbal and non-verbal communication, exploring how their particular body works, determining the overlaps between the sexual desires of the people involved and focusing on those areas, and paying attention to the meaning of sex for those concerned (Barker, 2013c). Tellingly, during their analysis of sex manuals, one of us (Meg John) was struck that the book they were most likely to recommend to anybody seeking such a text would be *The Ultimate Guide to Sex and Disability* (Kaufman et al, 2007). The advice given in this book is along similar lines and is in stark contrast to most of the mainstream texts they analysed (Barker et al, in press). Assuming that people are physically, cognitively, and sensorially diverse, and a centrality of sexual ethics, would be better for everybody, not just those who have been disordered or disabled by binary, medical models of sexual function, normality and disability (Barker, 2013b).

In addition to psychiatric classifications and popular advice-giving, this has major implications for the training of sexual health – and other related – practitioners. It would suggest physical and psychological diversity being addressed throughout such training rather than disability being tacked on in a tokenistic manner, or not addressed at all, as is currently the case (Coleman et al, 2013). It would also suggest that trainees be taught about sexual diversity throughout, rather than having separate training on sexual dysfunctions or paraphilias (for models that allow for such an approach see Barker, 2011a; Barker, in press).

Returning to the theme of this book as a whole, we hope that this chapter has illustrated that there is much to be gained by applying social models of disability to sexual distress, and by ensuring that social models of disability encompass sex and sexuality as one of many intersecting sets of identities and experiences.

Notes

[1] The ⋆ after trans denotes multiple possible endings (for example, -gender, -sexual, -vestite). Trans⋆ is an umbrella term which aims to capture the broad range of experiences of people who do not remain in the gender that they were assigned at birth.

[2] cis (short for cisgender or cissexual) is an umbrella term for people who remain in the gender they were assigned at birth.

ELEVEN

The social model of disability and suicide prevention

Helen Spandler interviews David Webb

(December 2013)

HS: Can you tell us about when you first came across the social model of disability? What impact did it have on you, as a psychiatric system survivor?

DW: Very briefly, it begins with what I now call my *four years of madness* in the late 1990s. It was not until after this time that I found out about and began to get involved in (mental health) consumer advocacy, activism and politics. I also started my PhD on suicide around this time. All this led to my first contact with the World Network of Users and Survivors of Psychiatry (WNUSP), and organisations like MindFreedom in the US, which opened my eyes to the global movement for radical change in how we think about and respond to madness (madness is my preferred alternative – not everyone's choice – to the harmful pseudoscience label of 'mental illness'). We had nothing like these organisations in Australia. The 'consumer' organisations that we had here at that time were pretty locked into the medical model of madness and focused on service delivery, not human rights. Which remains the situation today, sadly. I know because I made the mistake of chairing one of these organisations for a while. WNUSP also introduced me to the work being done at that time on the UN Convention on the Rights of Persons with Disabilities (CRPD), which further opened my eyes to what was needed and what was possible. It's been a breathtaking, exhilarating and incredibly rewarding journey for me, but also a demanding, frustrating and infuriating journey at times, which has contributed to the illness and disability (aka burn-out) that has led to my premature and unofficial 'retirement' from activism. Perhaps the most inspirational part of this wild journey has been to meet and work with some extraordinary people with disabilities who have taught me so much about what it is to be human – and even more about what human rights *really* means. I'd like to especially honour Lesley Hall who was not only a great leader of the disability movement here in Australia (and globally) but also great fun to be with – her sudden passing away just a few months ago was a great shock and a great loss. Vale, Lesley.

HS: In the book, some authors argue that we need to apply and extend the social model of disability to madness and distress. Others argue that we need to develop our own separate or equivalent framework, so that we can have a common dialogue with disability activists, on equal terms. What do you think?

DW: First of all, the social model of disability is not set in concrete and finalised, never to change. Second, although psychosocial disability (madness) is a relative newcomer to the disability movement, we have already contributed to the development of the social model and I'm sure this will continue in the future. Users and survivors certainly contributed to the work leading up to the CRPD which, in turn, was part of the ongoing refinement of the social model. We have also drawn attention to things like invisible disabilities, intermittent or episodic disabilities, mental as well as physical/sensory disabilities. So I don't think we need a separate model of our own, any more than we need a social model of blindness, or of deafness, or of physical disability. In fact I think it would be a disaster if we cut ourselves off from the general disability community in this way. For instance, if each sector of the disability community insisted on being different and separate then we would not have the CRPD today. One of the great achievements of the CRPD process is how it united people with disabilities on the common ground that we all share, which is discrimination and the struggle for human rights. So no, I don't think we need a separate social model of madness in that sense.

I do, however, support the call for a social model of madness, though for me this would be based on, not instead of, the social model of disability. The issue here, I believe, is about how we *interpret* and *apply* the social model – and, likewise, how we interpret and apply the CRPD – in the context of the specific issues we face in psych disability. Each different disability will have its own priorities or the most urgent needs. For instance, for some people it might be access to the physical environment, which is usually not such a big deal for people with psych disabilities. For psych disability, the most critical issue is the right to refuse unwanted medical treatment, which these days is usually not too big a deal for many other disabilities. Despite these large variations between different types of disabilities, what we all share is the right to be recognised – in law as well as in the community – as full and whole people, regardless of our particular disability.

So I think there's a lot of work to be done to interpret and apply the social model (and the CRPD) within the context of psych disability. But I really hope that this is done based on the social model rather than thinking that we need to re-invent that wheel.

HS: What would you say to people who are worried that situating their (mental health) experiences within a disability framework is imposing particular disabled identities on us/own experiences, that are not of our own choosing?

DW: My short answer is that this is usually another instance of discrimination against disability. It reminds me of some alcoholics I met at AA meetings who looked down on junkies. A slightly longer answer is that, yes, many mental health 'consumers' in Australia object to their situation being called a disability. A lot of this is about the power of language, in particular the negative power of some words or labels. For instance, I used to accept, albeit reluctantly, the tag of (mental health) 'consumer', which is the common label used here in Australia. But over time I've come to despise this awful label – and '(service) user' is only marginally less offensive. The only term that is acceptable to me these days is that I'm a (suicide) survivor, which I openly acknowledge includes a political statement of defiance against the status quo, including the status quo that wants to label me as a consumer.

So when I hear consumers objecting to the word disability, I ask them, "Do you ever experience discrimination because of your mental health 'condition'?" Invariably the answer they give is "Yes". To which I respond, "Then that makes it a disability issue." For me, disability is first and foremost about discrimination. If you experience discrimination because of some (notional) health condition then you experience disability.

There's much to unravel in this discussion, however, more than can be covered in even my longer answer here. For instance, the really insidious word in this discussion is not disability but 'impairment', or its partner in crime 'health condition' as it's used in the ICF.[1] Although the social model of disability (and the CRPD) represent a huge breakthrough, at the very heart of the concept of disability we still have a judgement based on a person's medical status. In the CRPD this is camouflaged in its use of 'impairment' in its vague definition of disability. In the ICF, which many regard as the more formal and precise specification of disability (most notably the World Health Organisation and many other UN agencies as well as many governments), it is the term 'health condition' that lies at the heart of the definition of disability. And 'health condition' is camouflage for medical status, or indeed, a medical diagnosis. Which is why I regard the ICF as the medical model in disguise rather than the 'best of both worlds' (social and medical) as the World Health Organization would like us to believe. So despite the great achievements of the social model and the CRPD, medical labelling still sits at the heart of the concept of disability for many people.

I don't know how we get around this problem. The best I can come up with (with thanks to Tina Minkowitz for our discussions on this) is to slightly modify the ICF definition of disability to include the notion of *imputed* health condition. There is much in the ICF that is really very good, such as the inclusion of social attitudes as an environmental barrier to inclusion for some people with disabilities. But the authors of the ICF (mostly medicos) refuse to recognise medical judgements as a potentially disabling and discriminating social attitude, even though that is frequently the experience of many people with disabilities, perhaps especially people labelled as 'mentally ill'. Returning to my consumer friends who object to being labelled as disabled, I do chuckle when they look down on people with disabilities but then willingly accept a Disability Support Pension (or DSP, as it's called here in Australia)

HS: You have suggested that we can apply a social model of disability to suicide? Can you tell us about this, and how you think it might work in practice?

DW: First of all, I see the social model as a potential antidote to the disastrous medicalisation of suicide over the last 20 to 30 years. It's got so bad that most people now just accept that people kill themselves because they're suffering from some sort of mental illness, despite no scientific evidence whatsoever to support this belief. There has been a massive propaganda campaign to promote mental illness as the cause of suicide which, I'm afraid, has been tremendously successful. So we've now reached the point where our efforts to prevent suicide are actually contributing to the suicide toll, I believe. Mostly this is due to our failure to respond to the real issues behind suicide as we focus solely on medical diagnosis and treatment. But it is also the harm that often comes with this medical response to suicide, which includes dangerous drugs, locking people up and forced treatment. For me it's a no-brainer that such violence towards suicidal people is not helpful and, indeed, often pushes people over the edge.

The social model is more than just a critique of the medical model, however. It includes the recognition of the social circumstances that may contribute to a person feeling suicidal, and also that a change in these social circumstance might be the key to healing and survival. A more social model of suicide would also challenge us to ask what can we do as a society to assist people struggling with suicidal feelings? Some of this exists already, of course, such as 24-hour crisis lines, but it is minute compared to what we waste on medical coercion and treatment. One critical area that I see is the urgent need for safe spaces where suicidal people can take time out to simply be with whatever they're going through – sanctuaries, refuges, even asylums (in the best sense of that word). I hear really good things about the Maytree Foundation in the UK as an example of this, though I've never visited them.

Most of all, though, a social model of suicide would fight for radical change in society's attitudes towards suicide. The phrase 'suicide prevention' has two meanings. First, preventing actively suicidal people from killing themselves – or what I prefer to call 'intervention', this is the ambulance at the bottom of the cliff. There is an urgent need for safer, more compassionate response to actively suicidal people, including sanctuaries. Second, the larger goal of preventing people from becoming actively suicidal in the first place. This is much harder but, I believe, is the only real hope for reducing the suicide toll. The real hope for real reduction in the suicide toll is what I sometimes call 'mentally healthy' communities. It's shocking that I have to use this awful language to convey this idea, so I have to put it in quotes, but most people get the gist of what I'm saying here in a kind of shorthand way. A big part of the challenge here is that I don't know what a 'mentally healthy' society looks like – and I've not found anyone who does (though some people have suggested I visit Bhutan). But I do know, for certain, that the society I currently live in is not a mentally healthy one, on the contrary. So for me, suicide prevention is a key element of a much larger (and equally urgent) discourse around creating communities where quality of life is a major priority. And the social model of disability, madness, suicide etc has a great deal to contribute to this discourse.

HS: In *Thinking About Suicide* (Webb, 2010) you have eloquently and powerfully argued that suicidal feelings are a legitimate human expression of suffering, and not a mental illness. If this is the case, is there an equivalent 'impairment' or 'disability' in suicide? To put this another way, some people might think that using the social model of disability in mental health implies that people who are suicidal or distressed are 'impaired' or 'disabled'. How would you respond to that?

DW: For this question, I'd first of all refer you back to the discussion above on some of the problematic language that you're asking me about here. I think it's nonsense to blame suicide on some notional, medical, 'mental illness'. And disability is primarily about discrimination so, yes, suicidal people certainly experience discrimination so they qualify as people who experience disability. And now we come up against that wretched word 'impairment'. But even here I think we can usefully think of impairment as relevant to the suicidal experience, so long as we don't define impairment using some shallow, meaningless medical label.

In my work I argue that suicide is best understood as a crisis of the self. And let's be clear, it can be an extreme and dangerous and even 'crippling' crisis. During what I now sometimes call my 'four years of madness' back in the late 1990s, I was really very dysfunctional much of the time. I was certainly unable to work, I was socially inept much of the time, including a lot of self-imposed social exclusion, I was often very stoned from 'self-medicating' the pain I was feeling, and I went dangerously close to serious injury and/or death on several occasions. No doubt about it, I was pretty damn dysfunctional by any measure you might apply. So in this sense, I think you can say that I was experiencing substantial 'impairment'.

It is, however, critical that we don't fall into a too simplistic notion of impairment, such as we find in the medical model and the ICF. Indeed I would prefer to avoid this word if at all possible because of its heavily loaded medical connotations. But whether we use this word or not, we need to look deeper and ask what kind of impairment is happening with and within suicidal people. We can begin by discarding the popular myth that it's about malfunctioning neurotransmitters. I think a useful starting point is to talk of distress, or perhaps despair. First of all, we all experience distress or despair at some time so this language unites us as people, as part of the same humanity, which helps break down the them-and-us prejudice that is part of the toxic taboo on suicide. Then, we can recognise that feeling suicidal arises from *extreme* distress or despair so we need to see that it's just a matter of the degree to which we feel something with which we are all familiar. Suicidality is not some altered 'state' that you suddenly jump into. It's on a continuum of perfectly normal and natural human experience and probably, most of the time, develops quite slowly over time. Indeed, looking back on my own history, I can see now that I was suicidal long before I was actually aware that I was at the time. I don't believe in another popular myth that suicidal is always an impulsive act (except in some, fairly rare, instances).

Talking about distress and despair takes us into the psychological (rather than medical) realm, which is a good start. I'd like to take the opportunity here to promote a term coined by one of the pioneers of suicidology, the great Edwin S Shneidman. As a psychologist, he argued that the common denominator in all the suicides he encountered was 'psychache'[2] – a wonderful, beautiful, meaningful, useful word. He defined psychache as unbearable psychological pain due to thwarted or frustrated psychological needs, which I think is a great starting point for the study of suicide. If you want one word for the 'impairment' that suicidal people might be experiencing, I would suggest that it is psychache.

I cannot finish, however, without challenging Shneidman's definition of psychache. During my studies into suicide I wrote to him requesting that he modify his definition of psychache as due to thwarted or frustrated psychological and/or spiritual needs. A small change that doesn't undermine the rest of his arguments, I thought. To my surprise he graciously replied to my cheeky letter, though rejecting my suggestion. When I had the great good fortune to briefly meet him not long before he died, I reminded him of my request, to which he replied, "Suicidology really needs a decent phenomenology of suicide." I had to laugh and wholeheartedly agree with him even though it was another rejection but one I had to accept as a big step forward.

Another central tenet of my work is the critical need for suicidology to hear the first-person voice of survivors – Nothing About Us Without Us, you might say. And I will keep arguing that the suicidal crisis of the self is often also a spiritual crisis of the self. As it was for me.

HS: Can you summarise what you think are the benefits for psychiatric survivors, and especially people who are suicidal and/or self-harm of using the social model of disability?

DW: I think I've already said a fair bit about this above but I'd also make the more general assertion that I regard the No 1 issue in mental health (I wish I could speak about psychosocial wellbeing – maybe one day) is discrimination. Sure, there's lots of other pressing issues, such as the availability and quality of services, but I honestly don't believe we'll get significant progress in these other areas until there's major changes in society's attitudes towards…psychosocial distress/disability, madness, mental health 'issues' (another common double-speak phrase), whatever, call it anything except 'mental illness', please. This discrimination is already recognised to some extent, though usually hidden behind another double-speak word, 'stigma'. It needs to be called by its correct name, which is discrimination. Plus most of the so-called anti-stigma campaigns I've seen are little more than patronising platitudes from those who oppress us – indeed many survivors see these anti-stigma campaigns as stigmatising. We know that the only real solution to discrimination, whether it's racism, homophobia, or prejudices against disability, is to meet and hear directly from those who are discriminated against. This is one of the key elements of that great campaign slogan 'Nothing About Us Without Us'. And I must say that one of the worst communities in this regard is academia who like to co-opt our slogan for their research proposals but somehow fail to see that it applies to their work as well.

Another point that's not been mentioned so far is the celebration of diversity that we find in the disability community and the social model of disability. This is really important for people who experience altered states of consciousness or who experience reality differently to some notional 'norm'. This is not really my area of expertise but I'm thinking here, for example, of people like the Hearing Voices Network. Taking this example, the issue should not be whether you hear voices that others don't but rather whether hearing these voices is distressing and, if so, what can be done to ease that distress. Personally, I link this to my ideas around the crisis of the self, I guess because I imagine that experiencing these very 'different' realities could sometimes challenge your sense of self in quite distressing ways. But the issue must be the distress experienced not whether someone's experience of reality is (very) different to mine. That's just more discrimination. I welcome a society that includes people who experience different realities, indeed I dread a society that seeks to eliminate this. And once again we find that people with disabilities (and the social model) are real pioneers and leaders in this celebration of diversity.

HS: Do you think there are any downsides for psychiatric survivors in adopting the social model of disability?

DW: It's hard to think of any because it is so superior to what we currently have, though I'm sure that some problems would surface over time. For instance, interpreting the social model (or the CRPD) too rigidly would be a hazard, I think. As I said at the top, it's not set in concrete, and it's not perfect either. For instance, as noted above, the definition of disability is flawed in some ways and there's certainly not universal agreement about it, which I think is probably as it needs to be at this time. So there's plenty more work that needs to be done to clarify and refine the social model, perhaps especially so in psychosocial disability (which is why this book is so important). Again, I'll mention the very influential ICF, which I regard as seriously flawed as the medical model in disguise, though still a vast improvement on previous definitions of disability out of the World Health Organization. Another downside, which we're already seeing, is the selective application of the social model (and the CRPD). This is particularly pertinent for psychiatric survivors, and especially in developing countries, when we see how selective the Mental Health Division of the World Health Organization (WHO) is in its application of the social model and the CRPD. Although the World Health Organization boast of their human rights focus, they're remarkably silent on forced treatment, the unmentionable giant gorilla in the room that is also the serious and urgent human rights issue for people who experience psychosocial disability, distress, madness or whatever). Here you find lots of tut-tutting about the terrible human rights violations of mad people who find themselves in prisons, or are neglected on the streets, or abused by families etc. But precious little comment on the abuses within (and intrinsic to) mental health facilities. Likewise, they assume the necessity of mental health laws that permit detention and forced treatment, the only issue here being that their *other* rights (privacy, healthcare and so on) are respected. The World Health Organization advocates for mental health laws in countries that don't have them. When I spoke at one of the conferences in Bangkok I urged countries without mental health laws not to copy what we have done in the west. Needless to say, I'm not one of the World Health Organization's chosen celebrity survivors.

For those fellow survivors (consumers) who object to the disability tag, I think, I hope, that this will wear off as the word disability loses its stigmatising discrimination. I've heard it said that disability will cease to be an issue when being blind or deaf, or living in a wheelchair, for example, is no more of a big deal than the colour of your hair. I like this idea and hope that we can one day reach this level of understanding for people who experience different, sometimes radically different, psychological realities. Maybe this dream is my own reality distortion but, like the Paris graffiti in 1968, 'I take my dreams to be reality because I believe in the reality of my dreams'. And I repeat, we have so much to learn – all of us – from people who live with disabilities.

HS: You have been a vociferous supporter of rights-based legislation like the United Nations Convention on the Rights of People with Disabilities (CRPD). What do you think it offers psychiatric survivors?

DW: I'm probably repeating myself now, but the main benefit is that the CRPD represents a game-changer in how we must now talk about madness. We now occupy the moral high ground when we demand our rights. More specifically, the CRPD points us towards the abolition of all mental health laws that authorise human rights violations on the grounds of some notional 'mental illness'. This is huge. And it will take a lot of campaigning and a long time to see this achieved where it really counts, in our national laws. But the writing is on the wall for those who want to maintain a regime of violence towards mad people. It's not right. It's wrong. It should be prohibited. With the CRPD, I'm now certain that this day is coming, though probably not in my lifetime sadly.

For my interest in suicide, the CRPD points to the day when we can have a mental health system (though preferably by a different name) that can actually support people through a suicidal crisis rather than making it worse. The CRPD also represents a blueprint, almost a checklist, of the changes society needs to make in its attitudes towards disability – including the disability that comes with a suicidal crisis.

I know that for some people this sounds like pie-in-the-sky fantasy but we can already see how the CRPD is changing the discourse, changing the culture, for people struggling with psych disability today. People with psych disability and their advocates are already claiming their rights much more assertively than was possible prior to the CRPD. They now have authoritative documents and language, as well as global solidarity, in their fight for their rights. This will only get stronger as the CRPD and the social model becomes more understood and accepted and more widely adopted. Until, ultimately, human rights abuse will be prohibited and punishable by law.

HS: Some people argue that while things like the CRPD is a crucial step forward for people with disabilities, it might leave some psychiatric survivors vulnerable. This is because it emphasises negative freedoms (the right not to be coerced and detained against our will) at the expense of positive freedoms (such as the right to alternative non-medical support of our own choosing). How would you respond to that?

DW: I don't agree. The CRPD does not especially emphasise negative freedoms, as you call them, over positive freedoms. The right to live where you choose, to education, to participate in society and many other so-called positive freedoms are equally emphasised in the CRPD. Indeed, I don't see this distinction between negative and positive freedoms in the CRPD, which I think is a good thing. It is true, though, that the positive freedoms you speak of all depend on the fundamental right to personhood on an equal basis with others. This is what makes Article 12 on the right to legal capacity so important for every other right in the CRPD – and this is true for all disabilities, not just psychosocial disability. And it is this right, the right to be your own person making your own decisions, that is the foundation of the CRPD's move to a supported decision-making model rather than the coercive, substituted decision-making model that we have at the moment. Again, this is not something special for or peculiar to psych disability but a core right for all people with disabilities.

HS: Yes, but the CRPD makes it clear that taking away someone's liberty on the grounds of disability is discriminatory. Do you think that there is any justification for detaining someone in a place of safety when they are actively but temporarily suicidal? Is this discrimination on the grounds of disability? If so, how?

DW: Ouch! OK, this is where I might get into trouble with my survivor comrades. I have argued that there are situations where it might be acceptable to detain someone to prevent them from killing themselves. At first glance, this might seem to contradict my human rights stance and, in particular, my support for the

CRPD. I maintain that this is not the case – though some strict conditions apply to my argument.

First of all, I think this situation represents the tension between collective versus individual rights, where a society asserts a collective right to override a person's individual rights. The clearest example of this occurring is the criminal justice system, which I think most people accept as appropriate and necessary (even if we may not like how it is implemented). So it already happens and is an understood and accepted principle in our legal system. It is also understood, however, that it is a practice that is fraught with danger and susceptible to abuse, often very serious and dangerous abuses. So great caution is required whenever we seek to limit or restrict a person's individual rights on the basis of asserting a collective right to do so. It is precisely this hazard that has led to the elaborate checks and balances, such as the separation of powers, the right to appeal and so on, in our criminal justice system. It is worth noting at this point that very few such checks and balances exist in our mental health systems even though the restrictions imposed on a person's individual rights are even more severe than is permitted in the criminal justice system – for example, you cannot force unwanted medical treatment on prisoners.

Within a human rights discourse, any collective claim to limit a person's individual rights is said to be permissible only if it is 'reasonable, necessary and justified' (and 'proportionate' is usually added here but this only comes into play if the claim passes the first three criteria). My understanding is that the United Nation's Paris Principles spell these out in precise legal jargon (though personally I found this document incomprehensible). Just a few human rights, most notably the rights to not be subject to torture or slavery, are regarded as inviolable or 'non-derogable', meaning that under no circumstances can a person have these rights taken away from them by a society. It's worth noting at this point that Tina Minkowitz, a psychiatric survivor and human rights lawyer, makes a compelling argument that involuntary psychiatric treatment satisfies all the recognised definitions of torture, and that this argument has now been favourably heard by the UN Special Rapporteur on Torture. Or in plain language, involuntary psychiatric treatment should be prohibited for the same reasons that torture is prohibited.

While keeping these principles in mind, I believe we need to commence a very important discussion on whether it is ever 'reasonable, necessary and justified' to intervene and detain a person who is in real and imminent danger of killing themselves as a consequence of their own behaviour – that is, deliberately self-destruct or suicide. Personally, I believe that a pretty strong argument can be made for this case, but only under very strict conditions.

The first strict condition is that the risk of death must be real and imminent, and not based on an arbitrary suspicion that there is a risk of suicide at some time in the future. Specifying criteria for determining how real and how imminent the danger is will be tricky – impossible actually, but some guidelines will be necessary if this intervention is to be permitted. So my second strict condition is that this determination must be based on real and actual *behaviour* rather than on some overall judgement about the person. Which leads to my third strict condition, which is that this determination must *not* be made on the basis of some medical diagnosis, which is not only particularly poor at predicting suicide but also notorious for harmful interventions based on these diagnoses. Detaining a person based on a medical diagnosis is exactly the sort of discrimination that the CRPD prohibits and my argument here does not contradict this important principle of the CRPD.

The most important of my strict conditions, however, is that if the collective is to claim a right to deprive a person of their individual right to liberty then this should only be permitted if it also comes with the obligation to ensure that the person is detained to a place of safety. This condition poses a huge challenge to our current mental health system because the psychiatric ward, which is where suicidal people are usually detained, is a distinctly *unsafe* and dangerous space. I truly believe that it's safer to leave people on the street than commit them to a psychiatric ward. Earlier on I discussed briefly the kind of safe spaces that I see as necessary at these times, places such as the UK's Maytree refuge – though how they might handle involuntary admissions is another tricky challenge requiring very careful consideration.

I know that this position is controversial and I don't pretend that my analysis is complete. I do, however, maintain that a case can be made for detention to prevent suicide but that this need not violate the CRPD in any way. I also maintain that we should abolish current mental health laws that justify detention and forced treatment on the grounds of preventing suicide due to 'mental illness'. There is no evidence that the current system helps and plenty of anecdotal evidence, along with a sound human rights argument, that it causes great harm, including increasing the risk of suicide. Furthermore, I say abolish mental health laws *now*! Yes, a long and careful discussion as outlined above is needed but this should not be an excuse for not getting rid of the harmful practices that we have today. As I said, doing nothing at all is better (less dangerous) than doing what our public mental health system currently does. Yes, we can do a lot better than nothing at all, and a proper, careful discussion will take us there eventually. Until then, we must stop beating up on suicidal people.

HS: We've covered a lot here. Is there anything else you'd like to say?

DW: Phew! Methinks that's enough. But I'm conscious that I've not said much about more constructive 'interventions' that might be of help to suicidal people other than the need for safe spaces and sanctuary. Very briefly, I totally support making a broad range of services available in these safe spaces, such as various psychotherapies and counselling services, and even medical services. But these must always be on a voluntary basis and always guided by the person's own wishes. I'd also like to see these spaces become a place where 'alternative' or 'complementary' services are available, including (but not limited to) Chinese medicine and acupuncture, naturopathy, dieticians, yoga and other meditation practices, physical exercise, the list goes on. This may sound rather grand and wishful thinking, and also expensive to provide, but I maintain that in the long run such proper and genuinely useful supports are not only more effective but more economical than our current disastrous and very expensive medical model for helping suicidal people.

A few years ago I was pretty despondent that the situation was bad and getting worse. But today I really do believe we're on the cusp of revolutionary change in mental health. Not quite a tipping point yet, though this is now in sight, I feel.

My final comment is that this revolution will only occur – can only occur – with the leadership of psychiatric survivors. Exactly as has happened with the wider disability community. We welcome supporters and allies from all sectors, but real change will only be possible if it's led by those directly affected by the urgent need for change. Or as the disability world has said again and again, now culminating in the CRPD – Nothing About Us Without Us.

Thank you so much for the opportunity to talk about these urgent issues.

Notes

[1] International Classification of Functioning, Disability and Health known more commonly as ICF, is the World Health Organization (WHO) framework for measuring health and disability at both individual and population levels.

[2] Edwin S Shneidman (1993). Suicide as psychache, *Journal of Nervous and Mental Disease*, 181, 147–49.

Part Four
Universalising disability policy

Advancing the rights of users and survivors of psychiatry using the UN Convention on the Rights of Persons with Disabilities

An interview with Tina Minkowitz

Eds: As a member of the World Network of Users and Survivors of Psychiatry (WNUSP) you have been instrumental in developing the United Nations Convention on the Rights of Persons with Disabilities (CRPD). Can you explain why you decided to use the Convention as an avenue to advance the rights of users and survivors?

TM: The opportunity that came about with the CRPD converged with preparation that I had inadvertently undertaken through my legal studies. In law school I studied disability rights law and concentrated on international human rights law in a third-year clinical placement. I began thinking about how to combine the two – disability non-discrimination and international human rights – to combat psychiatric oppression. One of my professors, Rhonda Copelon, had set an example through her work on women's human rights, which also required bringing a non-discrimination lens to human rights violations in order to make them cognisable in international law. In my third year clinic when we were researching the relevance of the norm prohibiting torture to the definition of rape and sexual slavery as international crimes, I began to apply the international criteria for torture to forced psychiatric interventions and found that it was a good fit.

When the World Network of Users and Survivors of Psychiatry (WNUSP) learned about the opportunity to contribute to developing the new treaty, I outlined a proposal for advocacy that was accepted by the WNUSP board. At the beginning of the process I had no expectations for success but felt strongly that the opportunity to speak also implied a responsibility. Since the treaty was about our rights (and the rights of other people with disabilities) our silence would have given up power that we had, and would have made us complicit with the failure to achieve our own goals. I have written elsewhere about the CRPD process and what made it successful from a user/survivor point of view in my article in *Psychiatry Disrupted* (Burstow et al, 2014), and in a paper entitled 'The emergence of a user/survivor perspective in human rights' (Minkowitz, 2012).

Eds: Can you explain why you specifically chose to work within a disability rights framework?

TM: I think the relevant issue is why does it make sense for users and survivors of psychiatry, and people who have experienced (or been labelled with) madness or mental health problems, to situate ourselves as people with disabilities and to advocate for our human rights within that identity group. I can answer in part by examining my own experience of forced psychiatry, as I did for a law school class in human rights. There were three elements that stood out as being significant from a human rights perspective. The first was being treated as someone who did not matter. Our individuality was obliterated in the institutional setting. This was exemplified by the provision of a drink that mixed coffee and tea, which tasted vile, explained as the solution to the problem of 'some people like coffee, and some people like tea'. The second element was a profound violation of physical and mental integrity, the effect of mind-altering drugs reaching inside my body and mind to alter me in ways beyond my power to control. The third element was the basis on which society and the law permitted such treatment to take place. We were classified and selected for segregation and violent intrusion into our minds and bodies on the basis of perceived disability.

The concept of perceived disability is not new; it is found in the Americans with Disabilities Act (ADA) and in a regional precursor to the CRPD, the Inter-American Convention on the Elimination of All Forms of Discrimination Against Persons with Disabilities.

For other survivors of psychiatry and for those who identify as users of mental health services, I am sure that there are other answers. In some of my further responses below I will amplify on the larger picture as to how the concept of psychosocial disability comprises various experiences related to being a user or survivor of psychiatry or as having experienced madness or mental health problems.

WNUSP became involved in the creation of the CRPD through its affiliation with the International Disability Alliance, a network of seven organisations (since expanded) that were primarily organisations of people with disabilities with a global democratic structure. WNUSP initially became involved with the global disability community as a member of the Panel of Experts of the UN Special Rapporteur on Disability. As a member of the International Disability Alliance (IDA), the advocacy of WNUSP was given equal weight with that of other constituencies of the disability community.

WNUSP identifies its constituency as users and survivors of psychiatry, as defined in the WNUSP statutes, that is, a user or survivor of psychiatry is self-defined as someone who has experienced madness or mental health problems or who has used or survived mental health services. This identity was brought forward into the CRPD work and has never changed, except that we give greater emphasis to the term 'people with psychosocial disabilities' which is preferred by members in the global south and is gaining currency everywhere. By specifying that the identity is self-defined, we reject any medical definition of ourselves; by including those who identify only as users or as survivors we preserve the privacy of choice as to whether to accept concepts such as madness or mental health problems that separate out certain kinds of human experience. A survivor identity can be brought into a disability framework through the concept of disability-based discrimination, which is an integral part of the CRPD and which does not depend on whether a person adopts a disability identity but on objective manifestations of adverse treatment based on a classification by others as disabled.

The Committee on the Rights of Persons with Disabilities (the group of independent experts designated under the CRPD to monitor compliance with the treaty) has consistently issued recommendations aimed at abolition of the practices of mental health detention and compulsory treatment, and has referred to persons with 'actual or perceived' disabilities in this context and generally in obligations relating to non-discrimination. The core advocacy points of the user/survivor movement that we brought to the CRPD (legal capacity to make one's own decisions; prohibition of discriminatory detention; and prohibition of non-consensual interventions/treatment) are not only integral to the treaty but represent its most dynamic and forward-looking legal contributions. The Committee's adoption of its first General Comment dealing with Article 12 on legal capacity demonstrates the priority and attention given to an issue identified with people with psychosocial disabilities and people with intellectual disabilities, and has been characterised by one Committee member as a 'legal revolution'.

In the CRPD process, we made the strategic decision to situate ourselves as part of the disability community and to frame our issues in general terms in order to avoid isolation and marginalisation within the development of the treaty. The choice in this context was not whether our rights would be affected by the CRPD – it was fairly clear that they would, irrespective of our own choices – but whether we would accept marginalisation of the rights of people with psychosocial disabilities as a 'special' issue with its own rules taken from mental health law, or whether our rights would be addressed comprehensively, on an equal basis with other people with disabilities, with the benefit of our own critical disability analysis.

In the CRPD process the principle of mutual respect between different sectors of the disability community developed into a working relationship that not only incorporated the advocacy agendas of each constituency but eventually allowed us to find commonalities that may not have been apparent before. This was particularly true for me as the designated representative of WNUSP, since our issues required me to articulate the underlying theory from a disability rights perspective in order to be framed meaningfully and effectively as an application of non-discrimination to specific human rights. Legal capacity in particular struck a chord with all constituencies as the emblematic right of self-determination and autonomy notwithstanding a person's need for some type of support or services; many people with disabilities also identified with the right to respect for physical and mental integrity which underlies the freedom from forced interventions, and we found that other sectors also related to experiences of abuse and privacy violation. Subsequent to the adoption of the CRPD each of the sectors at the international level re-focused on the rights that were most prioritised and valued by the constituency, while at a national level there sometimes continues to be a synergy in exploration of commonalities in disability experiences through CRPD implementation and monitoring.

The CRPD is unique and different from other rights-based legislation. The CRPD is the only legislation in international or domestic law that guarantees our rights on a basis of full equality with others, and that makes no exceptions to legitimise acts of violence and abuse. Mental health legislation that is purported to be 'rights-based' starts by acknowledging the right to liberty and the right to free and informed consent but then seeks to justify infringements of these rights so as to allow institutionalisation and treatment against the person's will; such legislation amounts to state acquiescence to the violations and as such represents an impediment to human rights and non-discrimination rather than a means to promote and protect human rights.

The CRPD conceptualises the human rights of people with a variety of experiences, which relate to the commonality of being treated as less than other human beings because we are seen as having a defect, that is, being different from a supposed norm in a way that is negatively valued. Before the CRPD we had law and policy at both the international and domestic levels that was based uncritically on a medical model of mental illness as disability – that is, as a defect that is identified by doctors and that marks the person for adverse treatment and inferior protection of rights and freedoms, all of which has been condoned by society. I dissent from the mental illness label that was applied to me by psychiatry and from the quasi-state power that has been given to psychiatrists to classify and select individuals for segregation, confinement, violation of their physical and mental integrity and inferior legal status.

Eds: Can explain your use of the term 'psychosocial disability'? It is not a term people tend to use in the UK.

TM: I first encountered this term when I became involved with WNUSP; a WNUSP leader explained to me that it gives us a parallel term to other types of disability (such as 'sensory,' 'intellectual,' 'physical') and that it was preferable to 'psychiatric' disability which links us to the psychiatric profession. On the other hand, many US activists use the term 'psychiatric disability' in recognition of the fact that it is only by virtue of psychiatric labelling that they experience disability in the sense of discrimination. After adoption of the CRPD I drafted a one-page explanation of psychosocial disability which was approved by WNUSP. We say that the term is meant to express the following:

- a social rather than medical model understanding of conditions and experiences labelled as 'mental illness';
- a recognition that both internal and external factors in a person's life situation can affect a person's need for support or accommodation beyond the ordinary;

- a recognition that punitive, pathologising and paternalistic responses to a wide range of social, emotional, mental and spiritual conditions and experiences, not necessarily experienced as impairments, are disabling;
- a recognition that forced hospitalisation or institutionalisation, forced drugging, electroshock and psychosurgery, restraints, straitjackets, isolation, degrading practices such as forced nakedness or wearing of institutional clothing, are forms of violence and discrimination based on disability, and also cause physical and psychic injury resulting in secondary disability;
- inclusion of persons who do not identify as persons with disability but have been treated as such, for example, by being labelled as mentally ill or with any specific psychiatric diagnosis.

In this characterisation we are using disability concepts and terminology and adapting them to our own situation. Many of us have come to believe that the disability framework articulated in this way is a good fit for our advocacy and lived experience. It is not necessarily the only theoretical framework we can use, but it is one that allows us to tell a story about why society tolerates violent practices meted out to us, and also to acknowledge and reclaim socially devalued aspects of ourselves and to assert needs that society has not accommodated. WNUSP often uses the terms in conjunction with each other, saying 'users and survivors of psychiatry and persons with psychosocial disabilities' so as to honour diverse self-identifications (just as the terms 'user' and 'survivor' are meant to honour diverse identities).

Eds: Can you recall when you first came across the social model of disability? What impact did it have on you, as a psychiatric system survivor?

TM: I encountered the social model of disability in 1997, when I met disability rights activists who attended a demonstration organised by survivors of psychiatric abuse to protest against a judge in Brooklyn, New York, who treated people with disrespect in commitment hearings. Two leaders of Disabled In Action became good friends of mine, and one of them was a teacher of disability studies. Through them I learned about the social model of disability as a self-consciously political stance that put the onus on society to accommodate differences. I studied disability law soon after that.

The concept of reasonable accommodation was helpful to me as a survivor because it conceptualised how it is acceptable to have different needs and different ways of being in the world. In the survivor movement, particularly at the time I became involved, in 1978, it often felt as if we had to deny any way that we might actually have challenging mental or emotional experiences, or else be placed in a role of mental patient, as a person incapable of managing one's own life or doing anything worthwhile. This is changing now for many reasons, but I think part of it is the influence of a disability perspective.

The possibility of reasonable accommodation helps me to look at ways that I might be different or might be perceived as different, and to articulate this so that it can be addressed rather than give rise to misunderstandings and frustration. On a collective level, the disability rights framework has the potential to speak to both those who identify as service users and focus on changing mental health practices, and survivors who emphasise the right to refuse any psychiatric intervention and the need to change the laws to fully secure this right.

The social model of disability is not any single thing nor does it belong to any one group or sector of the disability community. I do not agree with the formulation that is used in the UK which depends on the notion of impairment. While I respect the work of those who created the UK social model, it was never meant to apply beyond physical disability. Other sectors can adapt aspects of it that speak to us and articulate our own versions of a social model. During the CRPD negotiations, neither the disability community nor the governments involved could agree on a definition of disability, but we explored the issue in public and private discussions in an attempt to understand our commonalities. I consider disability to be a heterogeneous concept, one that comprises many distinct realities that do not all share a single common feature, but all of which share some common feature with some of the other realities that are encompassed.

Eds: What benefits do you think the social model of disability has for mental health service users and psychiatric survivors?

TM: I prefer to talk about a disability non-discrimination framework. Although I have sometimes referred to a social model of disability, people place their own meanings on that term. As I understand the social model, its main value is in placing the burden on society to accommodate differences and to meet a wide range of human needs without characterising them as 'special'. This approach to the social model emphasises the aspect of universal or inclusive design, which I apply to law and policy in order to address legal concerns of people with psychosocial disabilities as an integral rather than incidental aspect of legal doctrine.

I situate myself as a person with disability when I am including myself in the sector that has a right to be consulted on matters affecting my human rights, and also when I am relating myself to the commonality with other people with disabilities. My disability identity at those times is as a survivor of psychiatry; I create the space for this identity within the disability framework rather than seeing them as mutually exclusive.

Eds: We are interested in the consequences, for people with mental health problems, of being defined as disabled in law and specifically the abolition of separate 'mental health' law as inherently discriminatory. Might this lead to the criminalisation or neglect of people with mental health problems? Examples would be if someone commits a crime when experiencing a mental health crisis, or refuses help and support when they are in imminent danger of suicide or self-starvation.

TM: I do not understand the question about criminalisation. Literally, criminalisation of people with mental health problems would occur if a crime were defined based on behaviour that was perceived as a public nuisance because of its association with psychosocial disability (for example, if it were considered a crime to talk loudly in public without an obvious conversation partner).

A person who commits a crime when experiencing a mental health crisis first of all has the right to be presumed innocent until proven guilty beyond a reasonable doubt in a court of law. These due process guarantees are flouted in many ways in our existing system, including by transfer to mental health commitment regimes that impose custodial measures without such an adjudication, merely based on the allegation of criminal conduct and the opinion of psychiatrists that the person poses a 'danger to self or others'. Psychiatric inpatient and outpatient commitment have been referred to as criminalisation of people with psychosocial disabilities, since they impose control measures based only on a suspicion of future conduct that may not even be defined under the penal law, and on the existence of an actual or perceived psychosocial disability.

Neglect would occur if the state offered no support, or inadequate support, to people who are experiencing a crisis and whose needs are not being met. Many people experiencing crises that psychiatrists label as mental health problems prefer to avoid the public mental health system and may prefer to avoid services of any kind. There is a great deal of evidence to suggest that ordinary kindness and acceptance meets people's needs for practical support and emotional support during such an experience without violating their rights and while carrying much lower risk of lifelong trauma and lifelong dependency on services (see, among others, Robert Whitaker's *Anatomy of an Epidemic* (2010); Peter Breggin's, *Brain-Disabling Treatments in Psychiatry* (1997); Peter Lehmann's *Coming Off Psychiatric Drugs* (2004); and Loren Mosher, Voyce Hendrix and Deborah Fort's *Soteria: Through Madness to Deliverance* (2004)). Thus it can fairly be said that most if not all states are violating the rights of persons with psychosocial disabilities through neglect, by either maintaining a harmful and degrading mental health system that routinely violates basic human rights, or offering scanty services of any kind.

There is a great deal that can be done to support people who have suicidal feelings or who have difficulties with their food intake, by creating relational spaces where trust can develop to support self-expression and self-empowerment, rather than relationships of control, which foster deceit and resentment and are ultimately destructive to all concerned. We need also to create the opportunity for open discussions about suicide, and open ourselves to hear the pain – what suicidologist and suicide attempt survivor, David Webb, calls 'psychache' (see Chapter 11 in this book) – which cannot be done if people who speak honestly about suicidal thoughts and feelings are met with incarceration.

It is also somewhat disingenuous to frame this concern as being about the consequences of defining people with psychosocial disabilities as disabled in law. The abolition of separate mental health law, and in particular the abolition of commitment and compulsory treatment regimes, has been a goal of the movement against psychiatric oppression for decades. It was certainly the primary goal of the movement when I joined in 1978, long before the CRPD or even the Americans with Disabilities Act was envisioned. People labelled with mental health problems are already defined as disabled under many international and domestic laws. We can receive disability pensions and we are protected against disability-based discrimination under many general laws guaranteeing non-discrimination based on disability; we were included in the UN Standard Rules on the Equalisation of Opportunities for Persons with Disabilities, a non-binding declaration that was a precursor to the CRPD. The CRPD adds value to all these previous laws by explicitly bringing the violations named and experienced by survivors of psychiatric oppression under the framework of disability rights, so as to abolish them as acts of disability-based discrimination. To oppose the CRPD in this regard is to oppose the goals that have consistently defined this movement for social justice, on the grounds that it now has the legal tools to succeed.

The movement is growing worldwide. People with psychosocial disabilities in the global south and in smaller European countries have a better chance than we in the United States or United Kingdom of grasping and implementing the CRPD, because psychiatry holds less sway there and communities are not so reliant on psychiatry as a means of social control and paternalistic neglect. It is a movement whose time has come, it is consistent with the values and concepts of universal human rights, and it touches on the whole range of social justice issues bringing with it a profound acceptance of diversity and a call for more, not less, support for those who have unmet needs.

Eds: Can you say any more about how alternatives might be achieved in situations where people are experiencing a severe mental health crisis, where their capacity to make decisions may be temporarily challenged and they actually frighten, hurt or threaten other people, maybe, for example, at home or in the workplace. These can be extremely difficult situations, especially when the person is living or working with others who have limited choices and rights themselves.

TM: I am a human rights lawyer and a survivor of forced psychiatry. With regard to practical implementation, I can only speak of what I have learned from my own experience and from those in the movement who work actively on creating alternatives.

Parenthetically, from a human rights perspective it is somewhat misleading to talk about a person's 'capacity to make decisions [being] temporarily challenged'. The CRPD Committee in its General Comment on legal capacity affirms that fluctuations in mental capacity (a person's actual or perceived decision-making skills) do not justify a limitation of legal capacity (that is, the rights associated with legal agency). Furthermore, the concept of mental capacity itself is acknowledged to be controversial.

I have been part of the survivor movement for over 30 years. It is difficult for me to stay connected to a friend who is going through a crisis when she or he is relating to me in challenging ways. I feel frustrated when something that seems obvious to me is not obvious to them. What I have learned is that it helps to be as honest as possible, to say what I am seeing in the situation, but also to always acknowledge where they are coming from and not to get involved in a disagreement over how to characterise the reality we are looking at.

On one occasion I spoke with someone over a period of weeks who was seeking support to explore her feelings of wanting to commit suicide. This was one of the most challenging experiences I have had, since the communication stopped abruptly and I thought she had taken her life. It turned out she was fine and she needed time to let things settle for herself. I am grateful that my fears were unfounded, but I would most likely make the same decision I did then, to not alert the authorities since from our conversations I believed that the person, like myself, would prefer death to another round of forced psychiatry.

My ability to deal with people in crisis has been strengthened (though it's still not great) by the practice of Intentional Peer Support, which focuses on maintaining connection, acknowledging the relevance of each person's worldview, paying attention to mutuality in relationships, and moving towards what we want (such as the creation of a satisfying relationship).

If I do not speak of my own needs it is because I choose not to in this context, not that I think I am beyond needing support, as all human beings do.

We all have different skills and different levels of tolerance for physical risk; we do not all take on the role of public safety officers or first responders, though we should learn as much as possible to deal with crises of any kind. The creation of good practices to support someone going through crisis and is also behaving aggressively towards others is challenging, but I know activists who work on this. Unfortunately, the resources dedicated to such work, and to all support services other than mental health systems centred on biopsychiatry, are minuscule; furthermore, all existing alternatives, at least in the global north, operate within a context where commitment laws pose an ever-present threat to people with psychosocial disabilities who come to the attention of authorities for any reason.

Yet there are many instances demonstrating the power of relational skill and compassion to prevent violence. I am thinking of an instance where a young man walked into a school intending to shoot people, but a woman working in the front office reached out to him as a human being, sharing her own experiences of grief and loss and reminding him that he was not yet a murderer and did not have to be. He finally put down his gun and was taken into custody by police. The courageous woman had the benefit of training for this purpose as well as her own considerable skill and compassion.

THIRTEEN

UN Convention on the Rights of Persons with Disabilities: out of the frying pan into the fire? Mental health service users and survivors aligning with the disability movement

Anne Plumb

Introduction

This chapter will look at the United Nations Convention on the Rights of Persons with Disabilities (CRPD) and continue to ask whether or not mental health service-user/survivors are best served by becoming subsumed within a broader disability movement (Plumb, 1994; 2012a). I am concerned that the service-user user/survivor/mad movement, in trying to exploit the CRPD to address our situations, may leave us 'jumping out of the frying pan into the fire'. I will look briefly at some limitations of the social model of disability and identify some aspects of mental health service users' and survivors' experience, which I believe differ to people with physical impairments/disabilities and yet are central to the CRPD, namely autonomy (self-determination) and responsibility. I address these issues from my experience of 'extra/non-ordinary experiences' (what psychiatry calls religious psychosis), depression and suicidality and, also as a long standing ally of the disabled people's movement, and an activist in the survivor movement in the UK.

Limitations of the social model of disability

People with 'mental disorders' have been included in disability legislation in the UK alongside people 'substantially handicapped by illness, injury or congenital deformity or any other such disability' since the amendment, in 1974, of the National Assistance Act 1948. It is therefore fitting for mental health service users/survivors (with a psychiatric diagnosis, in particular) to join with disabled people/ persons with disabilities when making use of, or challenging, disability legislation as it can provide access to provisions, benefits and rights. My purpose, however, in writing 'Distress or disability?' in 1994 was to draw to the attention of disabled activists, eager to include us in their movement, the long history of, and distinctive issues facing, the mental health movement. I also wanted to highlight problems with the social model of disability (as derived from the social definition of disability proposed by Finkelstein, a member of the Union of the Physically Impaired Against Segregation (Finkelstein, 1975) which relates, by definition, to persons with *physical impairments* (UPIAS, 1981).

This issue is still pertinent as the CRPD includes us as persons with *mental impairments* (Article 1). The term 'psychosocial disabilities' is now being promoted by some mental health activists (WNUSP, 2008, 9), instead of impairment, but what is meant by 'disabilities' here? Most people today talk generally of disabilities, in the sense of the National Assistance Act definition above, which rather blurs Finkelstein's intention 'to turn the spotlight' placed by the medical and related professionals on individuals' conditions to society's responses to them, in order to expose exclusion and oppression (Finkelstein, 1975). I don't have space to say more on terminology here except that my late husband insisted that he was a 'disabled person' not a 'person with a disability'! Mental health service-users/survivors are divided on whether we individually accept a psychiatric diagnosis (medical condition) or not. Personally, I accept that our neurophysiology mediates between our environments (physical, personal, social, spiritual) and our psyche (self), but dispute that there is necessarily any physiological *impairment* underlying my experiences.

The position of the Union of the Physically Impaired Against Segregation regarding other oppressed groups was that:

> (t)he particular form which oppression takes in this society differ somewhat for each distinct group. Some, such as people who are called 'mentally handicapped', or those labelled 'mentally ill' clearly have a great deal in common with us. Full membership is however based simply on the fact of physical impairment. This is because we believe *the important thing is to clarify the facts of our situation and the problems associated with physical impairments.* But it is fundamental to our approach that we will seek to work with

> other oppressed groups and support their struggles…What
> *all* oppressed groups share is a vital interest in changing
> society to overcome oppression. (UPIAS, 1974, para 22,
> my emphasis)

It was clear to me that mental health service-users/recipients equally needed to 'clarify the facts of our situation'. I was drawn to Survivors Speak Out (SSO) which, along with other organisations in the UK in the 1980s, sought to expose psychiatry, challenge the medical model of mental illness by talking of 'emotional and mental distress and dissent' and recognise that life events 'took us into the system' (Plumb, 2012a).[1] From this perspective, the social model of disability has some major limitations.

Both the social model of disability and the CRPD focus on discrimination, which *follows* impairment/disability, for example Article 16 on Abuse, Exploitation and Violence. However, while we do experience discrimination (which oppressed group doesn't?), especially after contact with the mental health system, we often end up on psychiatric wards as a culmination of experiences *before* our admission. If survivors turn the spotlight onto our environments, in addition to challenging discrimination and exclusion we should also be highlighting the ways environments (personal as well as physical, social and cultural) affect people psychosocially (MHSS, 1987; Plumb, 1993). Possibly owing to a 'western bias', the disability movement has rarely addressed the causes of physical impairment/disability such as unclean water, toxic and dangerous work places, poorly funded health provision, or armed conflict.

Additionally, disabled people could insist that the spotlight be shifted from their medical conditions to their environment because, generally, they did not challenge their medical diagnoses as such but rather the control and influence of the medical profession and medical 'model' over their lives. In contrast, challenging psychiatric diagnoses and treatments have long been a part of the survivor movement (Plumb, 1999). Such challenges raise important *psychosocial issues* that should be reflected in any model we develop.

It is pertinent for disabled people/persons with physical disabilities to focus on discrimination, on environments not allowing them access. Mental health service-users/survivors, however, require a wider perspective, one that recognises the circumstances which give rise to our distress or madness in the first place, as well as the way that 'mental disorder' is perceived and acted upon in society. We need to insist on societies in which people may thrive emotionally and mentally. We could reduce oppression and repression to 'discrimination' but this illuminates little. We need to name sexual abuse, marital violence, bullying, exploitation, deprivation and so on. Likewise 'self-determination' is crucial to the social model of disability and CRPD but I will argue that it is not so straightforward for mental health service users/survivors.

UN Convention on the Rights of Persons with Disabilities

According to the Universal Declaration of Human Rights 1948, humans have rights, and legal status, because we are endowed with 'reason' and 'conscience' (United Nations, 1948, Article 1). Given the stereotypes around mental illness and madness, this wording perhaps explains why we have often been treated as lesser humans. It might also explain why the World Network of Users and Survivors of Psychiatry (WNUSP), negotiators in the drafting of the CRPD, insisted that, despite others deciding what is 'in our best interests', we do have reason and conscience. The WNUSP are celebrating attaining 'legal status' for us, as persons with 'disabilities', that is, a right to autonomy and liberty except where we contravene the rule of law (WNUSP, 2008; WNUSP and CHRUSP, 2013). For me, the really radical development in the survivor and service-user movement was our insistence on 'speaking out' when for so long our credibility had been denied, along with the validity of our experiences (Plumb, 1993; Plumb, 2012a). However, I do not see this as claiming that we fully understand our experiences. Rather, it challenges the assumptions made by people without our experiences who claim to know better.

I am going to look briefly at the following areas where I believe mental health service-users/survivors differ from people with physical disabilities and are not properly represented in the CRPD:

- self-determination
- intervention, risk and safety
- responsibility and criminality
- expressed wishes and consent
- alternative and replacement support.

Self determination

Autonomy (self-determination) is fundamental to the social model of disability. Why, after all, should a person with a physical impairment/ disability not be enabled to make, and act on, their own decisions (agency)? The CRPD negotiators sought recognition that service-users and survivors also have agency and can, and should, take responsibility – yet both 'mental *impairment*' (the term used in the CRPD) or indeed 'psycho-social *disability*' (favoured by the WNUSP) imply that our ability to be self-determining can be affected by emotional and mental states. I would argue that while we do have reason, conscience and agency, these are complicated by experiences categorised as 'mental disorder' that, *in some ways*, distinguish us from others.

In his book on suicidality, Webb has called for a broad community conversation and 'a collective story that is capable of communicating the *full depth and complexity* of the suicidal crisis of self' (Webb, 2010, 168 my emphasis).

Such a conversation is also imperative around what I call 'extra/non-ordinary experiences'. It is unfortunate that such *full* conversations appear not to have taken place before the drafting of the CRPD. The purpose of my chapter is to stimulate such a conversation as I am neither represented within, nor liberated by, this Convention, because of a restricted understanding of experiences like mine.

With limited space, I want here to look primarily at my own experience and that of Peter Campbell (a leading activist in the UK survivor movement). Campbell has recalled his experience:

> I believed that the earth was going to collide with the moon directly above my house, through a fault of mine. I lay under a bush in the street, mute, trying to keep out the rays of the setting sun in order that I wouldn't be seen and the collision wouldn't take place. (Campbell, undated, see also 1993)

Meanwhile, my 'first break' related to a Christian belief in the second coming of the 'Son of God' (Plumb, 1993; 2012a). I believed that Jesus had returned and was a sort of benevolent 1960s' Pied Piper[2] whose music would compel people to live in peace and love. My role was to identify him. In the middle of the night I sat in a Student Union building uncommunicative and unmoving, unsure what was expected of me, awaiting signs.

Both Campbell and I did indeed have agency. I could have refused to act on what I believed was a revelation from God (and thereby condemned myself to Hell?). Such experiences have been attributed to 'mental illness' and madness – but mine were not mere incoherent ramblings and we are long way from demonstrating the pathways between the functioning of neurotransmitters and actual mental images and thoughts. Nor was it some 'delusion of grandeur' I had concocted out of some personal inadequacy, another of psychiatry's claims. Most people have some questionable or unusual beliefs but there is something about ours that may make them more problematic. There is a parallel here with Marius Romme and Sandra Escher's findings from their first survey of voice hearers – that for some, voices enriched their lives, while others found voices negative, aggressive and incapacitating (Romme and Escher, 1993).

Both Campbell and I, in retrospect, know our beliefs were somewhat ridiculous – the 'Messiah' as a sort of Pied Piper? Some people are happy to simply view their beliefs as 'momentary madness' but I believe that a social model for mental health service-users/survivors requires us to look further into these experiences. For some of us it might be unhelpful, or even unacceptable, to talk of 'madness'. Some research seeking service-user views quotes one as saying: 'I stick to my guns and I don't like madness' (Beresford et al, 2010).

Questions arise as to what led Campbell to believe a celestial collision was imminent or that I was to witness a second coming and, more than this, that certain actions were *required* of us. At what point did our thinking become of no sense to anyone but ourselves? And under what circumstances did this happen? Emotional and mental exhaustion or alienation perhaps made our interpretations so real to us. A novel, *The Second Coming* by John Niven (2011), has recently been published in which the Son of God is a struggling musician in New York City trying to spread his hippy ethos and, in this story, overthrow evil in the music business. A similar conception, but for Niven a fiction, for me a reality.

What were the triggers? What were Campbell's and my circumstances at the time? What life experiences influenced our thinking and actions? To respond to situations we have to draw on our own past experiences and wider cultural understandings that inform, encourage and constrain our thinking and behaviour. Mine was a *response* to an unfamiliar transcendental experience that, for me, had *no ready explanation*. There was meaning in my apparent madness (Plumb, 1993) and Campbell has said that: '(I)t is actually extremely damaging telling people…that their deepest experiences are meaningless' (Campbell, undated, 3).

Contrary to common assumptions, I was clearly aware of what was going on around me. Indeed, my sensory perceptions were sharpened. Rather, because of my beliefs, I was not engaging with the people around me and because of my extraordinary experiences other things mattered more than the usual behaviours, preoccupations and routines of life. Unfortunately, valid as they may be, such experiences may not leave us in a good place. As the Hackney Mental Health Action Group stated in a Charter of Rights for People in Mental Distress: 'the severity and nature of their distress and the circumstances of their lives cause some people to seek help or be forced to accept treatment from mental health services' (HMHAG, 1986, 2).

I would have liked to have said something here about spirit possession but can only refer to the troubling memoir of Whitney Robinson who feels that she is possessed by a daemon (Robinson, 2011). In a review of Robinson's book, I concluded that I hoped it would leave readers with an imperative: 'to find better ways to help and support people through such terrifying, isolating and, yes, sometimes dangerous experiences – a change of paradigm and practice' (Plumb, 2012b, 22).

I would have also liked to explore what agency means in times of extreme depression. Will Hall, a host on 'Madness radio' in the US, for example, has talked of states of despair so deep that he could neither feed himself nor leave his apartment, but I only have space to point out that this again requires us to look more closely at 'agency' (Hall, 2013).

I do, however, want to say something more about suicidality. The CPRD is interpreted as recognising a person's right to take their own life (autonomy), perhaps in support of the demand of some persons with disabilities for 'assisted suicide' to be legalised (WNUSP, 2008, 15). Assisted dying, however, is seen as pain-free, dignified and taking place in the company of loved ones. Suicide is more often violent – involving severe injuries (if unsuccessful) and a lasting, if unintentional, trauma for surviving friends, family and witnesses. It is usually a solitary act. As I write this, I hear of two deaths on one rail track in the course of a single week; of two young people hanging themselves as a result of bullying and blackmail on the internet. Rather than brushing these aside as an individual's 'choice', should we, as a society, not be concerned? Will Hall has asserted that suicidal feelings are 'not the same as giving up on life. Suicidal feelings often express *a powerful and overwhelming feeling for a different life*' (Hall, 2013, my emphasis). This is echoed by David Webb who advises people to honour and respect their suicidal feelings as real, legitimate and important, *but without acting on them* (Webb, 2010, 3–4).

The question remains: should anyone intervene in situations such as ours?

Intervention, risk and safety

Here, I want to look briefly at the removal of people to a 'place of safety', under mental health legislation, on the basis of their being perceived as at risk to themselves or a danger to others. The CRPD presents liberty as paramount (Article 14). WNUSP, for example, have stated: 'The CRPD makes no exceptions allowing detention as a last resort or in exceptional circumstances' (WNUSP and CHRUSP, 2013, 8).

No action, it states, should be taken without the expressed wishes of the individual. A question for me is: were Campbell and I at risk if, being mute and uncommunicating, we were simply ignored? Or if I was simply forced out of a building that was due to be locked up? Rather than refusing to talk about risk and safety, something the CRPD negotiators have done and see as a victory (WNUSP, 2008, 5), we ought to have wrested the discussion *away from people acting on our behalf*, those deciding what is in 'our best interests', from those who assume to know what we are going through and how we should be responded to. We need that conversation among ourselves as to where we may have been at risk and what, *for us*, constitutes safety (Plumb, 1999). Service users in one recent research study (29 out of 60), for example, defended detention with the rest either opposing it or ambivalent (Katsakou et al, 2012). Where does the Convention leave these participants?

Although psychiatry's rationale, regimes, ward conditions, procedures, abuses, violations and relationship to 'patients' have frequently been challenged, and there are important issues here of *internalisation* and *self-stigma* (Chamberlin, 1987), these participants perceived themselves, in retrospect, as being at risk. They reported for example, 'feeling bewildered, behaving out of character, losing control over their behaviour...feeling distressed or frantic and elated'. Examples of risky actions include: a survivor who wrote on an on-line forum about lighting candles to keep evil influences at bay (her house burned down); a friend of mine who thought he could stop buses by standing ahead of them with his arms outstretched; and I very nearly stepped into a bath of boiling water in the belief that I needed to demonstrate faith in God (aka mystics running over hot coals). Authorities have responded to these risks in ways totally unacceptable to many of us, but should this mean that no-one should intervene? Despite this, WNUSP claim that '(i)t is well established that health care includes both physical and mental health, and there can be *no distinction between them* with respect to the right to free and informed consent, which protects both individual autonomy and physical and mental integrity' (WNUSP/CHRUSP, 2013, 8, my emphasis).

What about the situations mentioned above? Supporters of the CRPD have argued that Advance Statements/Directives and Crisis cards are a safeguard. Advance Statements, regarding mental health are, however, generally *retrospective*, based on an earlier experience. Additionally, they imply that, on occasion, a person *may not be able to give an expressed opinion*, a point, which has led some CRPD supporters to express unease, as the convention rests on the claim that, given support, we are *always* able to express our wishes.

In terms of intervention, I am reminded of a Christian parable – that of the Good Samaritan. A Jewish man, robbed and beaten, lies on the wayside. A couple of people just pass by but a stranger, of a different faith, tends to him and takes him to an inn to be further looked after. Setting aside the political question as to who should pay the inn keeper, our problem is – where is our equivalent of the inn? Today, in a medical crisis the arrival of an ambulance is generally welcomed and faith placed in the medical team. In a perceived mental health crisis many of us do not have such faith. The issue for me is not intervention as such; *it is the nature of that intervention and its consequences.*

Before moving on to another critical issue in the CRPD, criminality, I want to ask how important are words? Security and liberty are words that can be used in many ways. There is currently (2014) a consultation being carried out by the UN Human Rights Committee on 'liberty and security' (DOHR Article 3) to which supporters of the CRPD have responded insisting that the Convention, as they present it, is recognised. Their view appears to echo the libertarian psychotherapist, Szasz, who argued that the law should protect people's right to life, liberty and property – and from people who want to deprive them of these, but should not protect people from themselves (see Wyatt, 2012).

A different perspective is illustrated by the London-based Hackney Mental Health Action Group's *Charter of Rights for People in Mental Distress* (1986). Recognising that a fear of compulsory detention and treatment can undermine a right to personal *security*, they called for a full range of residential alternatives to hospital and for strategies to be developed to deal with the need to intervene in the lives of people actually in crisis. The charter argued that these alternatives should evolve from the experiences of people who have gone through crisis themselves, and those who have experience of assisting at such crises (HMHAG, 1986).

Responsibility and criminality

As controversial as non-intervention, the CRPD removes, according to the negotiators, separate secure unit provision and the 'insanity plea' (diminished responsibility) (CRPD Article 14; WNUSP, 2008, 16;

Minkowitz, 2011) as discriminatory. Furthermore, if service-users/ survivors commit any crime we should be treated no differently to any other citizen, though all should have an advocate of their choice.

Why, I would ask, were any distinctions made in the first place? While agreeing that these are underpinned by assumptions about 'madness' and 'mental disorder' I am very uneasy that a chief negotiator of the CRPD, Tina Minkowitz, has written that, '(t)he plea of not-guilty by reason of insanity…deprives individuals of a clear determination of their responsibility…The insanity defense violates the legal capacity of persons with disabilities (article 12.2) as well as Article 14' (Minkowitz, 2011, para 15). This seems to echo a libertarian ethos and explanation of 'mental illness' as presented by, for example, Thomas Szasz who argued that: 'there is no such thing as insanity only varying degrees of irresponsibility…[and] responsibility is, morally speaking, anterior to liberty…The issue becomes what…(the patient) is willing to recognise as his evasions of responsibility often expressed as symptoms' (see Wyatt, 2012, 6).

What underlies and defines criminality and the prison system are vast studies in their own right. As to why we may commit crimes when distressed or in an extra/non ordinary state is too big a subject to cover here. Nevertheless, I would pose a question about morality: do any of us, when in deep distress, let alone when in altered states, act violently or destructively or contravene laws *when otherwise we would not*? In other words, is our psychosocial experience affecting our agency? It has been said to me that 'acknowledging our wrongdoing helps with our healing' (personal correspondence). But where is the *social context*? On one occasion I could have put in the windows of a council office because no-one was hearing my complaint at a time when I was under great stress, but for someone noticing my distress and reaching out to me.

Furthermore, what should we make, for example, of the Judaeo-Christian story I heard many times in my childhood, where the patriarch Abraham, in being willing to sacrifice his son on an altar, is venerated for his faith and obedience to his God? How are people like myself to gauge the authenticity of any voices, revelations or signs, especially during our first encounters when they appear so real? Might we 'crack' because *too much responsibility* has been placed on us, through a lack of nurture, supportive networks or places to turn to for help? Dangerousness is grossly misrepresented by the media and authorities but, as with risk and safety, we need our own conversation about the psychosocial meaning of responsibility. Campbell, for example, could be seen as acting 'responsibly', both personally and socially (by protecting the planet).

I see the direction WNUSP and the CRPD have taken as a form of 'moral distancing' from people who 'don't behave well' during times of great distress or 'altered states', ignoring the social, political and cultural aspects of responsibility. Or, as Nev Jones has written, '"Sacrificing" the interests of individuals who have committed otherwise criminal acts due to temporarily but profoundly altered beliefs or states for generalised and decontextualised "right" to legal capacity is, at a minimum, an advocacy goal that should be subject to the highest level of critical scrutiny and ethical reflexivity' (Jones and Shattell, in press).Might there be the making of a new stigma here?

Challenging high security units, not least their use of indiscriminate and indeterminate detention and imposed treatment is certainly justifiable. It should not be forgotten, however, that in our prisons, when people are found guilty of a crime and sentenced, *but continue to protest their innocence*, they may not become eligible for early release, thus spending considerably more time in prison. Furthermore, if we have failed to change psychiatric units, how much more is required of us to change the prison system, with its increasing numbers of suicides and self-harming? Relating to the CRPD (Article 14), WNUSP's recommendations actually sound much the same as UK mental health legislation (WNUSP, 2008), for example, detention being proportionate to a person's circumstances, imposed for the shortest time. Police and prison cells bring to my mind Campbell's long campaign against seclusion: 'I have found myself locked up and abandoned in a cell, deprived of human contact, observed but not comforted.' (Campbell, 1993, 10).

Expressed wishes and consent

As mentioned above, the CRPD rests on an insistence that self-determination is paramount and the only issue is how to ensure individuals' wishes are made known and respected (WNUSP and CHRUSP, 2013). But, if people like Campbell and myself fail to express our wishes, what then? Moreover, even if we are engaging, how can we instruct an advocate when we ourselves may be bewildered by what is happening, especially if we have not encountered such an experience before? When, as survivor Alan Baker describes, '(o)ne is thrown into a turbulent river of change without knowing how to swim, one is in a strange and mysterious country without guide book or map, unable to read the signposts...' (Baker, 1991, 32–3).

I have only quite recently discovered that Buddhist practice aims to achieve the kind of transcendental experience I had – a kind of 'knowing' and a sense of being connected to all things – but, in the manner of so-called 'mental disorder', I ended up with a convoluted (but to me logical) interpretation, derived from a Christian upbringing and tales of Pied Pipers.

People with physical conditions may face bewildering situations in unexpected crises, but generally well-established and acceptable information about their situations will be forthcoming. My husband (a disabled activist) had little difficulty in describing what physical assistance he wanted or what changes were necessary in the broader environment and the public, in general, had few problems in understanding what was required (although they might resist provision).

For me, however, when I have been in emotional or mental distress or an 'extra-ordinary state', this is sometimes far from the case. In *hindsight*, I may know what I do *not* want (for example, removal to a psychiatric ward, psychiatric medication or some forms of psychotherapy), but it is much harder to express my immediate needs and not everyone is able to respond as easily to another's emotional needs or apparent 'madness' as to a request for physical assistance. And even if I do express my wishes, say for 'sanctuary', chances are such support is not available anyway. The WNUSP's focus on 'Choice' and 'Informed Consent' in Article 25d of the CRPD also has no meaning unless there are alternative options *readily available* (Plumb, 1999; Spandler and Calton, 2009). Even the WNUSP acknowledges that '(a)lternatives that respect the individual's autonomy and focus on meeting her or his expressed needs do exist, but they are most often marginalized and poorly funded' (WNUSP and CHRUSP, 2013, 5).

Some 30 years after I removed myself from the psychiatric system, I reflected on my struggle to survive. On my need, for example, to find a niche where I could be myself and find some security and direction; to deal with the trauma of the psychiatric system; to make sense of, and cope with, my experiences; to have money to get by and reflect on what had helped me. However, at the time, I was overwhelmed by confusion and indescribable despair (no imminent heaven on earth!) (Plumb, 1999).

Alternative and replacement support

How does my experience translate in terms of governmental or other support? Succinct descriptions of the requirements of people with physical and sensory impairments in order that they should not be discriminated against appear in the CRPD, such as Obligation 4, 'to undertake or promote research and development of universally designed goods, services, equipment and facilities and promote the availability and use of new technologies as well as other forms of assistance, support services and facilities' (UN, 2008, 6).

In addition, sections such as that on education, for example, are extremely detailed. The human rights' requirements of mental health service-users and survivors are, by contrast, only minimally included as in Article 16 of the CRPD mentioned above.

We have not yet pulled together our movement's vast reservoir of collective insight, experience, practical proposals and manifestos – reflecting our long mental health/survivor/mad activist history (possibly larger than the disability movement) – in the way the negotiators dealing primarily with physical and sensory impairment were able to. The WNUSP (2011) for example, have stated that, '(t)he serious adverse effects associated with psychiatric drugs…indicate that existing drugs should be carefully scrutinised for safety and efficiency with accountability to users'.

Yet such an obligation does not appear in the CRPD. Did the mental health negotiators involved in the drafting of the Convention see an opportunity to rid us of detention and forced treatment *before* our movement was at a point where we could detail a comprehensive replacement for current interventions? Since the adoption of the CRPD a lot of time and effort has gone into providing detail about how it should be interpreted and applied (for example, Minkowitz, 2011; WNUSP, 2008; WNUSP/CHRUSP, 2013), but this is in the context of legal capacity and non-intervention. How have sections of the service-user/survivor constituency, people like myself and participants in Katsakou's research, been so side-lined?

Is this an oversight, a lack of input from persons who may have flagged up the complexities of agency and responsibility that go beyond assistance with expressing wishes? Was it pragmatism, an opportunity taken to enable detention and forced treatment to be declared discriminatory if we tailored our agenda to that of the disability movement? Or was it a way to embed libertarian politics, echoing the influential libertarian psychotherapist, Thomas Szasz (Szasz, 1960; Plumb, 2013; Wyatt, 2012), in part because of the shortcomings of public provision, in part the growth of neoliberal politics? Should we welcome neoliberalism with its emphasis on individualism? Campbell, for example, writes of, 'ending up in hospital where my personal experience was denied and denigrated and demeaned' (Campbell, undated).

The WNUSP has highlighted the importance of models '(emphasising) the primacy of first person accounts, honouring thoughts and feelings, meeting practical needs, taking time for resolution or healing, and believing in every person's ability to transform his or her life' (WNUSP, 2011).

Are we, however, being pushed *uncritically* towards individual psychoanalytical/psychotherapeutic support (Wyatt, 2012)? There have been far fewer challenges in the UK to psychoanalysis/therapy, partly because we have been consistently denied these, but are we any better under, say, a psychotherapist like Szasz who has explained that '(modern) psychology is based on psychoanalysis...the psychoanalytic relationship...(being) based on the relationship between priest and penitent in the confessional. The crux of the confessional is *self-accusation on the part of the penitent*' (Wyatt, 2012, my emphasis).

As Szasz reveals, schools of psychoanalysis and therapy are as much institutions as psychiatry. In a free market we would be, to some extent, 'free' to choose but free-market politics also denies the regulation that might keep us from harm when we may be, dare I say, vulnerable? Much 'healing' therapy is inherently suggestive. Some activists point to 'trauma informed therapy' as a way forward but The Sanctuary Model© which aims to produce a Trauma Informed Culture, uses group pressure to 'encourage' members to abide by the sanctuary's norms, as was the case in the therapeutic hospital where I spent some time. This can easily become an oppressive practice.

A therapist with whom I briefly had sessions confided that, in her experience, people who did not pay for sessions did not work hard enough at personal transformation (echoing Szasz in Wyatt, 2012; Plumb, 2013). My retort that some of us have worked very hard for years just to survive, to stay afloat, before it all became too much went unheard. These efforts may be recognised but are presented by some therapists as acquired 'bad habits'. As for me, if I made a personal (and financial) *investment* for regular sessions for two years I could transform myself into *an amazing person*. This was a therapist who was familiar with abuse and discrimination but no mention was made of transforming environments, presumably because this is something I would have to undertake myself.

This issue returns my thoughts to the social model of disability. There is a place for developing resilience, distress tolerance, positivity and agency alongside recognition of events in our lives that have been damaging (for example, neglect, abuse and violence). However, what was radical about Finkelstein's social definition was not that it revealed social relations – these had already been recognised in rehabilitation, both physical and psychological (adjusting to the limitations of impairment), but that he shifted the *cause* of the handicap and thereby also where the *responsibility* lay for whatever problems were encountered (frequently illustrated in the example of a person having to use a wheelchair being confronted by steps). As with rehabilitation, it is notable that a founder of the Clinical Model of mental health had recognised social factors behind mental health (unemployment, pressure of work, deprived environments, 'nagging wife', 'psychopathic' husband) but saw the way forward, not in changing people's circumstances, but in enabling people to *cope*, through medical treatments (Sargant, 1967; Sargent and Slater, 1963). Their notorious treatments, such as insulin coma and leucotomony, have tended to conceal this aspect of the model.

The WNUSP see their 'biggest victory' as '[a] paradigm shift away from a model based on paternalism to one based on respect for our human rights' (WNUSP, 2008, 3). This is a marked challenge to the original Declaration of Human Rights which placed rights in the context of 'welfare' and acting 'in the spirit of brotherhood' [sic]. It is notable that those UPIAS members whose close look at their own situations, socially and politically, led to the social model of disability did not demand the removal of public provision, but argued that it should be transformed[3] (Plumb, 2012a). The disability movement has rightly condemned 'Charity' (Lumb, 1990) but I feel empathy towards service-users/survivors is important. Connecting with us might be a bit like producing a ramp for a wheelchair user. Will Hall has said that suicidal feelings are among humanity's worst forms of suffering and the response we give is a call to our greatest humanness (Hall, 2013). Much of my progress since my initial crisis has been through people who have reached out to me *unasked* (even the person I mistook for the Messiah!), restoring my faith in people, offering me hope and support and easing the burden of personal responsibility.

Conclusion: the politics of the CRPD

An international group of Mental Health System Survivors wrote in a draft policy statement many years ago:

> We are now, and always have been, fully human. We are
> not a different type from the rest of society...Rather we
> have been victimised by the mental health system because
> of our hurts and the hurts of those around. Because of
> trying to get help in the only places we know of, because
> we belong to certain oppressed groups, or refuse to fulfil

some of society's prescribed roles, or protest the wrongs of society...Our bodies and lives...have been damaged and constrained by interacting with the system. (MHSS, 1987)

With the ratification of the CRPD, many service-users/survivors/mad persons will feel that, at last, they have been included. However, it is clear to me that people negotiating on our behalf in the drafting on the convention, lost touch with some of their constituency. Perhaps this is not surprising given the extent of experiences covered under 'mental health'. But in my view, we need more collective dialogues, especially where these seem not to have taken place, and to pull together our considerable insights and experience into clear demands where none of us feel overlooked. This chapter maintains that the premise behind the CRPD that all of us are able at *all times*, given support, to express our wishes is flawed and that a focus on discrimination, while wholly appropriate for people with physical impairments/disabilities, is too limited for mental health service-users/survivors. It is reductionist, unlike the MHSS definition above. In my view, we now need our own Convention of Rights, complementing the CRPD, one that recognises the complexities of the 'psychosocial' experiences that separate us, at times, from others, including disabled people/people with disabilities. Looking more closely at the libertarian underpinning to the CRPD I find myself asking whether this Convention takes service-users/ survivors *out of the frying pan of psychiatry and state provision and into the fire of libertarian ideology* (Plumb, 2013). This is because it side-lines the situations of service-users and survivors, like Campbell and myself and the participants in the Katsakou study mentioned earlier, regarding risk and safety, and dismisses any distinction there may be between 'between the mad and the bad' (Wallcraft, 2002a).

Notes

[1] It is thought that the term 'survivor' was proposed following the earlier emergence of the international Mental Health System Survivors, an off-shoot of the re-evaluation/ co-counselling network.

[2] Robert Browning, 'The Pied Piper of Hamelin', a well-known story to children, like me, of the 1950s that is actually a legend going back centuries.

[3] For example the Derbyshire Coalition of Disabled People worked closely with the county authorities in developing the Statement of Intent (Davis and Mullender, 1993).

FOURTEEN

The global politics of disablement: assuming impairment and erasing complexity

China Mills

Introduction

In this chapter, I want to explore a particular aspect of the Movement for Global Mental Health that is relevant to the concerns of this book: how it situates what it calls 'mental disorders' within a wider global discourse of illness and disability. The Movement for Global Mental Health is an increasingly influential international network of individuals and organisations that, alongside the World Health Organization (WHO), aims 'to scale up the coverage of services for mental disorders in all countries, but especially in low-income and middle-income countries' (Lancet Global Mental Health Group, 2007, 87).[1] While what is meant by services here includes some mention of psychosocial and community interventions, in general, recommendations for first-line treatment in low- and middle-income countries seem to rest – for resource reasons (WHO, 2001b) – on psychiatric medications.

In an attempt to raise awareness of mental health internationally, the Movement for Global Mental Health points out the lack of resources dedicated to mental health in comparison to those for physical illnesses, such as for heart disease. To make this claim, it frames mental distress as 'illness' that is akin to physical illness, and all of these illnesses as disabilities. It calculates the high 'burden' of these different types of disability and then points out that many governments pay insufficient attention to mental health. Following this logic, a call is made for increased global equality both in terms of attention to, and funding of, healthcare for physical illness *and* mental illness, and in terms of access to treatments.

In some ways, this seems like an admirable attempt to raise awareness of the importance of mental health. However, I want to use this chapter to explore how the claim that mental distress is akin to physical illness is problematic in a number of ways. In an attempt to navigate some of these issues, this chapter will first explore the Movement for Global Mental Health's assumption that mental distress is caused by a biochemical imbalance that is chronic and disabling. It will explore how this may be problematic because it goes against much user/survivor advocacy that emphasises distress not 'illness' and calls attention to how experiences of distress are embedded within social contexts.

While the social determinants of mental health and disability are recognised within global disability discourse, the biological foundations of impairment tend to be assumed and prioritised. I will explore the problems this raises for mental distress, where there is little evidence of biochemical impairment. Some of the implications of this focus on biological causes will be explored through thinking about the high rates of suicides by farmers in India and the response to this by the Indian government, which tends to emphasise scaling up access to psychiatric medications. It will be argued that not only does this overlook the deleterious effects of social arrangements; it also enables medications whose efficacy and safety have been critiqued, to be imposed. I will suggest that a central issue in the move to scale up access to potentially harmful drugs is that of competency, an issue which also often divides those who experience distress from wider communities of disabled people.

After tracing some of the implications of understanding something as impairment, the chapter examines the issue of *cause* (of both distress and impairment). It will argue that the distress caused by societal conditions and/or trauma, the impairment caused by psychiatric 'treatment', and impairments caused by conditions of inequality and by persistent poverty are often erased in global disability discourse. Charting these myriad issues, the chapter ends by calling for approaches to both distress and disability that are embedded within social contexts. Attending to global discourse on mental distress is important within disability studies, for while the Movement for Global Mental Health can be critiqued from the perspective of the social model of disability, the social model itself can also be critiqued for similar reasons, particularly by transposing specific models of disability from high-income countries to other parts of the world. These are models that often frame distress as a 'disorder' that is chronic and disabling.

Neuropsychiatric disorders: 'Chronic and very disabling'

The mhGAP Intervention Guide (WHO, 2010, iii) is a set of guidelines specifically developed to aid treatment decisions in non-specialised healthcare settings in low and middle-income countries. Despite this, the guide is largely based on evidence from high income countries. Within the guide, mental, neurological and substance-use disorders are subsumed into one category – 'neuropsychiatric disorders' which includes 'Moderate–Severe Depression, Psychosis, Bipolar Disorder, Epilepsy/Seizures, Developmental Disorders, Behavioural Disorders, Dementia, Alcohol Use and Alcohol Use Disorders, Drug Use and Drug Use Disorders, Self-harm/Suicide, and "Other Significant Emotional or Medically Unexplained Complaints"'.

This move to subsume the above diversity of experiences and diagnostic categories into one category ('neuropsychiatric disorders') is made so that the 'burden' of these 'disorders' can be calculated and compared to other (often physical) disease categories, thus, enabling comparisons in the financing of resources for these conditions. The bringing together of diverse disabilities or impairment categories has also been a key strategic move within the wider disabled people's movement. It is evident, for example, in the cross-disability mobilisations and alliances that created the United Nations Convention on the Rights of Persons with Disabilities (CRPD). However these alliances were in part made to draw attention to a shared experience of social disenfranchisement, and of oppressive and disabling societal barriers, across groupings of impairment. This differs from the World Health Organization's groupings of 'disorders', which conflates experiences, such as depression and suicide, with 'disorders' that have an organic base, such as dementia and epilepsy. The World Health Organization clearly states that 'mental disorders…have a physical basis in the brain…they can affect everyone, everywhere' (WHO, 2001b, x). This implies that 'mental illnesses' have comparable underlying biological components and invokes parallels between access to psychiatric medications and to medication for epilepsy.

Such parallels are especially apparent in the mhGAP launch video, where a Chinese man explains that being diagnosed with epilepsy means that 'Everyone in my village, including my family, now knows I am normal', while a man diagnosed with psychosis in India explains 'they give me medicine. And I'm normal now, thanks to my doctors'.[2] Comparisons to HIV/AIDS are also made, with advocates of Global Mental Health arguing that 'Interventions for depression, delivered in primary care, are as cost effective as antiretroviral drugs for HIV/AIDS' (Patel et al, 2007, 44).

In the 2005 Global Burden of Disease Report the contribution of mental health problems to global disease was measured using the 'disability-adjusted life-year' (DALY): the sum of years lost to early death and years 'lost' due to disability. It was found that about '14% of the global burden of disease has been attributed to neuropsychiatric disorders' due to their 'chronically disabling nature' (Prince et al, 2007, 1). The comparison between disorders, enabled through the DALY, allows the World Health Organization to point out that 'Unfortunately, in most parts of the world, mental health and mental disorders are not accorded anywhere near the same degree of importance as physical health. Rather, they have been largely ignored or neglected' (WHO, 2003, 4). Similarly, the World Health Report 'focuses on a selection of disorders that usually cause severe disability when not treated adequately and which place a heavy burden on communities', and on economies (WHO, 2001b, 22). For example, for Patel (2007, 48), 'schizophrenia is a psychotic disorder of low prevalence, which is often chronic and very disabling'. Similarly, for Üstün et al (cited in WHO, 2001b, 33), 'Schizophrenia causes a high degree of disability...ranked the third most disabling condition, higher than paraplegia and blindness, by the general population'.

This 'official' story of schizophrenia situates the 'burden' of 'mental illness' within an ensemble of mortality/morbidity/disability, where it is the 'illness' that is disabling. Moreover, while burden is partly understood here in economic terms, the potential economic *causes* of mental distress are often overlooked. Yet the language of 'burden' stands in direct contrast to the sustained grassroots arguments by users and survivors (mainly within high-income countries) against psychiatric assumptions of lifelong pathology and deficit, and in favour of multiple, and sometimes more optimistic, conceptualisations of recovery. Users and survivors of psychiatry have historically pushed for a shift away from the language of 'illness' and 'defective mechanisms' and instead mobilise around frameworks of 'trauma/abuse/distress' (Cresswell and Spandler, 2009, 138). This emphasises people's relationship to society and locates the experience of distress within the social; where experiences such as hearing voices are often understood to have developed in response to trauma, rather than within people's 'disordered' brain chemistry (Herman, 1997; see the approach of the Hearing Voices Network, www.hearing-voices.org). This approach implies that disability is not only made possible by societal relations, often marked by unequal power relations, in response to an already present impairment. For oppressive social conditions may also provide the conditions for distress to come into being in the first place – that is, distress in response to trauma.

This poses a problem, or we could see it as an opportunity, in trying to understand distress within a social model of disability framework. However, distress is not the only issue that problematises the social model, for when we begin to think about many experiences of impairment, even when limbs are 'lacking' or mechanisms are 'defective', these often come about due to 'disabling', or we might say 'impairing', societal conditions. This becomes more acutely apparent when we consider the everyday reality of persistent poverty for many people globally, and particularly for people in low-income countries, discussed shortly.

Definitions of impairment and understandings of distress

It is worth noting that, despite being largely a biomedical organisation, not all World Health Organization policy employs a solely medicalised approach to disability. The International Classification of Functioning, Disability and Health (ICF), refutes a clear dichotomy between the social and medical models of disability, promoting a bio–psycho–social model as a way of understanding the dynamic interaction between the personal and the environmental. Using the ICF as its conceptual base, the World Health Organization and World Bank's *World Report on Disability* (2011, 3–4) recognises disability as 'complex, dynamic, multidimensional, and contested', and as an interaction, meaning it 'is not an attribute of the person'. The ICF (WHO, 2001a, 12) defines impairment as 'problems in body function or structure such as a significant deviation or loss': where body *functions* represent physiological functions, including the psychological, and body *structures* represent anatomy. The 'body' here 'includes the brain and its functions, that is, the mind', and thus, the psychological is subsumed under the category of body functions (WHO, 2001a, 12).

If we follow the World Health Organization's (2001b, x) assertion that mental disorder has a 'physical basis in the brain', then we can understand 'mental illness' as an impairment. But what happens when we confront the lack of evidence of impairment in people who are distressed. For example, critical psychiatrists, such as Moncrieff (2009, 10) point out, there is 'no convincing evidence that psychiatric disorders or symptoms are caused by a chemical imbalance'? Through the lens of the bio–psycho–social model, then, where is the 'bio' in much mental distress? Within the ICF (WHO, 2001a, 13) impairments (of both body function and structure) are classified by; (a) loss or lack; (b) reduction; (c) addition or excess; and (d) deviation. Here, then, distress could be understood as an impairment even without an organic or biochemical component, because it could be framed as a deviation in body function – a psychological deviation.

In the ICF understanding, all impairments 'represent a deviation from certain generally accepted population standards in the biomedical status of the body and its functions', the definition of which is undertaken 'by those qualified to judge physical and mental functioning according to these standards' (WHO, 2001a, 12). This makes clear that medical judgements in all areas of medicine (both physical and mental) contain value-judgements, a point that Sedgwick (1982, 17) feels is often missed by critics of psychiatry who at times assume a 'distinction between the natural-scientific, value-free language of physical medicine and the socially and politically loaded language of psychiatry'.

Yet the ICF's definition of impairment also raises questions about who is qualified to make these judgements, what knowledge counts as the 'evidence' base on which such judgements are made, and how do these 'standards' differ in different contexts and in different parts of the world? This raises further issues about what happens when these standards and judgements are transposed from one context to another. This is evident in the sometimes problematic application of the social model of disability in low- and middle-income countries (discussed shortly), and in the assertion that the mhGAP guidelines 'should become the standard approach for all countries and health sectors', meaning that 'irrational and inappropriate interventions should be discouraged and weeded out' (Patel et al, 2011, 1442). Yet while it pays attention to environmental barriers as disabling, the ICF states that the 'biological foundations of impairments have guided the classification' (WHO, 2001a, 12), which is of course problematic in the case of much distress where there is little evidence for any biological foundations.

The issue of 'cause'

While the World Health Organization assumes a biological component to 'mental illness', it readily acknowledges that '[e]pilepsy is not a mental problem', but explains that it is 'included it in the categorisation of neuropsychiatric disorders because it faces the same kind of stigma, ignorance and fear associated with "mental illnesses"' (WHO, 2001b, x). HIV/AIDS is also highly stigmatised, as is poverty (Leavy and Howard, 2013). Does this then imply that HIV/AIDS and poverty should be considered as 'neuropsychiatric disorders' too? While we might understand mental distress as a disability because those who experience it may also experience stigmatising and disabling societal practices – a framework that has helped build many cross-disability alliances within advocacy for the Convention of the Rights of People with Disabilities (CRPD) – what are the implications of categorising impairments based on similar societal reactions, rather than causes?

The inclusion of epilepsy as a neuropsychiatric disorder seems in accordance with the World Health Organization's 'neutral stand with regard to etiology' (cause) within the ICF (WHO, 2001a, 4). Thus the ICF 'does not distinguish between type or cause of disability, or between mental and physical health, taking the approach that 'Impairments are not contingent on etiology or how they are developed', whether genetic or due to injury (WHO, 2011b, 13). This approach seems desirable because it may help to avoid formulating hierarchies of impairment, where, for example, people with genetic impairments are treated differently from those whose impairment arose from injury. Yet, as we have begun to explore, it may be harder and potentially undesirable to remain 'neutral' about the causes of some forms of impairment, for example, injuries due to war or unsafe working conditions, or distress developed in response to living under occupation. Furthermore, a number of researchers (Angermeyer and Matschinger, 2005; Read et al, 2006a) have found that the stigma around distress increases if causes are attributed to brain disease, in comparison to explanations that emphasise psychological or social causes. While the ICF made an important step in explicitly acknowledging the role of environmental barriers with regard to disability, its approach somewhat overlooks the multiple socio-politico-economic causes of impairments. For example, the distribution of risk for AIDS is largely 'localized and non-random', because it is embedded, most often, in unequal social structures, constituting forms of structural violence (Farmer, 2005, 230).

Thus not only might we ask the question of what constitutes impairment within mental distress, we might further wonder what the implications are of understanding something as an impairment, and what interests does such an understanding serve. This is important because, for Sedgwick (1982, 31), medicine is 'not simply an applied biology, but a biology applied in accordance with the dictates of social interests, and thus always value-loaded'. In the case of the Global Mental Health and the World Health Organization's 'within brain' explanations of distress, the interests being served, intentionally or not, may well be those of the pharmaceutical industry that manufactures, markets and supplies the medications prescribed by psychiatrists (Thomas et al, 2005). There is an enormous financial incentive to expand the market for psychiatric medications, with low- and middle-income countries often seen as untapped markets. Because of these vested interests, Shukla et al (2012) argue that the Movement for Global Mental Health should not accept funding from the pharmaceutical industry.

The next section explores an example that illustrates why attending to the social conditions in which distress arises may change our understandings of what constitutes an ethical and appropriate intervention.

Pesticides and suicides

In India there have been over 200,000 farmer suicides since 1997 (Lerner, 2010). Many farmers commit suicide by swallowing pesticides. It is the farmers themselves, in the act of suicide, who call for a political reading of their actions, where '[a]n increasing number of suicide notes today directly address the Prime Minister…taking the form of a public statement accusing the state of betrayal' (The Perspectives Team, 2009, 2).

The research team from Perspectives (2009, 17), call for recognition that suicides 'are not individual acts of desperation but part of a systemic problem located in a much larger socio-economic-political context. It cannot be and should not be reduced to a phenomenon confined to the individual self.' This calls for analysis of farmer suicides to be grounded in an understanding of the 'agrarian crisis' – brought about through the rapid opening of cotton production to the world market, meaning increased precariousness and debt for farmers.

Yet, suggestions for reducing these suicides from within Global Mental Health tend to centre on reducing access to pesticides; improving medical care for pesticide poisoning; improving treatment for depression; and increasing use of anti-depressants (Patel et al, 2007, 50). Furthermore, the Indian government has responded to the suicides by sending out teams of psychiatrists, making anti-depressants more widely available (Sharma, 2004), and has launched a study that looks for genetic factors linked to suicide (Arya, 2007).

Considering farmer suicides in India, thus, directs our attention to the conditions in which what the World Health Organization conceptualises as 'neuropsychiatric disorders', including suicide, are embedded. It may be strategic and productive, at times, for disabled people to overlook the nature, and causes, of impairment, and form alliances across impairment categories to fight oppressive social barriers to their participation. However, identifying the causes of impairment and distress, may be necessary to focus activism on, for example, calls for redistributive justice. It is also important to ensure that any intervention does not reproduce the inequality or violence that may have led to impairment or distress in the first place. Indeed, a criticism often made of involuntary 'treatment' in psychiatry is that it repeats the trauma that may have initially led to distress through denying a person's power to speak about and define the meaning of their experiences (Johnstone, 1997).

Overlooking the causes of impairment, then, may be problematic for both distress and disability as it has implications for the focus of interventions, potentially moving these toward the individual body, instead of the context that the body inhabits. This approach also overlooks an urgent and contentious issue within psychiatry; that some psychiatric medications may cause impairment.

Disabling 'treatments'

Not only is there little evidence that 'mental illness' can be located in biochemicals gone awry, but there is growing debate from both within and outside of mainstream psychiatry about the efficacy and safety of psychiatric drugs. Many of these have been found to be at best little more effective than placebo, and at worst harmful, particularly in the long term (see Gardos and Cole, 1978; Breggin, 2002, 2008; Moncrieff and Cohen, 2006; Moncrieff, 2009; Whitaker, 2010; Angell, 2011; Timimi, 2011). Psychiatric drugs, like any psychoactive substances, alter brain chemistry through intoxication (Moncrieff, 2009), disrupting normal brain function and potentially constituting, for Breggin (2008), the 'brain-disabling' principles of psychiatric medications, confronting us with 'an epidemic of iatrogenic brain damage of large proportions' (Breggin, 1990, 456).

We may well resist descriptions and prescriptions of a fictitious 'normal' person, which assumes that drug interventions will restore people to a 'normal' condition (Lakoff, 2005). But what happens when the 'treatments' issued to restore this fictional normality actually cause people's brains to function in a manner that is 'qualitatively as well as quantitatively different from the normal state' (Hyman and Nestler, 1996, 161), that is, when medications cause impairment? Here, then, the reconfiguration of distress as an 'illness' located within people's so-called chemically imbalanced brain not only denies the potentially personal and social meaningfulness and causes of distress, but also denies the potential psychiatric and iatrogenic causes of impairment. That psychiatric 'treatment' may cause impairment is something which the ICF's (WHO, 2001a) lack of focus on the causes (etiology) of impairment overlooks, and potentially erases, despite this having ethical implications in terms of where to focus interventions.

Research that analyses the potential harm caused by psychiatric medication shifts what is seen as 'disabling' from the 'illness' to the 'treatment'. Yet, despite the potentially harmful effects of many psychotropic drugs, the World Health Report states that,

> Essential psychotropic drugs should be provided and made *constantly available* at all levels of health care. These medicines should be included in every country's *essential* drugs list... These drugs *can* ameliorate symptoms, reduce disability, shorten the course of many disorders, and prevent relapse. They often provide the first-line treatment, *especially in situations* where psychosocial interventions and highly skilled professionals are unavailable. (WHO, 2001b, xii, emphasis added)

While it may be the case that many drugs *can* reduce disability, the evidence referred to above suggests that such drugs, especially if used long-term, may also cause impairment. Furthermore, the 'situations' where professionals and psychosocial interventions may be unavailable are often in low-income countries, and so, because these countries are constructed as resource poor, the use of psychotropic drugs as first-line treatment appears to be 'especially' advocated. Here, drugs that may have brain disabling effects and thus *increase* impairment, are re-framed as 'essential' treatment to *reduce* disability, and included in the World Health Organization's *Model List of Essential Medicines* (2011b, 2011c) for children and adults.

This reconfiguration of potentially harmful interventions into 'essential treatment' seems to be enabled through the category of 'mental illness' and through the image of the 'poor country'. One thing that both these categories share is an assumption that those who experience them, that is, the distressed and the 'poor', are assumed to be, either momentarily or more permanently, incompetent and in need of others to act in their 'best interests'. The issue of competence is also often a point of division between those who experience distress and the disability community more widely. It is thus of central importance, and is worth exploring further here.

Competency and 'best interests'

The recognition that all judgements of 'illness', whether physical or mental, are value-laden, and that impairment is neither a 'presocial nor pre-cultural biological substrate' (Thomas, 1999, 124), is key to navigating the place of distress within disability studies. There has been enormous global activism within and through the UN Convention of the Rights of People with Disabilities (CRPD), with many psychiatric survivor and user organisations in low- and middle-income countries identifying as psychosocially disabled, and forming alliances across impairment categories with disabled people's organisations. In fact, the CRPD is often used as a basis on which to critique and resist the Movement for Global Mental Health's scale-up of psychiatry in low- and middle-income countries, and to speak back to World Health Organization global initiatives. This is evident in the Pan African Network of People with Psychosocial Disabilities' (PANUSP) response to the World Health Organization's 'QualityRights Tool Kit' – a set of tools developed to assess and improve human rights in mental healthcare facilities. PANUSP critiqued the tool kit on the basis that it 'does not adequately reflect the ethos of the CRPD which has embraced the social model of disability' (2012, 2).

Some, however, such as Ann Plumbe (2012a), ask whether something fundamental to the survivor movement has been lost in the framing of distress as disability, particularly in the bending of survivor demands to fit the disability discrimination agenda, underpinned by the social model of disability. The concern here is that the social model's assumption of impairment may potentially let the medical model, and biopsychiatry, in through the 'back door' of global disability advocacy, allowing the assumption of 'unsound mind' within mental distress to slip in alongside it (Spandler, 2012). This remains a key issue in need of interrogation within any global projects based on disability and/or distress, for while we may come to recognise that all impairment is contextually and socially embedded, it is usually only 'mental illness' as well as intellectual disability that carries an assumption that those being 'treated' are irrational and not competent to make decisions about their own treatment.

This could be read as being reflected in the fact while a key element of the CRPD has been the involvement of disabled people, this stands in stark contrast to how priorities are set within the Movement for Global Mental Health. The research priorities underlying the 'Grand Challenges in Mental Health' initiative (Collins et al, 2011) were decided by a group of 'experts' (the Delphi panel) selected and nominated by the US National Institute of Mental Health, through a process that did not involve collaboration with local communities or user/survivors (Shukla et al, 2012).

We could read the assumption of incompetence as being one of the rationales behind this, alongside perhaps the fact that much of the focus of Global Mental Health is within low- and middle-income countries. For like those constructed as 'mentally ill', 'the poor are also assumed to be 'momentarily at least deprived of their capacity to define their own interests', meaning that outside experts diagnose both the problem (lack of income) and prescribe the 'cure' (economic reforms) (Rahnema, 1992, 163). It seems important, then, to explore this use of the language of disability as it differs in the ways it is spoken within a global arena by the World Health Organization, and more locally by Disabled People's Organisations, as they may be using it to outline very different agendas, which at first sight seem to be the same.

In fact, thinking not only about distress but also about impairment in contexts of low and middle-income countries may begin to push further the boundaries of mainstream disability studies. This is because, a) many people in these contexts may not understand themselves to be disabled, or impaired, and, b) impairments may always and already be politicised from being a result of, for example, war or industrial disasters. This has parallels with how the 'symptoms' of much mental distress might be understood to be due to trauma or social inequality.

Global norms of disability and distress

Like the Movement for Global Mental Health's aim to establish a global norm, a single story of mental distress as 'illness', mainstream disability studies has been criticised by some for imposing a particular disability framework within countries where many people do not understand their experience in the language of disability and/or impairment, or contest the very concept of disability (Meekosha and Soldatic, 2011), and where impairment and disability are not easily disentangled (Meekosha, 2011). Grech (2009, 771) argues that the diverse lived experiences of disability in low and middle-income countries, and of indigenous groups within high-income countries, are 'at worst excluded or at best included in piecemeal fashion in the mainstream disability studies literature'. Even when these experiences are included, the literature often overlooks the social production of impairment (see Connell, 2011; Meekosha, 2011). In part this may have come about due to the push for 'positive' representations of disability within high-income countries, to move away from a medicalised language of disability prevention, yet it glosses over and disallows discussion of the social production of impairment in contexts of oppression and poverty (Gorman, 2013).

Mainstream disability studies also tends to overlook how unequal power relations between low- and high-income countries 'produce, sustain and profit out of disability' – how high-income countries may 'disable' low-income countries (Meekosha, 2011, 668) – and how racism systematically disables indigenous peoples, in both high-, middle- and low-income countries globally (Hollinsworth, 2013). This calls for an understanding of impairment in the context of the historical and contemporary violence of colonialism (Connell, 2001). And furthermore to how models of disability, and global norms in relation to mental health, from high-income countries can operate as a colonising discourse as they impinge upon and seek to discredit complex lived realities in low-income countries (Meekosha and Soldatic, 2011; Summerfield, 2008).

Conclusion: the social complexity of all illness

This chapter has tried to mobilise a critique of the Movement for Global Mental Health that goes further than questioning its problematic assumption that distress is a disabling 'illness'. Rather than assuming that mental distress is not an illness, or a disability, because it lacks a physical impairment and because it involves social and political judgements, it is possible to see the sociopolitical complexity within which *all* illness and impairment are embedded. This questions the presumption that physical illness and the medicine that intervenes upon it is somehow objective and value-free. The politicised nature of much impairment seems to become even more apparent not only when we try to think about 'distress and disability' but when we further shift our gaze to the multiple lived realities of impairment within many low- and middle-income countries (and in many areas of high-income countries). Here impairment may be more often associated with poverty, war, malnutrition, environmental degradation, poor quality housing, dangerous work and/or displacement. However, just as the social complexity of mental distress may be overlooked or erased by the global norm of mental illness as located within brains, promoted by the Movement for Global Mental Health, the global complexity of impairment may be erased by dominant mobilisations of the social model of disability from high-income countries.

Thus, attempts to put mental and physical illness 'on exactly the same footing' (Sedgwick, 1982, 29) need not necessarily strategically frame distress as having 'physical' causes within the brain, for, instead, they could attend to the socially constructed nature of all conceptions of health and illness. In this framework mental illness could be seen as an illness like any other, without implying biological determinism, and 'mental illness' could be a critical concept used to draw attention to the unequal organisation of societies. This links to Farmer's (2005, 210) call to resocialise medical ethical dilemmas, for example, around vaccines or HIV/AIDS medications, because 'their full social complexity is our best vaccine against the erasures' of the social and economic rights of the poor and of global inequalities. This is something that – despite the Movement for Global Mental Health Commission on Social Determinants of Health (2008), which sees inequality as a major cause of ill health – is often overlooked.

While the social production of impairment may be somewhat overlooked in mainstream disability studies within high-income countries, in some contexts impairments are recognised as always politicised, for example in those whose impairments are the results of the chemical disaster in Bhopal (Hoskins, 2011), or amputees from the civil war in Sierra Leone (Berghs, 2011). Thus, any form of disability studies needs to be alert to the 'the collective, reflexive process that embroils bodies in social dynamics, and social dynamics in bodies', where 'disability' refers to the ways bodies are entangled in social dynamics; and 'impairment' is the way social dynamics affect bodies (Connell, 2011, 1370–1) –including the power to refuse to recognise responsibility for this disablement.

Highlighting the social complexity of impairment and distress is important because it helps direct us to where interventions might be most useful, for example, in resource distribution or poverty alleviation. Thus, considering the entanglements of poverty and disability, it could be argued that a global redistribution of power and resources may be more effective than increasing access to psychiatric drugs. This is important, and provides a sense of hope, because many transformations in global wellbeing have occurred because of social and structural change, such as sanitation, and not due to expensive medical technologies (Farmer, 2005; Sedgwick, 1982).

In fact many user/survivor groups in low- and middle-income countries explicitly reject the export of psychiatric technologies from high-income countries. Groups such as the Pan African Network of People with Psychosocial Disabilities make this clear when they say that '[t]here can be no mental health without embracing our [people with psychosocial disabilities] expertise. We have always remained the untapped resource in mental health care' (2014, 385). When people who experience distress are seen as central to improving wellbeing for themselves and others, for example, through self-advocacy and peer support, then this shifts assumptions about low-income countries being 'resource poor'.

There is thus a need to question the global relevance of models from high-income countries and to develop frameworks that are 'grounded in and conversant with local contexts' (Grech, 2011, 98). This means that understandings of distress and support systems should be 'home-grown' within local contexts and not solely imported from the global north (Fernando and Weerackody, 2009, 205). Furthermore, in order to generate useful data, mental health work should not employ 'western' templates and 'pre-formed notions of what is "mental health" or "health"; and local definitions from the "bottom up" should be the starting point for research and policy' (Summerfield, 2012, 528).

This has implications for thinking about distress and disability locally and globally, enabling encounters where distress may not be understood as illness or as disabling, and where impairment may not necessarily translate into disability, and may be already understood as socially and politically meaningful.

This calls for a 'disability politics' that is entangled in, and not divided from the 'politics of impairment'. This could enable more alliances between disabled people's groups (Meekosha and Soldatic, 2011). Such a project would grapple with taking global wellbeing seriously and responding ethically, while retaining an understanding of the complexity and politicisation of distress, impairment and disability. Alternatively, perhaps a space could be created where these three categories are no longer relevant and where other ways of knowing take their place in our imaginations.

Notes

[1] See also www.globalmentalhealth.org

[2] WHO Mental Health Gap Action Programme's launch video, 2008, Directed by Iqbal Nandra, www.youtube.com/watch?v=TqlafjsOaoM

FIFTEEN

Disabilities, colonisation and globalisation: how the very possibility of a disability identity was compromised for the 'insane' in India

Bhargavi V Davar

On 1 October 2007, the Government of India ratified the United Nations Convention on the Rights of Persons with Disabilities (CRPD). In doing so, it made a commitment to the people of India and to the international community on its obligation to *respect, protect* and *fulfil* the equal enjoyment of all human rights and fundamental freedoms of all people with disabilities, on an equal basis with others. For large sections of the disabled population in India, the CRPD augurs a brand new future, and is seen as a wonderful opportunity to combat the discrimination that exists within Indian society, provided that new proposed legislation in mental health and disability complies with the CRPD.[1] Unfortunately, colonialism and post colonialism, in India as well as other commonwealth nations, continue to create barriers to people with psychosocial disabilities; preventing them from gaining the full enjoyment of human rights and social inclusion envisioned in the Convention. In this chapter, I will describe the evolution of this situation in India and the Asian region and explore how people with psychosocial disabilities are beginning to adopt a disability identity and framework to argue for their human rights. I argue that mental health laws in India, and their histories through the last 200 years of colonialism and beyond, have prevented people with psychosocial disabilities from identifying or defining themselves as disabled, and therefore, any chance of their being fully included within the new proposed disability legislation.[2]

Their identity has been framed historically within common law, as being 'of unsound mind' or as 'mentally ill', or more recently, as 'persons with high support need'. The 'incapacity' provisions in civil, family and common laws that work in tandem with mental health legislation have exacerbated the situation of facelessness for people with psychosocial disabilities (Davar, 2012). I argue that this situation prevails today, despite the CRPD ratification. The reasons are historical; like other commonwealth countries, India was colonised for a couple of centuries by the British. Notions of 'incapacity' which were embedded in colonial laws continue to frame the status of the psychosocially disabled in India today. The policy environment for persons with psychosocial disabilities in India is complex, involving multiple ministries, over 200 exclusionary legal provisions, archaic legislative provisions and poor political will to reform the mental health sector.[3] At the time of writing this chapter, two pieces of legislation have been brought before the Parliamentary Cabinet for approval: the Rights of Persons with Disabilities Bill and the Mental Health Care Bill of 2013. The former has evolved from a human rights based policy in India, the Persons with Disabilities Act 1995. The latter is a new formulation, but yet another variation on the pre-human rights lunacy acts that have prevailed since colonial times, namely, the Lunatic Asylums Act of 1858, the Lunacy Act of 1912. See Davar (2015 a; b) for an exploration of more recent changes relating to the new proposed Mental Health Care Bill of 2013.

This chapter argues that the question of personal identity is befuddled due to this complexity wrought by the changing ways in which personal status has been determined throughout history and different, even incompatible, disability laws. This situation is compounded by the impact of the Global Mental Health Movement's vision for 'modernity', which is imposing psychiatric treatment on the populations of low- and middle-income countries (Prince et al, 2007; Patel et al, 2011), developments that are critically discussed elsewhere in this book (China Mills, Chapter 14).

Shifting discourses around madness

Identity questions are complex for people with psychosocial disabilities in India because of epistemic shifts in the discourse surrounding 'mental illness' or 'madness' over time. Concepts of madness have changed at least three times in India between the 1850s and now. The 'lunatic' of the Lunatic Asylums Act 1858 became the person of 'unsound mind' of the Indian Lunacy Act 1912 and this was replaced by the 'mentally ill person' of the post-colonial Mental Health Act and is now poised to become the 'person of high support need' in the proposed new Mental Health Care Bill 2013. These changing definitions of people with psychosocial disabilities are *legal* definitions and continue to have a huge impact on the lives and experiences of people diagnosed with a 'mental illness'. Ironically, however, despite these shifts in terminology in line with 'modernisation', persons with psychosocial disabilities in India continue to be non-persons in law. While the letter of the laws may have changed, their spirit remains the same.

People with psychosocial disabilities do not ask, "How should I describe my disabled identity?" Rather, their question is, "Do I even have an identity?" Their question is not, "What development benefits[4] can I receive?" Rather, it is, "Have I a right to enter the Development arena, being a non-person?" (WNUSP and Bapu Trust, 2013). They share this lack of personhood along with people in other Commonwealth nations which were British colonies, and struggle with both frameworks of incapacity laws and colonial penal mental health laws. Their entry into the arena of disability policy and legislation is compromised due to this state of affairs. Since they remain non-persons in law, they are excluded from social entitlements and more generally, from inclusion in the Development enterprise, that could bring them within the scope of socio-economic progress. There is a hope that with the new 'paradigm shift' enshrined in the United Nations Convention on the Rights of Persons with Disabilities, there will be new opportunities for identity development and inclusion within socio-economic process. The proposed new Rights of Persons with Disabilities Bill 2013 holds out promise in that direction. The Mental Health Care Bill 2013, by contrast, continues to be an 'incapacity' law, which denies human rights and provides for involuntary civil commitment for persons with 'mental illness'.

The impact of colonialism on mental health law

Indian mental health policies and laws are founded on colonial principles of control by segregation (Ernst, 1991; J Mills, 2000; 2004; Fernando, 2014; C Mills, 2014). Despite this, there is an assumption among mental health professionals that 'modern nations' have always had (or should have) mental health law with elements of civil commitment and deprivation of liberty (see, for example, Patel, 2013; Pathare and Sagade, 2013). Jacob et al (2007), taking a south Asian perspective, write that many low- and middle-income countries lack mental health legislation to direct their mental health programmes and services, and have expressed special concern in the case of Africa and South East Asia.

In the last decade, the World Health Organization (WHO) mapped countries of the world on the basis of whether or not they had a mental health law. It was reported that 'many countries fail to put them in place: 40% of countries have no mental health policy and 64% of countries do not have any mental health legislation or have legislation that is more than 10 years old' (WHO, 2005, 1). The WHO put out a document to help support countries to 'develop mental health and human rights oriented mental health legislation'.[5] In their more recent Draft Comprehensive Mental Health Action Plan of 2013,[6] the WHO's Mental Health and Substance Abuse department developed the target that '50% of countries will have developed or updated their laws for mental health in line with international and regional human rights instruments (by the year 2020)'.

Guided by the World Health Organisation activities in the South East Asian region, Indian governmental service providers see mental health law, involuntary treatment and institutionalisation as legitimate ways to provide care and treatment to the 'mentally ill', especially those found on the streets and homeless. Mari and Thornicroft (2010) propose a 'balanced care' model, arguing that institutions should not be shut down and must play an important role in providing 'acute psychiatric' beds for emergency situations, requiring the intervention of civil law and civil commitment procedures. Civic resistance by users and survivors of psychiatry to the new version of a coercive mental health law (Mental Health Care Bill, 2013) in India is seen as a regressive step, setting up a barrier to providing much needed care and treatment (Gopikumar and Parsuraman, 2013; Patel, 2013).

In the last decade, many Indian psychiatrists have felt the need to reclaim the 'scientific' history of Indian psychiatry. For example, they have often been enthusiastic about the coming of the 'golden age' and the modernisation of psychiatry (Kumar and Kumar, 2008; Nizamie and Goyal, 2010). Somasundaram (2008), in his 'memoirs' about the Kilpauk Mental Hospital in Chennai, has spoken in exalted terms about a new wave of 'modernising' care for the 'mentally ill' with the discovery of psycho-pharmaceuticals in the 1950s. These histories have ignored the complex insertion of colonial ideologies, and the exclusivity of asylum based care and treatment, in reshaping contemporary mental health practice. I have argued elsewhere that certain elements from colonialism including the lunacy law, the asylum architecture and segregation practices which are still in place have become so inextricably mixed into the project of providing mental health services, such that the Indian imagination cannot separate care giving from asylum practice (Davar, 2015a).

The claim that modern nations have always had, or should have, mental health laws, is in itself worthy of examination. In most low- and middle-income countries of Asia, Africa and South America, at present, there are no mental health laws or, for that matter, institutions. The countries colonised by the British, between the 1850s and 1940s, do have mental health laws based on old colonial British law (this includes Commonwealth countries like Burma, Sri Lanka, Brunei, Borneo, Singapore and Malaysia). This situation pertains too in erstwhile British colonies (such as those in Africa) and French colonies (such as Korea). The situation is different, however, for countries that were never colonised (such as Nepal and Thailand) and for those that were colonised or occupied by other nations. There is no large legacy of mental health and incapacity law, nor of institutions, in the Philippines (colonised by Spain); nor in those countries colonised by the Dutch and Portuguese, nor yet in those occupied, but not colonised, by Japan in the post-war period. China, occupied by the French and later Japan, and with its history of communism, has a different political context. Though it didn't have a mental health law until recently (Phillips, 2013), it does have closed door institutions for a variety of their citizens including those deemed to be 'mentally ill'.

The impact of colonisation helps to explain the variety of institutions and legislation in different countries. Thus, the question of whether a country has a mental health law should be placed in a historical context and not assumed; it is not a 'scientific' claim about psychiatric care and treatment, nor 'progress'. Rather the 'modernisation' of 'mental healthcare' which can be traced back to the 1850s (and later in some places) along with mental health laws and asylums were introduced by colonising nations, particularly Great Britain.[7]

Mental health law: incapacity and civil death

In the old British colonies, mental health law existed in tandem with 'incapacity' provisions within all common law (family, civil, criminal). Effectively, the British developed a normative framework for the legal disenfranchisement of a variety of people, including the 'idiots', 'insane', 'paupers', 'nomads', 'lepers' and 'criminal tribes'. These constituencies were 'non-persons'; they had no legal rights within society and special institutions were created for them. They were brought within penal laws (for example, the vagrancy laws, laws to punish and incarcerate the 'criminal tribes' and the 'nomads'), leprosy legislation; and laws for the penal incarceration of the 'insane' and the 'idiots' (Kannabiran and Singh, 2008). Even though no special institutions were created for women, and those who renounced material lives in favour of a spiritual life (the *sanyasis*), these people were also considered as 'civil dead' or as 'non-persons'.

The courts evolved criteria for declaring the insane as 'civil dead' even though not physically dead. These provisions continue well into the post-independence period, even today. No legal rights accrue to the 'insane' and the courts can treat them as legally 'dead'. At the last count, there are over 150 legal provisions found in a variety of laws which can be mobilised to deny their legal personhood and capacity (Davar, 2012). Many groups of people with disabilities are also included within the regime of 'incapacity' with respect to some provisions and some aspects of life (including the 'deaf mute', 'leprosy cured', 'deaf', 'physically and mentally infirm', 'handicapped').

Only the 'insane' are completely excluded from having *any* legal rights. Another group of 'non-persons', the vagrants, continue to be criminalised through civil commitment laws, but they are not declared civil dead. The 'lepers' and the 'idiots' got relief from penal laws and from civil death: in 1988 the Indian Leprosy Act was repealed and people with intellectual, cognitive and developmental disabilities were released from the penal laws when the National Trust Act was created. An overarching disability law, the Persons with Disabilities Act 1995, was also created at this time. Unlike the mental health laws, these protected the rights of persons with disabilities and were inspired by the United Nations Human Rights agendas.

So, contrary to the stated views of policy makers, contemporary mental health law, and the institutions created under it, are not 'modern'. The disability laws (National Trust Act and Persons with Disabilities Act) were created in the post-independence and in the human rights era, and unlike mental health laws, embody positive rights. The 'disabled' person in disability legislation has a more positive presence than the person in mental health law. In a similar way, I have described how the 'patient' of the mental health system got legally determined through the colonial period in a very different way than did the general healthcare patient (Davar, 2015b).

What are the implications of being a 'non-person' before law in the context of contemporary mental healthcare, where service delivery is driven by a mental health law? Such a person can be admitted against their will into a mental asylum regulated by the Mental Health Act 1987 and they will not have any of their legal rights as a 'patient' of the healthcare system recognised. As I have argued elsewhere, the judicial procedures adopted by the colonialists, through the Indian Lunacy Act 1912, to protect personal liberty are greatly diluted, or even caricatured, in the Mental Health Law 1987 (see, Dhanda, 2000 for a comparative analysis). Further, following a great human rights violation that happened in an institution in 2001, designated the 'Erwady tragedy', the Indian Supreme Court has directed the construction of *more* mental asylums in each and every state of India (Krishnakumar, 2001; Murthy, 2001; Davar and Lohokare, 2008).

The Mental Health Act 1987 allows coercive psychiatry, that is, admission by use of force. The courts do not use due diligence in arbitrating any forcible admission or forcible extension of stay, because those admitted on grounds of 'insanity' are legal non-persons and are not recognised to have any legal rights to representation. Upon reading 20 judicial orders for admission and extension of the last five years, I found the orders were just repeated word for word, with only the case number changing, which suggested that a judicial inquiry had not been conducted. The person who was being institutionalised was referred to as 'Non-applicant' in the papers; and the State was the 'applicant'. The case of persons with mental illness is the only one in the country where decision on the legal deprivation of personal liberty is conducted by the court without legal representation for the person whose rights are deprived. The recent proposal for a new Mental Health Care Bill 2013 does not alter this situation; in fact it builds law on a premise of incapacity. Even the minimal safeguards and justice procedures found in the 1987 Mental Health Act are to be dismantled, and a constitutional right to liberty is proposed to be treated as merely an administrative procedure of admission by doctors.

Due to the above situation, not many people with a psychosocial disability disclose their identity or status in India (Davar, 2015b). It is also often difficult for people in many Asian countries to have associations of our constituency, due to these social, legal and other barriers. Struggles to access justice and their own legitimate space in society are barely recorded (Minkowitz and Dhanda, 2006).

Identity struggles in India

In India, in the period leading up to the advocacy around the CRPD, activists like myself were influenced by historical critiques of psychiatry, but it took a while for us to make sense of being a 'person with a disability'. Throughout the 1980s and the 1990s we were influenced by the 'mad liberation movements' of the west and the anti-psychiatry critiques. I was among a group of women in the country who self-identified as 'mad' who started to mobilise around our rights. We were inspired by many of the earliest leaders of the mental patients' liberation movement and some of us travelled, despite severe economic hardships, to visit and learn from the second generation leaders of the movement, such as David Oaks, Mary O'Hagan, Sylvia Caras, Iris Hoelling, Chris Hansen, Ron Unger, Judi Chamberlin, Peter Lehmann and others. I recall that at this time, we defined alliances around the question, "Are you 'a mad woman' too?" The question of identity and representation was so important (Davar, 2008a; 2008b).

We did not 'know' that we were 'users and survivors' nor did we ever imagine that we were 'disabled' people. That latter term was repugnant for us, as it signified impairment and deficits. These were all concepts that emerged much later in the late 1990s and, more forcefully, with the entry of the CRPD. I was the only Asian to attend the General Assembly of the World Network of Users and Survivors of Psychiatry (WNUSP) at Vejle, Denmark in 2004. But before my entry into the Board of the WNUSP, the then Board members asked me if I was a 'user' or a 'survivor', which would have qualified me for the post; and I could not answer that question with a simple 'yes' or 'no'. But, coming back home, we collected oral histories of women who went 'mad' (Bapu Trust, 2010). Through *Aaina,* a mental health advocacy newsletter, we started to publish people's stories and policy critiques. By the time the CRPD started getting articulated as a formative discourse in human rights in 2006, I had identified myself as, not a person with a psychosocial disability, but as a 'survivor' of psychiatry. Several peers were articulating this question for themselves and arriving at a variety of responses. These identity choices are described in more detail in a forthcoming book (Davar and Ravindran, 2015).

It was with this identity as a 'survivor of psychiatry' that I went on to create a national platform for CRPD advocacy. From 2005 onwards, users and survivors of psychiatry in India led efforts to bring all stakeholders together on a common platform, called the *National Alliance on Access to Justice for Persons living with a Mental Illness* (NAAJMI). NAAJMI was active from 2005 until 2012, with the specific purpose of advocating around the CRPD, particularly on the right to liberty, life in the community and recognition of our full legal capacity. Several regional consultations were held, and finally a national one in New Delhi, consolidating a list of human rights for our constituency. This is described in full in NAAJMI (2009). Collaboration with Gabor Gombos, survivor and, later, an CRPD committee member, enabled us to fine-tune our dilemmas on articulating and negotiating different identity possibilities; and we learnt a new identity category, 'self-advocate' (described in Gombos and Dhanda, 2009). The participants in all these local and national dialogues discussed whether we should be called 'mentally ill' or 'persons with psychosocial disabilities' or 'users and survivors' of psychiatry. Doctors who were present in these dialogues were against a social paradigm and argued that there was no 'disability' element in 'mental illness' because it was a medical/health issue. They also argued that such identity questions were western concepts, as was the whole notion of human rights.

As described in Gombos and Dhanda (2009) the confrontational approach of the Indian Psychiatric Society to human rights concepts was highly disturbing. It was finally decided by the NAAJMI leaders that, like persons living with HIV/Aids, we could name ourselves as 'persons living with a mental illness'. At the time, we could not relate to 'psychosocial disability' as there was no experiential content to this concept. NAAJMI came to an end in 2012, following serious differences of core beliefs among the leaders who began the movement, including myself, on the questions of identity and personhood. Some believed strongly in the legal regime of coercive psychiatry, but with 'humane safeguards'; while others, like myself, believed that the CRPD entailed the repeal of the mental health law and argued for the inclusion of all our human rights within universal disability law.

An important learning from the NAAJMI consultations was that the CRPD can lend support to arguments for the human rights of persons with psychosocial disabilities. The groups which met and deliberated wanted the inclusion of such rights as to 'self and personhood', to 'be listened to' and to 'spirituality'. These had more personal and subjective dimensions than the largely socio-economic rights spelt out by people with physical disabilities. Rights to personal liberty also fetched a higher 'talk time' in the consultations than socio-economic rights (NAAJMI and Bapu Trust, 2010).

Psycho-social disability alliances in the Asian region

In May of 2013 an important event was organised by the Bapu Trust. A consultation called the *Vision and Strategy for Transforming Communities for Inclusion of people with psychosocial disabilities*[8] brought together a group of 27 disabled activists, mostly people with psychosocial disabilities from the Asian region. It included people from Nepal, Philippines, China, Bangladesh and India.[9] The aims were to explore the possibility of a common framework for policy advocacy in the Asian region; discuss questions of identity (whether persons with mental health problems are persons with a psychosocial disability); and to plan for community mental health services. Attendees were invested in the implementation of Article 19 of the CRPD, which provides for the right to independent living and be fully included in the community. Finally, the conference aimed to foster links with cross-cutting disability and development discourses across the region.

During the event it became apparent that many Asian countries have, at the most, a single institution in their capital city for the whole country, which was considered a good thing; no mental health law, about which there was some ambivalence; and meagre community-based mental health services, which was considered a bad thing. In the Philippines, civil commitment into the single mental asylum that exists is governed by a recently created Code and a few incapacity laws are found in a general civil Code. Nepal's sole institution is an open door hospital, which does not look like an asylum, and no 'asylum' law exists. Likewise, Indonesia has no mental health law and only one 'asylum' in Manila. In some countries, especially Indonesia, serious violations of human rights were happening within families and neighbourhoods. In several countries, for example Bangladesh, Nepal and the Philippines, a skeletal/draft mental health law has been waiting for further process by the government.

The Indian situation was quite different from many other Asian countries. At the time of Independence (1947), there was only a rudimentary infrastructure, mostly for institutionalising the 'insane', including around 35 or so mental asylums left behind by the British. In contemporary India, by contrast, there are over 600 mental asylums, both public and private, run on penal principles and over 200 incapacity provisions: modelled upon colonial legal and architectural designs.

Disability identity and the CRPD

The question of identity, which seemed closed off by extant laws, has been opened up for us in India through discussions around the CRPD. Most Asian countries have ratified this convention since its adoption in 2007. Following this development, disabled people's organisations in the Asian region are mobilising to advocate for an inclusive disability policy within their respective countries. Inclusion of 'marginalised' groups, especially 'persons with psychosocial disabilities', is increasingly on the agenda in such mobilisations of cross-disability organisations.

In the Asia event described above, people with psycho-social disabilities, along with some key cross-disability leaders who participated, intensively debated the question of the 'disabled' identity versus the 'mentally ill' identity. Parallel brainstorming sessions were held on how we 'are' for ourselves, and how we 'are' for others (that is, people in the cross-disability mmovement).[10] In this meeting, against the background of the CRPD, we agreed that we were in a situation of 'identity crisis'. We agreed that 'mentally ill patient' is a term linked to a medical diagnosis, applied to us when there is no support and self-coping fails; and in some cases, refers to someone who is incapacitated by society and law. 'User and survivor' identity also, it was felt, came with baggage of western history and framed us within the medical context. In addition, in many regions of Asia, there were no services, so there was no question of 'using' or 'surviving' a service. On the other hand, people from India and China, with strong experiences of oppression within the medical system, identified as a 'user and survivor' and not as a person with a disability. I and others felt that the term 'disability' emphasises societal discrimination and also chances of recovery of personal identity.

The question remains of how to reconcile these differences, and whether there is a need to reconcile them. While, in the west, there has been a struggle to shift from a 'mentally ill person' to that of a 'disabled' person, in many low- and middle-income countries, though not all, a user survivor identity was largely absent, and being 'psychosocially disabled' is a newly forming identity, inspired by the human rights vision of the UNCRPD. This debate intensified during the drafting of the UNCRPD and later, and many of us campaigned hard to be included in the wider disabled people's movement. Yet, when we came face to face with cross-disability networks, our identities become even more complex and challenging. In recent times, we have elicited an identity as 'the most marginalised', 'people with high support needs', and so on, within the cross-disability movement. However, many people in the room identified, not as a 'person with high support need', but rather as a 'person with psychosocial disability'.

Conclusion

I have argued that mental health legislation continues to reflect colonial practices of segregation and seclusion and is in conflict with the CRPD and emerging disability rights discourse. While new proposed legislation – the Disability Rights Bill and the Mental Health Care Bill – does recognise the constituency of persons with psychosocial disabilities, they are still handed over to the Ministry of Health and Family Welfare which regulates the asylums. This effectively cancels out most of our rights. It is a curiosity that the Law Department, whose job it is to reconcile conflicting laws, did not identify contradictions between these two legislations.

In the realisation of the CRPD, people with psychosocial disabilities in the Asian region have an opportunity to extricate themselves from the traditional framework of 'incapacity'. The concept of 'psycho-social disability' (especially as it is articulated in the Convention) comes with the promise of human rights and empowerment, rather than deprivation of liberty. It normalises human experiences, within a range of problems faced by human beings in general, at times of vulnerability. Life is not limited to medical pathology and there is no 'civil death'. Arguably the disability concept brings people with psycho-socially disabling experiences within the spectrum of human diversity, thus potentially minimising our exclusion.

Although the policy situation in India and other countries in the Asian region is extremely complex and contested, persons with psychosocial disabilities have imbibed the 'spirit' of the CRPD. We are coming together, mobilising and forming associations and self-advocacy organisations based on an emerging disability identity.

Notes

[1] indiatogether.org/uncrpd-health

[2] Writing this paper was enabled by a book writing grant received by me from the Karl Jaspers Center for Excellence, Department of Anthropology, University of Heidelberg, in the year 2010; my grateful appreciation for the continuing patience, support and mentorship provided by Prof William Sax.

[3] In fulfilling those obligations persons with psycho-social disabilities and DPOs in India are having to advocate with at least two separate ministries with key roles (the Ministry of Health and Family Welfare; and the Ministry of Social Justice and Empowerment); several 'physical and mental incapacity' laws; three human rights orientated disability laws and disability authorities at the national level (National Trust Act, 1999; Persons with Disabilities Act, 1995; Rehabilitation Council of India Act); one colonial/neocolonial mental health law (Mental Health Act, 1987); a handful of health and disability policies among other general social policies; drafts of various new proposed laws in the context of the UNCRPD, relating to full enjoyment of all freedoms and human rights of people with disabilities (The Rights of Persons with Disabilities Bill; Mental Health Care Bill); and several budgets, plans and programmes documents.

[4] There are no disability support payments in India. However, there are a number of schemes and programs on education, livelihoods, healthcare, social security, food, housing and other where persons with disabilities could be included. These are broadly referred to as 'developments'.

[5] www.who.int/mental_health/policy/legislation/2_HRBasedMHLaws_Infosheet.pdf?ua=1.

[6] Draft Comprehensive Mental Health Action Plan of 2013, World Health Organization, Executive Board, 132nd Session, Provisional agenda Item 6.3, EB 132/8, January 2013, apps.who.int/gb/ebwha/pdf_files/EB132/B132_8-en.pdf?ua=1.

[7] It is of course a historical curiosity that such asylums, which admitted patients by the deprivation of personal liberty, were built in precisely those times when 'liberty' became a core part of western political theory and emerging Constitutions, aka John Stuart Mill and his phenomenally influential treatise, *On Liberty*.

[8] May (2013) *Transforming Communities for Inclusion: A Trans-Asia Initiative Transforming Communities for Inclusion of persons with psychosocial disabilities: A Trans-Asia initiative*, 30 April-4 May, Conference held in Pune, organised by the Bapu Trust for Research on Mind and Discourse, at Hotel Holiday Inn, Pune, India, http://camhjournal.com/advocacy/transforming-communities-for-inclusion-a-trans-asia-initiative/.

[9] Report on *Transforming Communities for Inclusion: A Trans-Asia Initiative Transforming Communities for Inclusion of persons with psychosocial disabilities: A Trans-Asia initiative*, 30 April–4 May 2013, Holiday Inn, Pune. Supported by the Open Society Foundation, New York and organised by the Bapu Trust for Research on Mind and Discourse, Pune, http://camhjournal.com/advocacy/report-transforming-communities-for-inclusion-of-persons-with-psycho-social-disabilities/.

[10] See note 9.

Part Five
Meeting places

Neurodiversity: bridging the gap between the disabled people's movement and the mental health system survivors' movement?

Steve Graby

Introduction

This chapter traces the origins and evolution of the neurodiversity movement, which consists of people with conditions (such as autistic spectrum 'disorders', AD(H)D, dyspraxia, or dyslexia) which have been positioned somewhere between the traditional categories of 'disability' and 'mental illness'. The neurodiversity movement has roots in, and, as will be argued, has new insights to offer to, both the disabled people's and survivor movements.[1] Therefore, it should be of interest to those seeking to bridge conceptual gaps between the disabled people's and survivor movements – such as the sticking point between them over the concept of 'impairment' (Plumb, 1994).

Writers and activists within the neurodiversity movement are acutely aware of, and concerned with, the social construction of both 'distress' and 'disability', and have developed their own distinct analysis of these concepts. This chapter gives an overview of some of that thinking. It draws on my own experience within the neurodiversity movement, as well as on published literature from all three movements, to illustrate the convergences and divergences between them, and finally offers some suggestions for ways forward.

Disabled people and mental health system survivors: two movements

The relationship between the disabled people's movement and the survivor movement is complex. In its early stages, the modern disabled people's movement was overwhelmingly focused on physical impairment. This is reflected in the names of seminal groups such as the Union of the Physically Impaired Against Segregation (UPIAS), in whose founding policy statement 'people who are called...mentally ill' were classed among 'other oppressed groups' with which it was felt that the physically impaired ought to ally, while retaining a separate identity (UPIAS, 1974). The movement's 'big idea' was the social model of disability (Hasler, 1993). As a broader understanding of this was developed, however, survivors increasingly became considered part of the movement and of the category 'disabled people'. Included within this group were other 'non-physically' impaired groups such as d/Deaf people and people with learning difficulties, which groups have also notably remained somewhat separate in their self-organisation from the 'broader' disabled people's movement.

Reactions to this from the survivor movement have been mixed. Some survivor activists have welcomed the social model because of its attribution of disability to social exclusion and oppression, rather than to something inherent in individuals. For many, however, the concept of impairment as distinct from disability has been a major stumbling block, with some survivor activists arguing that to categorise mental distress as an impairment is to return to the medical and pathological models of 'mental illness' from which their movement seeks to escape (Plumb, 1994; Wilson and Beresford, 2002). Other survivor activists, such as McNamara (1996), regard the 'impairment debate' as divisive and detrimental to the movement, arguing that survivors are 'disabled' by the stigma and material oppression they experience, whether or not they are regarded as having an impairment. This does, however, raise the question of the limits of the term 'disability': as Plumb (1994) points out, if disability is defined solely as oppression and impairment is not regarded as a prerequisite for it, many other groups could be considered 'disabled' who would not ordinarily be defined as such.[2]

Neurodiversity: a new perspective on the debate

A more recent development potentially provides a new and significant intervention into this debate: the neurodiversity movement. This movement encompasses people with a variety of diagnostic labels (such as autistic spectrum conditions, dyslexia, dyspraxia and AD(H)D), and arguably has roots in both the disabled people's and survivor movements. The neurodiversity movement grew primarily out of self-advocacy by autistic people, which began to emerge in the 1990s in response to the growth of a parent-dominated 'autism advocacy' lobby. In response to the latter's search for a 'cure' for autism, neurodiversity activists argued that it and similar conditions should be seen not as pathologies needing a 'cure' but as natural differences which should be accepted and accommodated.

Significantly, the diagnostic categories generally put under the umbrella of 'neurodiversity' fall somewhat between the broader categories of 'mental illness' and 'disability/impairment'. Like the former, they are included in the Diagnostic and Statistical Manual of Mental Disorders (DSM) and primarily diagnosed by psychologists and/or psychiatrists. However, they are also linked to the latter; first due to their overlap with categories of 'learning difficulty'/'learning disability', and second due to being typically defined as congenital and permanent. This contrasts with most categories of 'mental illness' which are typically regarded as first occurring in adolescence or adulthood, often caused by traumatic life events, and episodic and/or 'curable'.

The term 'neurodiversity' started to be used around the late 1990s, primarily by the emerging generation of autistic adults writing first-person accounts of their experience. It possibly had more than one independent origin at around the same time (Meyerding, 2002). One often-cited 'first published usage' is Judy Singer's chapter in the 1999 book *Disability Discourse*, edited by Marian Corker and Sally French. Drafts of this chapter were circulated among online autistic spectrum groups before its publication, leading to online usages of the word pre-dating the book and generating other usages which may be traced back to Singer (1999), despite earlier publication dates (Savarese and Savarese, 2010). Moreover, neurodiversity perspectives were articulated by autistic activists, such as Jim Sinclair, Larry Arnold and Martijn Dekker, before the word itself was used. Sinclair's 1993[3] article 'Don't mourn for us', for example, despite not using the term 'neurodiversity', is often regarded as one of the founding documents of the neurodiversity movement (Boundy, 2008; Sinclair, 2012a).

While people with diagnoses on the autistic spectrum were certainly the main originators of the term and the concept – and the neurodiversity movement continues to be centrally focused on autism, with many regarding it as synonymous with the 'autistic rights movement' – other conditions such as AD(H)D, dyslexia, dyspraxia, and in some cases the broader field of 'developmental disabilities' or 'learning difficulties' were acknowledged as being part of neurodiversity from the start. The representation of people with such diagnoses in the neurodiversity movement has increased in more recent years.

In addition, some people are beginning to identify with the concept of neurodiversity who have been classified by psychiatry in categories more commonly associated with 'mental health' than with 'disability' (such as 'schizophrenia' and 'bipolar disorder'). For example, Suzanne Antonetta, who was diagnosed with 'bipolar disorder', gave her 2005 book *A Mind Apart* – which describes her experience, and that of autistic author, Dawn Prince-Hughes, as well as those of friends with diagnoses such as 'dissociative identity disorder' (formerly known as 'multiple personality disorder') – the subtitle 'Travels in a Neurodiverse World'. An online community of self-defined 'multiples' also exists, who see their separate 'personalities' not as a dissociative pathology but as different 'people' sharing a brain and body, each of whom has a right to exist. This has links to, and overlaps with, the autistic and broader neurodiverse communities (Baggs, 2006).

A core principle of neurodiversity is that conditions such as autism, AD(H)D, and so on, are 'real' and neurological in nature. This contrasts with the view held by many in the 'anti-psychiatry' and 'critical psychiatry' communities that AD(H)D is a category constructed by pharmaceutical companies to pathologise behaviour in children who may previously simply have been seen as 'naughty', in order to promote the sale of drugs such as Ritalin (see, for example, Timimi, 2002). Similarly, the neurodiversity movement opposes the beliefs, held by many 'autism parents' and 'alternative' medical practitioners, that autism is an 'epidemic' caused by any number of factors such as diet, environmental pollutants or, most notoriously, vaccinations such as that against measles, mumps and rubella (Waltz, 2013).

These conditions are seen as constituting a variety of minority 'neurotypes' of equal validity to the majority (so-called 'normal') human neurotype, which should be neither pathologised nor 'cured'. In fact, if minority neurotypes are not 'illnesses', by definition no 'cure' for them can exist. Therefore, some of the movement's most visible activism has been in opposing charities such as Autism Speaks whose objectives are to 'cure' or eliminate autism. Alongside public bodies such as the New York University Child Study Center, these charities' advertising campaigns portray autism (and, in the latter case, other psychiatric diagnoses) as a monstrous, villainous entity, requiring a metaphorical 'war' to 'defeat' it (Kras, 2010; Gross, 2012; Sequenzia, 2012). This parallels the portrayals of disabled people by, and the disabled people's movement's activism against, charities such as Leonard Cheshire in the UK and the Muscular Dystrophy Association's Telethon in the US (Johnson, 1994; Clark, 2003; Withers, 2012).

Neurodiversity activists thus seek social acceptance and equal opportunity for all individuals regardless of their neurology (Ventura33, 2005), believing that neurological diversity should be celebrated and appreciated, and there is no one type of neurology which is 'the best and the only way' (AS-IF, 2007). People who experience difficulties in society due to their cognitive or behavioural differences from the norm therefore need to be recognised and accommodated, with an emphasis on the need to change society rather than the individual.[4] Boundy (2008, unpaged) regards 'the desire to be freed from forced behavioural conformity' as the 'most central concern of the neurodiversity movement and community'. The neurodiversity movement, like the disabled people's movement (Oliver, 1994), is thus strongly critical of 'normalisation' paradigms, and prioritises 'subjective well-being' (as defined by the individual) over functioning in normative ways (Kapp et al, 2013).

Neurodiversity is often described as comparable to ethnic diversity and to the diversity of sexual and gender identities (Antonetta, 2005; AS-IF, 2007). As neurodiversity activist Nick Walker (2012, 156) writes, 'there is no "normal" state of human brain or human mind, any more than there is one "normal" race, ethnicity, gender or culture'. Thus the term 'neurotypical' was coined by neurodiversity activists to refer to the majority neurotype without reinforcing its privileged status and the marginalisation of others (Singer, 1999; Walker, 2012).[5] While a group or a society can be 'neurodiverse', it is generally considered inaccurate to call an individual person 'neurodiverse', as neurodiversity encompasses both the typical and the atypical; however, 'neurodivergent' can be used as a generic adjective to refer to people of minority neurotypes.

It has been argued that the neurodiversity movement was influenced by, and rooted in, the disabled people's movement and, in terms of its identity-construction, particularly the Deaf identity movement (see for example, Dekker, 2004). Others have also argued that it is rooted in the survivor movement and ideas associated with it, such as the 'anti-psychiatry' of critical authors such as RD Laing and Thomas Szasz (Boundy, 2008).[6] For those with an interest in bridging conceptual gaps between the disabled people's and survivor movements, such as the sticking point over whether the concept of 'impairment' applies to survivors, the neurodiversity movement should therefore be of great interest as an already-existing fusion of both.

Activists in the neurodiversity movement seek to reclaim impairment labels (such as 'autism') from the authority of the medical and psychological professions, and to re-value them, in positive terms, as components of a self-determined identity (Sinclair, 2012b; Meyerding, 2002). In this, the neurodiversity movement takes a stance similar to the 'affirmation model of disability' proposed by Swain and French (2000), and further developed by Cameron (2008; 2011). The latter argues that an affirmative model of 'disabled' identity that is consistent with, and complementary to, the social model affirms not disability but impairment. Impairment, in turn, is re-defined as 'difference to be expected and respected on its own terms in a diverse society' (Cameron, 2008, 24). This position is associated with movement slogans such as 'celebrate difference with pride' and closely parallels the 'Mad Pride' stance of some radical strands within the survivor movement (for example, Curtis et al, 2000). The affirmation model offers a way of understanding disability as oppression, without necessarily assigning negative value to the physical or mental differences conventionally categorised as 'impairment'. This would mean that Plumb's (1994) warning that 'admitting to an impairment' means 'legitimising and maintaining the link with "illness"' (p 18) does not necessarily hold true.

Trauma, oppression and the problematics of distress

The experience of distress is, however, difficult to fit into an affirmation model. Arguably, by definition, the term 'distress' can only describe something bad and unwanted. For this reason, the concept of 'Mad Pride' is one with which many survivors do not identify, and there are considerable tensions within the survivor movement between, on the one hand, those who see their 'madness' as positive or neutral and, on the other, those who consider 'distress' as a problem requiring a solution, albeit not a medical or psychiatric one. It could be easy to dismiss the neurodiversity perspective as not at all helpful for the latter group, who may see their experiences of distress as rooted in trauma, oppression and the impossible demands of life in a profoundly alienating society, rather than to do with any 'difference' to which a positive value could be ascribed. However, writers and activists within the neurodiversity movement are acutely aware of, and concerned with, issues around distress, and have developed a considerable analysis of it, within a framework that distinguishes it clearly from (unproblematic) 'difference'.

Neurodiversity activists are also keen to point out that many people with conditions such as ADHD or 'high-functioning' autism go undiagnosed into adulthood – particularly if they present in ways that do not fit psychiatrists' stereotypes of those conditions – and that this experience very frequently results in mental distress and/or involvement with the 'mental health' system. This can include misdiagnosis, with labels such as 'schizophrenia', which also has gendered aspects, as women are arguably more likely than men to be misdiagnosed or to go undiagnosed (Baker, 2004). Neurodiversity activists contend, however, that the distress experienced by these people is usually not a product of their actual neurotype, so much as a (fully reasonable) reaction to being continually misunderstood and rejected by a neurotypical-normative society; an example of what Thomas (1999) describes as psycho-emotional disablism (see Reeve, 2012a; and also, Donna Reeve, Chapter 7, in this volume). Thus, what is needed to alleviate distress is not 'medical' intervention, but a transformation of society. This position fits well with Plumb's (1994) conceptualisation of distress as 'dissent', as well as with the central contention of the social model of disability: that a disabling society, rather than a disabled individual, is 'the problem'.

In a vicious irony, this distress may then itself be regarded as 'pathology' by society, resulting in the involvement of the psychiatric system, where it is then further pathologised within a 'symptom'-focused 'illness' paradigm. Indeed, some neurodiversity activists suggest that many of those characteristics currently considered to meet diagnostic criteria for conditions such as autism are – rather than markers of 'innate' difference – the traumatic effects of on-going psycho-emotional oppression experienced by neurodivergent people. Such reactions are even more likely to be pathologised if that 'innate' difference results in reactions to trauma that are different enough from those of neurotypical people not to be easily recognised as such – and seen instead as 'unintelligible' behaviour (Pilgrim and Tomasini, 2012) – and/or if situations are experienced as traumatic that a neurotypical person would be unlikely to recognise as such; for example, an autistic person with hypersensitivity to sound may find the noise of crowds or traffic unbearable, and might therefore react to it in similar ways to physical pain, such as crying or screaming, running away from the noise in apparent panic, or using repetitive movements (such as hand-flapping or head-banging) as a counter-stimulus to help cope with it.

From a neurodiversity perspective, therefore, the concept of 'mental illness' can be seen as a socially constructed category including both 'neurodivergence pathologised' and distress experienced as a result of psycho-emotional disablism or other forms of oppression.

Proponents of neurodiversity would tend to accept that certain aspects of some divergent neurotypes may be distressing (for example, the sensory intolerances and/or auditory processing difficulties experienced by many autistic people, or difficulty following a conversation as experienced by someone with ADHD).[7] They would simultaneously question whether these differences are 'inherently' distressing, however, or more a matter of social and environmental surroundings not being suited to the individual. Most would also accept the possibility that, for some (although certainly not all) people who experience mental distress, that distress may be caused by some form of physical or chemical factor, and thus not originate from, though it may well be exacerbated by, social or environmental conditions. In such cases, however, self-definition and self-determination, rather than paternalistic medical authority, would still be regarded as the preferred basis for any social response to distress. Therefore, the neurodiversity framework can enable the inclusion of both those who identify their mental distress as purely biochemical, and those who regard it as purely 'socially reactive'. It is not necessarily mutually exclusive to conceptualise distress both as part of some 'impairments' and as the result of unfair and oppressive social conditions.

Neurodiversity activists tend to accept that wide-ranging social change is too ambitious and long-term a goal to be useful to an individual in acute distress, of whatever origin. They thus generally support a pragmatic, libertarian response to individual distress, based on whatever 'treatment' a given individual determines to be useful to them. For example, while neurodiversity activists oppose the routine prescription of psychotropic drugs for 'normalising' purposes (such as stimulants like Ritalin for ADHD), and non-consensual drugging (either directly against the will of the 'patient' or of children too young to give informed consent), most would support the right of the individual to choose to take such drugs, if they find their effects useful. This position fits well with ideas supported by the survivor movement, such as the 'drug-centred model' of psychoactive drug action, which has been proposed by the critical psychiatrist, Joanna Moncrieff (2007), as a replacement for the 'disease-centred model' of mainstream biomedical psychiatry. By conceptualising drugs in terms of the effects that they produce and whether they are helpful, rather than as the 'cure' or 'treatment' for a 'disease', Moncrieff's model empowers people experiencing mental distress to make their own decisions about whether or not to use drugs (or other 'treatments').

Convergences and divergences

The neurodiversity movement's idea of a spectrum of equally valid neurotypes, deserving of recognition and accommodation rather than pathologisation, are echoed by those of some authors within the survivor movement. For example, the American feminist survivor, Kate Millett, author of *The Loony Bin Trip*, an autobiographical account of her experience of coercive treatment in the US and Irish mental health systems, wrote:

Let sanity be understood to be a spectrum that runs the full course between balancing one's checkbook on the one hand and fantasy on the other. Possibly higher mathematics as well. At one end the humdrum but exacting work of the mind, at the other, surrealism, imagination, speculation…A spectrum. A rainbow. All human. All good or at least morally indifferent. Places within the great, still-unexplored country of the mind. None to be forbidden. None to be punished. None to be feared. If we go mad – so what? We would come back again if not chased away, exiled, isolated, confined. (Millett, 1990, 314)

This could be seen as 'foreshadowing' of the concept of neurodiversity almost a decade before it was invented. However, one significant difference remains. While neurodiversity activists focus on their 'differences' being permanent and biological in nature, many mental health system survivors strongly reject the idea that there is any fundamental neurological difference between them and other ('normal'/'typical' or non-psychiatrically-labelled) people; arguing rather that they have 'natural' reactions to traumatic and/or oppressive experiences that they have lived through. Plumb (1994), for example, cites an analogy used by the survivor activist, Mike Lawson, who deemed the mental state pathologised as 'paranoid schizophrenia' to be like a hedgehog curling up into a ball in response to danger; yet this is actually an analogy to which many autistic people who experience 'shutdown' as a response to stress, including myself, can definitely relate to! Some of this difference in perspective may have to do with the particular experiences of people placed in different diagnostic categories. Many autistic people, for example, have suffered greatly from assumptions that either they themselves, or their families, are 'to blame' for their differences and/or difficulties, or that there must be a traumatic cause, which needs to be 'uncovered' and 'processed' by psychoanalytic or other forms of 'talking therapy', aimed at 'healing' this non-existent 'damage'.[8] For some people, it can be a massive relief to find out that their divergence from the social norm is due to an innate neurological difference; that they are not a formerly 'normal' person who has been 'broken', but were a different – and equally 'whole' – type of person from the beginning.

Conversely, many mental health system survivors associate ideas of biological difference with medical models, and biologically-based 'treatments' such as psychotropic drugs, by which they have often been profoundly oppressed and violated (harms of which, it should be noted, the neurodiversity movement is also keenly aware). Many survivors have never had their social environments examined as a 'cause' of their distress, the label of 'mental illness' being used to deny the reality of their experiences of violence and oppression. While some in the survivor movement regard psychoanalysis or other 'talking therapies' as much more positive responses to 'problems in living', autistic activists – such as Judy Singer (1999) and Mel Baggs (2006)[9] – are often strongly critical of such paradigms as unhelpful and inappropriate responses to their needs. This critique is, in part, because of the 'parent-blaming' paradigm mentioned above – shared by some 'anti-psychiatry' authors, such as Alice Miller (1991) and Peter Breggin (1994) – but is also in part due to fundamental issues with the paternalistic and unequal therapist–client relationship. Similarly suspicious perspectives on 'talking therapies' are shared by other strands of the survivor movement, such as therapy survivor groups.

The experiences and perspectives of people in the survivor movement and the neurodiversity movement may here seem opposed to one another. However, both result from having been misunderstood and mistreated by a paternalistic psychiatric system, which assumes that it knows and understands the minds, experiences and needs of its 'patients' better than they do themselves, and focuses on 'curing' or 'normalising' the person, rather than changing the society in which the person lives into one in which they can be happy and accepted. Some people may find psychotropic drugs harmful and 'talking therapies' useful; others may find 'talking therapies' harmful and drugs useful; yet others may find both equally harmful and prefer to be simply 'left alone'. The most important issues, however, regardless of such individual choices, are self-determination over what (if any) 'treatment' or 'assistance' is appropriate for individual needs, and an understanding of difference, distress and dissent as all being located within social and political contexts (rather than simply being 'pathologies' of the individual). If such self-determination and understanding was available for all then the question of whether the origin of a person's social or emotional difference is 'traumatic' or 'congenital' – while it may 'matter' profoundly to the individual in terms of self-perception and self-understanding – would not necessarily 'matter' to society in terms of how that person should be 'treated' or responded to. In all cases, the person's own understanding of their needs would be accepted, and their needs accommodated.

Conclusions

I believe that the ideas of the neurodiversity movement can provide a useful 'bridge' across some of the conceptual and practical divergences between the disabled people's movement and the survivor movement. Some members of both older movements may disagree – with one another and with the neurodiversity movement – over some of the ideas and terminology used. I believe, however, that insights from neurodiversity can enrich the perspectives of both in ways that illuminate the common ground they share with each other. This is particularly the case if it is approached with the recognition that all terms and definitions are imperfect and can be contested.

I think that activists in the neurodiversity movement, by virtue of their identities and experiences overlapping with both the disability and survivor movements, have an important role to play in expanding possibilities for dialogue and collaboration between them. The fact that there is overlap between the people and experiences involved in all these movements is also a reminder that categories such as 'disabled' and 'survivor' do not necessarily have strict, definable boundaries. However, this does not mean that these categories are not 'real' or important in terms of both theorising and actively fighting inequality and oppression.

I suggest that the neurodiversity movement is particularly well placed to bring together broader categories of marginalised people(s) into a (necessarily loose, but nonetheless potentially hugely important) solidarity network of movements fighting for radical acceptance of all types of human diversity, under a broad banner of 'anti-normalisation' (Bumiller, 2008) and challenges to supposedly 'universal' assumptions about 'human nature' that privilege majority and historically dominant groups. In the current political and economic climate, in which welfare cuts driven by neoliberal ideology threaten the very survival of disabled or otherwise underprivileged people in the UK and many other 'western' societies, and the segregation of 'the poor' into separate categories is used by governments and the mass media to 'divide and rule' and prevent effective opposition, such networking and collaboration is ever more acutely necessary.

The experiences of people placed in different categories, or who identify with different movements, necessarily differ, and their differences should not be erased in the name of unity; however, nor should they be essentialised in ways that lead to divisive separatism. A fundamental principle of the neurodiversity movement is that people and their perspectives can be radically different from one another, but that all can be part of an inclusive society that recognises the – sometimes difficult, but often positive – reality of such differences without stigmatising or pathologising them. This realist but anti-essentialist respect for difference and diversity can, I believe, be the basis of working together for all our liberation.

Notes

[1] There are a large number of different terms used to refer to the social movement of people who have been labelled with 'mental illness' which, as Peter Beresford (2004) points out, are all opposed or regarded as offensive by some sections of the movement. I have somewhat arbitrarily decided to use the term 'survivor movement' in this paper, mostly for the sake of simplicity – my apologies to those who prefer other terms.

[2] It is worth noting here that there is some disagreement within the disabled people's movement on the subject of impairment, with some, particularly feminist and post-structuralist, disabled writers arguing that the distinction between impairment and disability is not as clear-cut as it seems in simplistic readings of the social model; particularly given that impairment itself can be regarded as socially constructed (see, for example, Thomas, 1999; Thomas and Corker, 2002; Tremain, 2002).

[3] Sinclair's article 'Don't Mourn for us' was originally published in 1993 in the Autism Network International newsletter, *Our Voice*, Volume 1, Number 3, www.autreat.com/dont_mourn.html

[4] This is of course also a core element of the social model of disability.

[5] This is parallel to the usage of terms such as 'cisgender' as a contrast to 'transgender' in the LGBT community. While outside the scope of this chapter, the LGBT and/or 'queer' rights/liberation movement is also concerned with the acceptance of identities as valid parts of human diversity which were previously pathologised as 'mental disorders'. As such, it has significant overlap with the neurodiversity movement (see, for example, Lawson, 2005; Bumiller, 2008).

[6] It should be noted, however, that – while parts of the survivor movement, particularly in North America, certainly have been inspired by anti-psychiatry – the anti-psychiatric body of theory was primarily developed by academics and dissident members of the 'psy' professions, rather than by survivors themselves. It cannot therefore be regarded as the theory of the survivor movement.

[7] Within the framework of the social model of disability, these would be examples of what Thomas (1999, 42–3) calls 'impairment effects' (as distinct from disability, including psycho-emotional disablement).

[8] The most notorious, and arguably the most influential, such theory in the field of autism is that of the mid-twentieth-century child psychologist, Bruno Bettelheim, who argued that autism was caused by emotionally neglectful 'refrigerator mothers' (Waltz, 2013). While, in the English-speaking world, his theories have been largely superseded by biomedical paradigms, they are still arguably dominant in some other countries, such as France (Jolly and Novak, 2012).

[9] The autistic writer and activist, Mel Baggs, previously wrote under the names Amanda or AM Baggs, under which names she is still arguably better known (in particular for her writings on the website, autistics.org, and her video 'In My Language').

SEVENTEEN

Distress and disability: not you, not me, but us?

Peter Beresford

Introduction

The relationship between distress and disability has continued to be a vexed and controversial one at all levels. This was helpfully illustrated by the Lancaster University seminar and the follow-up report, which led to this publication.[1] These tensions are also embodied in their different conceptualisations, internal and external definitions, cultures and movements. For some time it has even seemed that there might be an impasse in relationships between distress and disability because of the clear lack of consensus among mental health service users/survivors about the issues involved. There has also rightly been a reluctance to ignore or override conflicting views because of the damage it could do to survivors individually and collectively. It has sometimes seemed that there might be insurmountable difficulties in the way of developing increased understanding, solidarity and unity between survivors and disabled people's movements (as well as individuals), undermining either or both of them through trying to impose some kind of uniformity and common framework.

Recently, however, in this author's view, there have been developments which may offer a way past the roadblock that there has seemed to be between disability and distress; between disabled people and mental health service users/disabled people's movements and mental health service user/survivor movements. They relate to a flurry of new, emerging, exciting and important discussions which are taking place associated with both neurodiversity and mad studies, which this book also itself reflects. In this chapter, I will seek to explore some of the historic issues that have related to the state of the relationship between disability and distress and also consider the implications of such more recent and current developments.

Disability and distress: links and differences

To begin with, I need to make my own position clear. I write as a mental health service user/survivor and academic who has been actively involved for a long time in survivor organisations and the psychiatric system survivor movement. This began with Survivors Speak Out and Mind Link and has embraced other survivor liberatory and research organisations since. I have also engaged with and been involved with the disabled people's movement and formed links and relationships with people actively involved in it. Some of the survivors I have known and been close to over the years have also been people with physical and sensory impairments. Perhaps it is not surprising given such a personal history that I have always felt that building links and relationships between disabled people (understood in terms of people with physical and sensory impairments and more broadly) and psychiatric system survivors, can only be helpful. Obviously there can be many differences between the two – in experience, understandings and so on, but equally there are overlaps – even to the point, as I have said, of some people combining both identities. Because both identities, that of mental health service users and disabled people, are subject to oppression, discrimination, negative stereotyping and stigma, it has also seemed important to me to try and gain strength from each other, build solidarity and emphasise our overlaps and common oppression and experience, while respecting our differences (Beresford et al, 1995; Beresford and Gifford, 1996; Beresford et al, 1996; Beresford, 2000; Beresford et al, 2002).

I have to say that my early concerns and writings about survivor issues in relation to disability and the disabled people's movement were influenced by worries I had that the mental health service user/ survivor movement (more than the disabled people's movement) was a reformist movement that sought to bring about change within the psychiatric system, often from within it. I was also concerned that we were beginning to see the emergence of hierarchies and the subversion of its liberatory goals as some survivors began to occupy key roles within the structures of the psychiatric system and its systems for 'user involvement'. That of course meant that the more radical voices could expect to be marginalised. What made this a particular concern was that the psychiatric system seemed to have an infinite capacity both to undermine and to resist the efforts for change made by survivors and their organisations – especially from within. To make the issue even more difficult and more painful, there were also radical but wise voices, like that of Louise Pembroke, who warned us against standing away from the psychiatric system, saying, that if we did, what would happen to 'our brothers and sisters in the back wards'? At the same time in terms of the activities and agendas of the mental health service user/survivor movement, there did seem to be a relatively narrow preoccupation with the psychiatric system, although increasingly it was becoming apparent from early survivor research like that undertaken by the Strategies For Living project at the Mental Health Foundation, that many service users saw key ways forward *outside* the psychiatric system, for example, through work building relationships, supporting people's empowerment and skill development, through complementary therapies, peer support and user-led services and so on (Faulkner and Nicholls, 1999; Faulkner and Layzell, 2000).

At the same time non-survivor academics like Marian Barnes and colleagues, were drawing distinctions between the UK mental health service user/survivor movement as consumerist in nature and the disabled people's movement as citizen rights/empowerment based (Barnes et al, 1999). This highlighted existing tensions between the two, although it didn't do justice to competing strands in the survivor movement. Not only did it over-simplify, but it also ignored radical elements in the survivor movement.

I was therefore keen to draw on what I saw as the strengths of the disabled people's movement for the survivor movement; benefits of it being more independent of the service system, separatist and also prioritising the development of its own alternative understandings of support and services and its explicit commitment to individual and collective rights and an inclusive model of citizenship (Campbell and Oliver, 1996; Oliver, 1996; Barnes and Mercer, 1997; Oliver and Barnes, 1998; Barnes et al, 2002). This did not mean that I discounted the principles and values that survivors had developed and highlighted. These have included speaking for yourself, offering each other mutual support and prioritising a humanistic approach to understanding and action (O'Hagan, 1993; Campbell, 1996). At the same time, I have consistently believed that closer links between mental health service users/survivors, disabled people and their movements were likely to be beneficial for both.

Important tensions

This approach has had its critics. Anne Plumb, the survivor activist, has perhaps been the most coherent and longstanding of these, offering counter arguments (Plumb, 1994). She has been a consistent survivor voice, unhappy with the survivor movement getting closer to the disabled people's movement, while having knowledge of and links with both. Anne has argued that such a strategy could result in the independent identity of survivors being undermined and the particular history and culture of our movement being overshadowed. Meanwhile many mental health service users have expressed a reluctance to identify as disabled people, seeing it as an additional source of stigma, while some disabled people have articulated similar views about being associated with mental health service users. As a result over the years, there have been some collaborations between survivors and disabled people, some links established between their organisations and indeed some user-led organisations which included both mental health service users/survivors and disabled people (and other groups of social care service users, like my own Shaping Our Lives). However active collaborations, joint projects and partnerships between the two movements have remained limited.

At the same time both the disabled people's movement and the social model of disability that it developed have come in for criticism for failing to address issues of diversity. These criticisms have been longstanding and include suggestions that they have not adequately addressed the situation, rights and needs of mental health service users/ survivors and people with learning difficulties, or issues of difference in relation to gender, sexual orientation, age and ethnicity (Morris, 1996; Shakespeare, 2006; Thomas, 2007).

Philosophical differences?

Beyond the kind of principles identified above, the mental health service user/survivor movement in the UK has tended not to be clearly ideologically driven. The reasons for this are complex and uncertain. They appear to include concerns that this might be used further to invalidate and exclude them on grounds of their perceived 'unreason'. Thus if they reject the medical interpretation of their experience, this might be used to mean merely that they don't want to acknowledge they are really ill. Many mental health service users also seem reluctant to develop their own theories about their experience in case they create another orthodoxy, having already suffered at the hands of medical orthodoxy.

The picture has been different in the UK disabled people's movement. From its early days, it has had clear links with broader political ideology. This was reflected in the demands made in the formative document produced by the Union of Physically Impaired Against Segregation (UPIAS) in 1976, one of the pioneering disabled people's organisations,

Fundamental Principles of Disability (UPIAS/Disability Alliance, 1976). From this developed the social model of disability, whose architects were associated (often by their critics, sometimes by themselves) with leftist and Marxist politics (Campbell and Oliver, 1996; Oliver, 1996). The social model of disability which became the philosophical underpinning of the disabled people's movement in the UK and in some other countries is essentially a political idea. It posits the perceived *impairment* of the individual (physical, sensory, intellectual) – which has been the basis for medicalised individual modern definitions of disability – against the social reaction, discrimination and oppression – *disability* – experienced by people included in the conceptualisation. Critics have suggested that impairment has been inappropriately subordinated and the focus been overly on disability; the relationships and overlaps between the two has been inadequately explored and the disabling effects of impairment underplayed (Crow, 1996b; Shakespeare, 2007; Thomas, 2007). However, the social model has had enormous importance in disability politics, policy, studies and disabled people's lives. Many thousands of disabled people have experienced it as liberatory. It has underpinned disabled people's conceptualisation of independent living. They have reconceived independent living as not about managing on your own, but about having the support and mainstream access needed to live life on as near equal terms as possible as non-disabled people (Campbell and Oliver, 1996). The social model of disability has also been the basis for disabled people's proposals and pioneering provisions for support, from direct payments and peer support, to user-led services and user controlled/emancipatory disability research.

The impact of 'recovery'

The reluctance of mental health service users/survivors and their organisations to develop their own equivalent independent model or philosophy, however, seems to have left them vulnerable to being co-opted to accept someone else's. This has happened with the model of 'recovery' which has become central in UK mental health policy and practice. It has been presented as a social movement, as well as gaining the support of many survivors and their organisations. The attraction of 'recovery' lay in it seeming to reject conventional ideas of writing off mental health service users/survivors as permanently damaged and pathologised. As a professional model imported from the United States, the model offered sufficient ambiguity to gain service user interest and support. The emphasis on 'recovery' was meant to improve life chances, but service users want better quality help from recovery services and don't define it as professionals do (Gould, 2012). Ownership of the idea of recovery seemed to lie with dominant policymakers, in medicalised understandings and over-arching political ideology. Recovery is essentially based on a medical model – 'getting better' (Harper and Speed, 2012). Thus unlike the idea of independent living, pioneered by disabled people, which took account of disabled people's ongoing need for support, recovery suggests that it would be possible to withdraw support as people 'recovered'. This ignores the reality for many mental health service users/survivors that their need for help and support may be varied, continuing or recurring. Ultimately the idea of 'recovery' creates barriers rather than a basis for understanding between mental health service users/survivors and disabled people because it is inherently antagonistic to a social understanding.

The associated emphasis on 'reablement' has encouraged a notion of 'throughput' in services, with support withdrawn when people are regarded as sufficiently 'recovered' rather than its importance being recognised in maintaining their well-being. While as part of this move, the political talk has been of 'improved access to psychological therapies (IAPTs)', a London School of Economics study found that many local commissioners were are not using the £400 million government funding 'for the intended purpose' (Mental Health Policy Group, 2012). Service users have also raised concerns that in practice IAPTs have sometimes resulted in over-mechanical, inadequately skilled and too short-term provision, narrowly based on 'cognitive behaviour therapy' (CBT), rather than the supportive range of counselling services for which many mental health service users/survivors have long hoped and campaigned.

Interest in social approaches

Over this same period, an increasing interest in more social approaches to mental health issues has also emerged in the UK. This has been reflected in the establishment and development of the Social Perspectives Network (SPN). The SPN describes itself as a coalition of service users/survivors, carers, policy makers, academics, students and practitioners interested in how social factors both contribute to people becoming distressed, and play a crucial part in promoting people's recovery (www.spn.org.uk). SPN has also shown a particular commitment to addressing issues of diversity and inclusion in mental health and has shown a preparedness to challenge policy which fails adequately to address these issues (LDC/SPN, 2006; Griffiths and

Allen, 2007). This interest in more social approaches, has also been associated with the production of a growing number of publications concerned with such approaches in mental health (for example, Sayce, 2000; Ramon and Williams, 2005; Tew, 2005b; 2011; Tew et al, 2012). However, such sources, while interested in and exploring social factors relating to mental health, tend nonetheless generally to accept essentially medicalised understandings of 'mental health' and the diagnostic system associated with them. These tend to be taken as given, while there has been a concern to extend the search for causation beyond the individual, to their social circumstances.

Continuing dominance of medical models

Despite increasingly evident rhetoric about 'recovery' and this broader interest in social approaches to mental distress, the medical model of mental illness continues to dominate in the UK and indeed internationally (Pilgrim, 2009). To some extent in disability policy, policymakers have acknowledged and in some ways taken account of the social model of disability, for example, in taking forward policy and provision for direct payments and the last government introducing an 'independent living' strategy and making commitments to support a national network of user led/disabled people's organisations. However the same has not happened in the context of mental health (ODI, 2008). The prevailing medical model has remained essentially unchanged for at least half a century. If anything it has extended its influence with the creation of a plethora of new judgemental and behaviour based diagnoses and an increasing preoccupation with bio-ethics (Beresford and Wilson, 2002). The corollary of this medicalisation of madness and distress has been the use of drugs as the default treatment response, with an over-reliance placed on them and a disproportionate role and influence appropriated by the pharmaceutical industry in the conceptualisation, treatment and research of 'mental health'. While government rhetoric gets grander, with talk of 'new horizons' in mental health (Cross-Government Strategy: Mental Health Division, 2009), based on a broader 'well-being' approach and talk of 'completing the revolution' in mental health (The Centre for Social Justice, 2011), if anything, the response to people's mental health conditions gets punier and also seems more controlling. While Labour and coalition governments have competed with each other in their apparent aspirations (Burnham, 2012), so it seems, under the traditional mental illness paradigm, people's actual mental health services/support are deteriorating and widely condemned.

What survivors say

In the context discussed above, of limited engagement between survivors and disabled people and their movements; the continuing dominance of medical models of mental illness, of less support and more control, and yet an emerging interest in more social approaches to mental health, a small group of us sought and gained funding for a small-scale project to explore mental health service users' views on models of 'mental health'. This was a survivor-led project and we particularly wanted to explore such models with mental health service users/survivors (as well as some disabled people and some people who shared both identities). We wanted to position the project outside a medical model of mental illness, so we called it *Towards a Social Model of Madness and Distress?* (Beresford et al, 2010). There were some clear key findings. These included that:

- Most service users believe that a medical model based on deficit and pathology still dominates public and professional understanding of mental health issues, shaping attitudes and policy.
  They largely see such a medical model as damaging and unhelpful.
- The labelling and stigma following from a medical model of mental illness emerge as major barriers for mental health service users.
- Service users see social approaches to mental health issues as much more helpful. They feel that broader issues need to be taken more into account to counter the individualisation of mental health issues.

The emerging picture became more complicated, however, when we asked people what they felt about the social model of disability and how it might relate to madness and distress.

Most participants in this project were familiar with the social model of disability. But there was no agreement about whether it related helpfully to mental health issues. Instead service users were *divided* in their views. Some service users feared that the association of the social model with disability would add to the stigma they faced. There was also a feeling that disability and mental health issues were different and that the idea of 'impairment' underpinning the social model misrepresented the experience of mental health service users. Some mental health service users felt that they and other mental health service users/survivors might not have an impairment and that it might therefore be unhelpful to apply this idea to them. As one put it:

'I think instinctively, at a gut level I've felt, no, my mental health problems are not an impairment. I don't see that they are an impairment for a range of reasons. So I think that's a limitation in the way I understand the social model of disability at the moment, I don't actually feel that the impairment bit accommodates my experience.'

I have often encountered this rejection of the idea of impairment, even externally perceived impairment, among mental health service users/survivors, who may see their perceptions/emotions as something positive, even illuminating, rather than negative, and their experience in terms of diversity rather than necessarily as a problem.

The project also highlighted another related issue which divided mental health service users/survivors: the matter of terminology. While some participants in the project valued the words 'mad' and 'madness', many did not and felt more or less uncomfortable with them. This is perhaps not surprising given the contested and frequently stigmatic nature of language in this field, especially of terms like 'mad', 'crazy', 'loony'. Thus there were comments like: 'I stick to my guns and I don't like the word "madness". I think it ought to be done away with. It's labelling and stigmatising.'

Thus our project offered a picture of mental health service users/survivors who rejected medicalised interpretations of them as damaging and destructive; who valued more social approaches, yet where many felt that the use of anti-medical language like 'madness' could make things worse! This project suggested that any efforts to impose conformity between distress and disability was unlikely to be unhelpful. We are currently carrying out a second stage to this project, following up and exploring these findings with a diverse range of mental health service users/survivors to check out their views about them and what they see as helpful ways forward.

Learning from the neurodiversity movement

In the meantime, as signalled at the beginning of this chapter, there have been two key developments which may have an important bearing on models of disability and mental health and on the relationship between disability, madness and distress. The first of these is the development of first hand discourses about neurodiversity. In Chapter 16 of this book, Steve Graby, one of the contributors to these discourses, suggests that the neurodiversity movement may offer a new and helpful intervention in the debate about the relationship between disability and distress: the disabled people's and survivor movement. As he says, the neurodiversity movement includes 'people with a variety of diagnostic labels (such as autistic spectrum conditions, dyslexia, dyspraxia and AD(H)D), and arguably has roots in both the disabled people's and survivor movements'. As Graby puts it, the neurodiversity movement has grown primarily out of the self-advocacy of autistic people themselves, which has developed as a challenge to the growth of 'a parent-dominated "autism advocacy" lobby', concerned with finding a 'cure' for autism.

The neurodiversity movement, in contrast see autism, AD(H)D and similar conditions as natural differences to be accepted and accommodated. A core principle of neurodiversity is that such conditions are 'real' and neurological in nature; they embody human *diversity* rather than representing pathology or deficiency. Thus the movement seeks to celebrate neurodiversity and for it to be recognised and valued. It similarly seeks acceptance of identities previously pathologised as mental disorders, as a valid part of human diversity, aiming to 'reclaim' and 'revalue' impairment labels. Building on the affirmative model of disability as developed by Cameron, the idea of impairment no longer has to be a block in the way of survivors' relating to a social model, because impairment is now reconceived as difference (Cameron, 2008, 24). At the same time, as Graby observes, this is not to deny that 'some divergent neurotypes may be distressing'. Thus the experience and ideas of those mental health service users/survivors who see their experience as negative, is not ignored or devalued. While the ideas developed by the neurodiversity movement, may be seen by some to be unfinished, leaving some issues raised by mental health service users in relation to disability unresolved or un-agreed, they nonetheless provide a basis for making better sense of the shared issues and common causes that there are for disabled people and mental health service users/survivors. They provide further opportunities to explore possible meeting points. Thus for survivors and disabled people alike, there is food for thought here; reasons to reassess their understandings of themselves and of each other and, a possible route out of confinement within traditional medicalised understandings and models of themselves.

Graby sees the neurodiversity movement as having a potentially 'bridge building' role between the survivors' and disabled people's movement, highlighting overlaps between them and challenging simplistic assumptions that these identities have 'strict and easily defined boundaries'. In his chapter he makes what I believe is a key point for taking forward both understanding and action around disability and madness and distress. He highlights the importance of bringing:

together broader categories of marginalised people(s) into a (...loose, but...important) solidarity network of movements fighting for radical acceptance of all types of human diversity, under a broad banner of 'anti-normalisation'... [While t]he experiences of people placed in different categories...necessarily differ...[a] realist but anti-essentialist respect for difference and diversity can, I believe, be the basis of working together for all our liberation.

Mad studies

We have seen how many survivors have been discouraged from aligning themselves with the terminology and framework of madness, even though they feel damaged by the dominant medicalised paradigm. Now, however, there are developing discussions which may have the power to change this. This same issue of working towards greater solidarity to challenge the threat from ruling right-wing market-driven neoliberal ideology and politics (committed to reduction in state support and services) is also highlighted by this, the second of the key developments which I want to explore here. This is perhaps the critical one and in my view offers a new way forward for mental health service users/survivors and those who identify with them and seek to support their rights and needs. In my view, it also makes possible the development of a new, more equal relationship between disability and madness and distress. This is the emergence of mad studies.

Mad Pride is an international development, which had its origins in Canada in the early 1990s. By the late 1990s similar events were being organised as Mad Pride in England and around the world from South Africa and the United States to Australia.[2] In the UK this tended to be a high profile but *minority* activity among mental health service users/survivors. However, in recent years we have seen the emergence of a number of discussions and organisations which associate themselves explicitly with the idea of madness. Now there are also major publications which are doing the same (Coles et al, 2013; Staddon, 2013; Burstow et al, 2014). The most significant of these in my view is the book *Mad Matters* which brings together experience and ideas from Canada (LeFrançois et al, 2013). While it claims only to speak for the Canadian experience, I believe that it has much greater international significance and highlights the contribution that developing debates about madness may offer for negotiating issues relating to disability and distress. I believe that this is the case and that *Mad Matters* specifically may have a pivotal part to play in this task for two reasons.

The first reason is that the text offers a basis for and possibility of solidarity. It has often seemed to me that the struggle that was taking place and had to take place over people's minds and lives was one of survivors against psychiatry. This was a struggle where battle lines were drawn, with psychiatry committed to a pathologising and damaging model of mental health service users, operating in close alliance with powerful international pharmaceutical companies, whose economic interests such medicalisation strongly served. This has often felt like a lonely and one-sided struggle. But we can get a different sense from *Mad Matters* and the emerging domain of mad studies that it demarcates, of what can be possible. Here we can see a wide range of interests coming together, linking up and working together. The book offers a definition of mad studies, its central focus, as:

> an umbrella term that is used to embrace the body of knowledge that has emerged from psychiatric survivors, Mad-identified people, antipsychiatry academics and activists, critical psychiatrists, and radical therapists. This body of knowledge is wide-ranging and includes scholarship that is critical of the mental health system as well as radical and mad activist scholarship. This field of study is informed by and generated by the perspectives of psychiatric survivors and Mad-identified researchers and academics. (LeFrançois et al, 2013, 337)

So the book includes many chapters written by people with direct experience as recipients of mental health services (psychiatric survivors and Mad-identified people) and also others written by academics and allies with personal or professional interest in this area. People here are not speaking for others but offering their own different contributions and understandings. But they are doing it within a framework of madness, which rejects medicalisation and its plethora of associated and ambiguous ideas and structures, from diagnosis to recovery. And here we can get a sense of the value, the strength and the possibilities of such solidarity. We can see the benefits of developing a plurality of resistance rather than on emphasising divisions. Suddenly this feels like a struggle that can gain widespread support, both from survivors and others; a struggle that can be won.

Second, what gives this book and the movement of which it is a part, significance for the present discussion, is that it has the potential to change relationships with ourselves, with psychiatry and with disability. One of the difficulties that has always faced mental health service users/survivors and others working to challenge psychiatry, to which I referred earlier, is that they did not want to replace one orthodoxy with another; one monolithic theory with another. They did not want yet another dominating explanation or set of ideas imposed on them or risk imposing them on themselves. This, however, has also seemed to weaken them because it did not offer a clear marker and value base on which to found their actions, as, for example, the social model of disability has done for many disabled people. It could leave our experience and viewpoints as survivors susceptible to the interpretations and theories of others, as we have seen with the idea of 'recovery'. However, it has long been clear that for survivors more social approaches both to understanding and responding to their situations make much more sense and feel much more positive than their experience of the damaging and stigmatising medical models that have long been attached to them. *Mad Matters* takes us further forward on this journey. I can't sum up my thoughts better than I did in the book's foreword:

> This book is a vital sign of these times. It has delineated a new subject of study and in doing so offers us all much greater hope of making sense both of what goes on within us, what impacts from outside, how the two interact and how their relationship may be made a much more positive and humanistic one.
>
> It is a *for*, not an *against* book. Not only does it offer critiques of psychiatry and associated law, public policy, media and propaganda, as well as subjecting psychiatry's questionable 'treatments', knowledge production, pedagogy and academic activities to serious and necessary scrutiny. Not only does it examine longstanding tendencies to criminalise and pathologise madness and associate it with violence and individualised irrationality and deviance. More important, perhaps, it also explores the history, culture and language of madness and mad people. It highlights the diversity of mad experience and understandings, the violence of psychiatry, the ambiguity of its reformism and the emergence of survivor research and academic engagement. As the editors say, the book:
>
> combines the more established understandings of mad matters, including anti-psychiatry approaches and long-standing psychiatric survivor narratives, with an exciting and burgeoning form of activism and conceptualisations,

emanating from a new generation of people…engaging in
a variety of forms of radical and mad activist scholarship.

Within these pages we do not find a new orthodoxy, something that
activist psychiatric system survivors have long guarded against. Instead
there is food to nurture different social understandings and strategies
in response both to madness and distress and to the psychiatric system.
There are strategies here for the future both to challenge psychiatry
and the psychiatric system and beyond and for conceiving and building
something radically different for all of us.

I had always thought that as survivors we needed a clearer
underpinning model and ideology – our own social model. That
might be true, but perhaps in a different way to what I had expected.
What *Mad Matters* highlights is the groundbreaking role that our joint
development of our own strong, comprehensive body of knowledge,
equally valuing lived experience alongside other knowledges, framed in
terms of madness, can play in offering a way forward. It demonstrates
that having our own strong body of knowledge, framed outside a
medical model, can be better than seeking an overarching monolithic
theory which can overshadow us. This book offers such a diverse and
holistic body of knowledge from many sources – so many insights, so
much experience all in one place. *Mad Matters* demonstrates that such
knowledge has already developed critical mass. Framed in terms of 'mad
studies' it represents a clear and unambiguous break with medicalised
models. Just as with 'queer' studies and social model based disability
studies, it leaves no doubt that traditional dominant individualised
discourses are being both challenged and rejected. Of course, as we
saw in the Joseph Rowntree Foundation study, this may create tensions
for some survivors, but it also provides the opportunity for them to be
able to think and work through alternative understandings.

At this stage, it is difficult to know whether mad studies will develop
as a separate discipline or framework, sitting alongside disability studies
on equal terms, or whether it will become part of a broader, more
inclusive disability studies. Doubtless it will prompt as much discussion,
disagreement and dialogue as disability studies and the social model of
disability already have done.

The book, *Mad Matters*, and the activities it reports and out of which
it grows, have certainly delineated a new subject of study and in doing
so offer us all much greater hope of making sense both of what goes on
within us, what affects us from outside, how the two interact and how
their relationship may be made a much more positive and humanistic
one. *Mad Matters* melds insight and understanding with making change.

Here's 'praxis' and 'conscientisation' as the radical social reformer, Paulo Freire, would understand and argue for them (Freire, 1972). I believe that it makes it possible for us to engage with disability with more confidence and on more equal terms. Mad studies offers us a rallying cry and a rallying point to inspire and energise. It also provides a detailed and diverse intellectual basis for shared understanding and collaboration between traditional bounded areas of disability and distress. I don't think that this has ever been possible for us trapped within psychiatry and its medical model – either conceptually or physically. But outside psychiatry's dominance and frameworks, in equal alliance, I believe it becomes a real possibility, even in the present difficult times of coalition between neoliberalism and an expanding psychiatric empire. Indeed this coalition gives added impetus to the building of such alliances, based on our own understandings of ourselves. It also helps break down the artificial barriers that have developed between disability and distress and their associated movements, which have made it more difficult to address their overlaps and commonalities.

Notes

[1] See Anderson, J, Sapey, B, Spandler, H (eds), 2012, *Distress or Disability?*, Lancaster: Centre for Disability Research

[2] See more at www.mindfreedom.org

'It's complicated': blending disability and mad studies in the corporatising university

Kathryn Church

Introduction

> Let's say you accept the principle that all study of past cultural practice is a contribution to the history of the present. And let's say that you also accept the testimony of your exhausted body that the present is a time of struggle. (Marc Bousquet, 1998)

Across their diversity, the contributors to this book address the question of whether and how 'mental distress' and disability do/ might come together in theory, policy and/or practice. I am pleased to be included in the collection although, at one point, I thought I might have to deliver my text in short hits of email. It was a wry nod at what has been happening to me since I became director of the School of Disability Studies at Ryerson University, Toronto.[1] After just three years, the enforced discipline of providing brief, objective and functional communications – *pressed* by relentless reporting deadlines and *compressed* into unyielding electronic templates – has eroded my ability to think and write in more fulsome ways; to complicate rather than (over) simplify; to make problematic rather than make nice (Smith, 1987). This chapter is a chance to fight back. In that spirit, I draw eagerly from the politicised word play of the psychiatric survivor activists who surround and inform me: mad; mad-identified; mad-positive.[2] The shock of these terms make you STOP...and say... 'WHAT?' And in that interruption, that space of sudden confusion, we can invoke a strand of human experience and history that pre-dates and challenges psychiatric dominance. We can seize an opening into 'something otherwise' – something we could call Mad Studies.

My task is to think about how madness became an identifiable and substantive part of the curriculum, instructional and student life in disability studies at Ryerson. Within our programme, how or where does madness fit in relation to disability? How do the two exist within the faculty/staff team of the programme itself? Are there tensions in the relationship? And can we talk about them? In the absence of much literature on this topic, I will draw from practice in the school (Miettinen et al, 2009), keenly aware that the broader context for my description is the long downsizing of education in western capitalist nations (Leitch, 2005). In the past few years, the university that hosts our programme has rapidly, explicitly and almost unquestioningly embraced 'innovation and entrepreneurialism' as the wave of the future (Gee, 2010; Levy, 2011; 2012). As the process intensifies, my practice is increasingly about the struggle for Disability Studies: as an organisational entity, and as an exemplar of older traditions of critical social analysis. It is about fulfilling administrative duties while continuing to act as an ally of the psychiatric survivor and disability movements. It is about keeping my balance as a person while living with the deep contradictions of these subjective locations. It is therefore also an emotional experience fraught with confusion, worry, discomfort, panic, disbelief, frustration, fear and rage interrupted by spurts of elation, triumph, wonder, pride and hope.

I am a feminist methodologist, which means that I take seriously my lived experience of corporate reorganisation and the re-narration of universities. Regardless of job title, my task is to analyse reflexively my compliance with – and resistance to – the redeployment of material and intellectual resources around me (Michelson, 1996). Feminist academics may indeed constitute a 'community of disagreement', as Bouchard argues (2012), but we are a community roused against these transformations (Eyerman, 2000). I draw strength from the ways that we put ourselves and our bodies on the line in our analysis: laying bare the 'melancholic exhaustion, depletion and demoralization' (Bondi, 2014) that accompany managerial roles; 'breaking the silence' around the hidden injuries of 'agency, injury and transgressive politics' (Gill, 2009; Madhok and Rai, 2012). Yet I know that our 'unwanted female bodies' are lodged within a 'masculine symbolic order' (Fotaki, 2013) that is likely to continue.

What is the relevant literature for this problematic? I have been drawn again to sociology and organisation studies, and drawn into the newer fields of critical management and academic labour studies. I read about neoliberal reason and politics (Peck, 2010; Corbett and Walker, 2013; Parker, 2014), gravitating to sources that will help me understand them as a 'controversy in action' (Belgrave et al, 2012), or a bureaucratic performance (Woolford and Nelund, 2013). I attend to 'new managerialism and higher education' (Deem, 1998), the rise of 'the schizophrenic university' (Shore, 2010) and practices of surveillance within it (Lorenz, 2012). Situated in these relations, I find it useful to read ethnographic contributions to the sociology of organisation (Morrill and Fine, 1997; Wadham and Warren, 2013; Lampei et al, 2014), ethnographies of work, and workplace ethnographies (Jordan and Dalal, 2006; Brannan et al, 2007; Edwards and Belander, 2008). Puzzling over contact with senior administrators, I read about studying elites and penetrating the 'dark side of organization' (Conte and O'Neil, 2007; Linstead et al, 2014). These disciplines and debates inform me – and this chapter – as I struggle in and against managerialism.[3]

Structure matters

The School of Disability Studies at Ryerson was established in 1999 with 25 students and the intention of improving services and support to disabled people in Ontario's educational and community service sectors. It was designed as a two-year degree-completion programme that would enable full-time workers with community college diplomas to earn a Bachelor's degree through part-time study. Some of our students live in Toronto but many come from smaller cities and towns in the province. Primarily a distance education programme, we deliver courses all year round using on-line, on-site and blended modalities. At present, about 350 students are making their way through the programme. Racially and culturally diverse, almost all of them are women aged 20 to 55. Most are also directly connected to disability worlds: through personal experience, as a sibling, a partner/spouse and/or a parent.[4] We value that connection as a form of expertise but not all of our students choose to disclose – particularly a learning disability or a mental health history.[5]

Several years ago, Disability Studies created a Minor for students from other programmes in the Faculty of Community Services: Social Work, Early Childhood Studies, and Child and Youth Care. A new Certificate in the Accessibility for Ontarians with Disabilities Act (AODA) is extending our reach into profit and non-profit organisations who must comply with the Act. With these exceptions, our basic structure has not changed. After 15 years, we remain a small school with three full-time faculty members, a shifting roster of sessional instructors, and a relatively small budget. 'A small school': what an unfortunate phrase! It leaves the impression that running Disability Studies is simple compared to other university programmes. In practice, I am almost overwhelmed by its complexity, if only because the programme operates in a zone of administrative anomalies that defies resolution.

If we are to grow – and we want that to happen – we need new appointments for early career faculty who can carry the programme into the next generation. But without significantly higher revenue, our case is not persuasive. In response to the 2013–14 university-wide budget cut, I was instructed to increase our new admissions by 50 more than the historical yearly average.[6] When I agitate with the Dean over this situation and others like it, I speak only about Disability Studies. I cannot risk provoking confusion or resistance – common reactions to madness – when I am advocating for the school. Disability Studies is the name by which we are known; it marks the issue that has most currency in the university's equity profile. I tinkered with this strategy recently in updating our marketing flyer. Now, tucked quietly into the text, is a claim that the programme is 'recognized internationally for catalytic leadership in disability arts and culture, and the recent emergence of Mad Studies'. I could go no further without a substantive discussion with my colleagues.

A disability-centric curriculum

In the historical layering of the school's development, disability came first, and remains central to how we perceive and market ourselves. Early promotional materials advertised the school as the first programme in Canada to offer a Disability Studies curriculum independent of the medical and/or rehabilitation paradigm. A sociopolitical model of disability is one of our primary theoretical alignments. Quoting the American Society for Disability Studies, our website asserts that our purpose is to examine 'the policies and practices of all societies to understand the social, rather than the physical or psychological determinants of the experience of disability…to disentangle impairments from the myths, ideology and stigma that influence social interaction and social policy'. Grappling with disabling social relations rather than individual impairment is a synthetic point for all of our instructors regardless of disciplinary training or topic area.[7] Required courses include *Rethinking Disability* (DST501), *Disability and the State* (DST502) and *Rethinking Images of Embodied Difference* (DST 525). Our most recent advertising suggests that students will receive instruction in new theoretical approaches with an orientation to disability justice.[8]

Launched in 2004, *Mad People's History* is both a variation on this theme and a break from the pattern. Popular from its inception, this course works against the dominant psychiatric paradigm by placing the perspective of the 'mad, insane, or mentally ill' at the centre of knowledge formation. Early on, we moved it from an on-site Disability Studies offering to an on-line course that is 'tied' to the School of Continuing Education (Reville, 2012; Church, 2012). This move made the course available to other programmes and the general public. The ensuing flexibility opened some interesting opportunities for community development as well as teaching: locally, through community-based workshops entitled *Talking Back to Psychiatry*, and internationally.[9] About 80 students take *Mad People's History* on-line in any given academic year. In a parallel process, the programme reinvented *Mad People's History* under the title *A History of Madness* and made it available as an upper-level Liberal Arts elective. The three sections we offer each semester draw students from across the campus: from engineering and business, theatre, journalism, and image arts, nursing and social work. Since out-of-programme/faculty courses at Ryerson earn more money per student than in-programme courses, *A History of Madness* is convincing on the bottom line.[10]

It is difficult to view these two courses as anything but a success for Disability Studies. In just a decade, using standard classroom and distance teaching modalities, the programme reaches more than 400 students a year with counter-hegemonic reinterpretations of 'mental illness'. Some of the course readings are so fresh they are being written – often by the instructors – almost simultaneously with the delivery of lectures. In our programme, mad-identified students find an intellectual and relational home which is sufficient to grow their scholarship while students with more classic disability backgrounds encounter mad course content as a new perspective. It is a heady mix, and, for the most part, everything goes along swimmingly. But how sustainable is this arrangement? Mad courses are potent offerings from Disability Studies but they are spicy alternatives not secured as part of a full-time faculty member's teaching load. Instead, as a historical artefact of the programme's development, they are boxed into Electives attached to the precarious labour of sessional instructors. Steady earners in terms of student registrations, these courses are more vulnerable to budget cuts than our core curriculum.

One of my late night worries, then, is watching exciting mad-identified doctoral candidates launch their teaching careers in the programme's mad courses, observing them build our capacity and reputation for Mad Studies all the while knowing that we will lose them to 'real' jobs unless we secure some positions that will ensure their livelihoods and future contributions. What worries me further is that the university might offer the school one position when we really need two: one identifiable as a Disability Studies hire; and one to continue inventing Mad Studies. Failing that strategic generosity, current faculty will be forced to make some difficult and potentially divisive decisions about which part of our programme to feed with fresh leadership.

Blurring the binary

What I am teasing out (at) here is a differential relation between disability and madness that is structural rather than conceptual, one that resonates with discussions of managerialism in the academy (Deem, 1998) and the casualisation of academic labour (Leitch, 2005). Currently a tension, it could become a schism. I have not narrated it that way because teaching/learning in our programme is complicated along so many other dimensions: across disabilities, for example; and between disability and race/culture in relations that are shot through with social class. There are many schisms in this matrix – real and potential – as my internal behavioural check-list testifies. 'Is it too early in the morning for that meeting? Does she read ASL (American Sign Language)? Have we ordered an interpreter? Is the interpreter certified? How are people getting there? Are we providing transit tickets? Is that building accessible – and the washroom, too? Is there room for people to pace if they need to? Could we arrange these desks in a square? Is that light too bright? Are there batteries for the microphone? Did we send that agenda electronically? Are those images described? Who is missing? Who have I overlooked? Who should speak? What wording should I use with this group? How often should we take a break? How will that action be received?'

At the same time, there is a strong tendency for practices to leap the fence. Disabled students march in the Mad Pride Parade; mad-identified students learn how to caption web-docs; deaf/Deaf students provide large-font hand-outs for class presentations; everyone learns to talk in tandem with ASL interpreters. And then there is the cross-hatching we have built into curriculum. The student debate assignment for our introductory course includes dilemmas drawn from the mad community. *Strategies for Community Building*, a required course currently taught by a disability scholar, is organised around seven steps derived from mad movement organising. Recently, using the elective called *Disability and the Law*, the school created a forum for visioning how the right to legal capacity should be recognised and supported in Ontario. During an on-site weekend, the course hosted a conference that featured panels highlighting the lived experience and expertise of three groups: people with intellectual disabilities, psychiatric survivors and people living with HIV/AIDS. Many of the disability/mad stories told that day were also stories of racism directed at Aboriginal people and immigrants.[11] In this process, participants not only identified regimes of control operating across groups, we used disability as a form of intersectional analysis.

Methodology counts

My favourite zone of disability/mad cross-over is methodological. I am thinking specifically about *Research Methods for Disability Studies*, a course I designed for the school and have taught many times. It is organised to side-step the quantitative/qualitative divide by attending to the ways in which words, images, objects and numbers can all 'count' in the production of social inquiry. As a further challenge to conventional approaches, I lead with the interpretive paradigm (a zone of student comfort) and arrive two semesters later at the dominant quantitative paradigm (a zone of fear). 'What counts as knowledge?' Working from that question, I use readings, popular movies and hands-on exercises to guide students into an unfamiliar subject matter and a set of practices. I teach the same research traditions and techniques to all of them, regardless of embodiments or subjectivities, life or work situations, community affiliations or activisms. The studies they eventually produce share a common orientation.

Of course, I am seasoned enough to know how much variation emerges in implementation. One of my colleagues conducted important research that surfaced the organising efforts of women she termed 'accidental activists' in the disability movement (Panitch, 2008). Now quite elderly, all are mothers of children with intellectual disabilities who were motivated by their children's lives to become instrumental in large scale change: deinstitutionalisation, policy-making and the development of new organisations and living arrangements. For these women, activism was situated 'naturally' as part of the work of mothering in the context of family life; not one of them comfortably identified as a disability activist.

This study is important for students in our programme, especially those who are themselves mothering children with disabilities, and who are fighting still for inclusion within and across a range of segregating systems. It does not work quite so well for mad-identified students, particularly where family trauma is at the root of individual breakdown. Nor does it translate well to the mad movement. Historically, psychiatric survivor leaders have struggled with the language, interpretations and positions taken by families of 'the mentally ill' in Ontario and elsewhere. Over the past decade, family-based organisations have led campaigns for forced hospitalisation and psychiatric treatment; they have secured legislation to facilitate Community Treatment Orders ('leash laws') that ensure medication compliance through professional surveillance in community settings (Fabris, 2011).

So, here is a place where two social movements – the family movement around intellectual disability and the mad movement – separate rather than converge and this separation makes for differential research dynamics. I have always been struck by the welcome that my colleague received from her key informants. She was not bluntly confronted over being an outsider to the lived experiences she elicited, nor was she called to account for speaking authoritatively to the history she constructed from their accounts. By contrast, as an early researcher of the mad movement, I was confronted immediately, repeatedly and justifiably over my presence and positioning as a woman of academic and other kinds of privilege (Church, 1995; Cresswell and Spandler, 2012). Still engaged and 25 years along, I no longer assert myself as a knower of the movement. I speak only to research that is collaborative in production and to my positioning as an ally in the inquiry (Costa et al, 2012).

Conclusion

> You might even say that at this historical moment, there are no 'careers' in the academy – only struggle – and activism is the modality of living with struggle...Activism improves your work. (Marc Bousquet, 1998)

I began this chapter with writer's block linked to an overdose of managerialism. That block eased somewhat as I described some key features of how one school of Disability Studies is blending disability and madness. It receded dramatically as I connected that description to literature that analyses critically the widespread corporatisation of the university. Proceeding from practice, I located a division in the academy between 'disability and distress' that is not fully addressed by discussions of identity or experience. Rather, it is an organisational separation produced by the stratified positioning of instructors during an ongoing crisis in academic labour. In other words, the tension of blending disability and madness in our programme is a neoliberal dilemma. Thinking things through in writing has crystallised an analysis that I did not set out to make. It has renewed my appreciation for the school's activist positioning with disability/mad movements, and alerted me to the possibilities for a wider array of allies than I had previously considered. Still, any way you look, 'it's complicated'.

Acknowledgements

My gratitude to the editors of this collection for their skilful guidance and almost infinite patience. As always, thank you, Timothy Diamond, for knowing how to listen.

Notes

[1] I have been a faculty member in the School of Disability Studies at Ryerson since 2002. My five-year term as director began in 2011.

[2] I refer primarily to several instructors associated with mad courses offered by the school over the past ten years: David Reville, Danielle Landry, Jijian Voronka, Jenna Reid and Sarah Snyder; also to the group associated with the event called Recovering our Stories which adds Lucy Costa and Becky Macfarlane to the group; and finally to the mad-identified students who are building scholarship in our programme year by year. These people constitute the circle of continuous dialogue, learning and action for me in this area.

[3] Ironically, in reading to understand 'directing' as a form of work, I find it difficult to stay current with the burgeoning literature of Disability Studies. My sense of separation from the field is part of the subjective experience of managerialism.

[4] Our application form asks people to describe why they are interested in Disability Studies. Most applicants narrate some aspect of personal history as their spark and ongoing motivator. We do not keep statistics that account for students by disability/illness.

[5] There are a further 350 who, for a variety of life and job-related reasons, were admitted but did not stay with the programme. The total (700 people) is a rough measure of how large the programme could be. We have more than 100 graduates many of whom have moved on to advanced degrees.

[6] We have not yet reached the target and there is a further budget cut in 2014–15. Meanwhile, a sign over the door of the University's Vice President of Finances reads: 'Not one penny more.' Point taken.

[7] The social model is also part of the 'shock' that students experience during our introductory course. At the request of the school's Student Advisory Committee,

Kim Collins, our Student Engagement Facilitator, recently crafted an FAQ entitled 'What to expect from DST 501'. Advice included: 'Expect to be challenged physically, emotionally, politically and academically…You might feel overwhelmed by the material.'

[8] In one of my many drafts of the 2104 marketing flyer for the programme, I used the term 'inter-sectionalities'. The Dean's office red-flagged it for removal as too complex for popular understanding.

[9] In consultation with Disability Studies at Ryerson, a group of service users in Edinburgh developed a course entitled Mad People's History and Identity which is by, about and for people with experience of mental health issues. It happened this way: on two occasions, they registered one group member as an international participant in Mad People's History in our programme. These students, most notably community history worker, Kirsten Maclean, not only learned our syllabus, they taught it to the larger group. From there, it was a relatively short step to a syllabus that connects more directly to the history of service users in Scotland. With the support of NHS Lothian (National Health Service) and academic allies, they filtered that course into Queen Margaret University. Free to participants, the course ran over six weeks in March 2014. More are planned.

[10] This statement belies the complexity of funding here. Several years ago, a one-time-only lump sum addition to our base budget recognised our contribution to the larger university curriculum. The ongoing course-generated registration fees go to the university and not directly to the school.

[11] We hosted this event with the Institute for Research and Development on Inclusion and Society (IRIS). Seizing an opening created by the United Nations Convention on the Rights of Persons with Disabilities, IRIS was seeking to create a new framework for the right to legal capacity with the Law Commission and the Government of Ontario.

NINETEEN

Solidarity across difference: organising for democratic alliances

Mick McKeown and Helen Spandler

Introduction

Ideas which help bring mental health users and survivors together with the wider disability movement are increasingly important given the current threats to welfare provision and the need to defend (and sometimes extend) support, both to mental health service users and disabled people. Questions arise, however, over the extent to which such understandings, and the means by which they are arrived at, might foster solidarity – both within the survivor movement itself and between the movement and potential disabled allies. This chapter will not critique the merits or otherwise of particular models and theories of distress and disability (attended to elsewhere in this book). Rather, we will explore how individuals and groups might take part in discussion and debate to arrive at a better informed politics of mental health and disability (and understanding of the links between them). This should, in turn, lead to more productive alliances within and between mental health and disability movements. This is not to say that separate and autonomous organising within specific disability groups is always ill-advised. However, a broader politics of social change also requires alliance-building across difference.

We recognise that any aspirations for alliances or consensus ought to be tempered by an appreciation that relations along the way are likely to be unsettled and unsettling (Church, 1995). As in any context where ideas and strategy are open to debate, there is an ever present possibility of the sort of acrimony or 'splitting' that can be the enemy of collective action. We suggest that ideas about deliberative democracy and relational organising might help frame strategic debates between or within different user groups about contested issues such as who is more 'deserving' of support or whether we need more or less professional intervention. We start by outlining these ideas, then explore particular settings where critical dialogue among and between psychiatric survivor activists and disability activists can be worked with. Building on our experiences of community campaigning and trade union struggles, we explore their possibilities for forging productive alliances.

The need for new dialogue

Neoliberal austerity politics and policies have created an impetus for users of welfare services to come together. Mental health service users and survivor activists are thus increasingly likely to pursue their interests within a broader disability framing (Beresford et al, 2002). Developments in welfare can, moreover, rarely be divorced from the ascendancy of the neoliberal. In a mental health context, DSM5 – aimed at the categorical definition of madness and maintenance of the professional status of psychiatrists – can be seen as arising from an unholy alliance between the latter and the American insurance industry (Lacasse, 2014).

In the UK, disabled people and people with mental health problems are disproportionately affected by cuts in support services and by measures such as the 'bedroom tax' and Work Capability Assessment. These have provoked resistance from broad-based community coalitions. Groups such as Black Triangle and Disabled People Against the Cuts present a radical framing of disability politics as protest, purposively inclusive of other welfare user groups (Scott, 2014). The catch-all nature of these initiatives is welcome and necessary but can sometimes overlook differences of identity, perspective and objectives. If these differences are not acknowledged and addressed they can undermine solidarity, particularly where one group is singled out by a government wedded to divide and rule tactics. For example, the widespread stigma against individuals deemed to have mental health problems is exacerbated by the promotion of negative public attitudes towards so-called 'welfare scroungers' or 'malingerers' (revisiting the old deserving and undeserving poor distinctions). Without more nuanced deliberations, even critical disability groups may contain members who share such views and any potential solidarity could be lost.

Arguably, the UK government – wedded to neoliberal policies – has manipulated radical movement ideas (such as the social model of disability and independent living) to undermine state provision of welfare (Morris, 2011). For example, while the independent living movement demanded support from the state for disabled people to be able to participate equally in society, on their own terms, the idea of 'independence' has been used to justify cuts to people's support budgets and to narrow eligibility for disability benefits. According to Morris, 'this mind-set is integrally linked to the promulgation of the idea that an increase in the number of people receiving 'disability' benefits is a sign of increasing 'welfare dependency' rather than a sign of...a society which makes resources available to attempt to create a level playing field' (2011, 6).

A similar fate has arguably met 'recovery' approaches in mental health. From its origins as a radical survivor-led concept, recovery can become a stick with which to beat service users (Spandler, 2014). For example, proponents of a radical notion of 'thriving' – a threshold set above mere recovery – suggest that those who do not thrive are to blame for their predicament: 'lingerers rather than recoverers...stuck in cycles of dependency, jumping on the disabled bandwagon'.[1] This phraseology unfortunately echoes the government's more general reference to welfare benefit recipients as 'skivers not strivers' and wilfully ignores the structural reasons why people may find themselves stuck with a low quality of life; not least, the iatrogenic effects of psychiatric treatment itself.

These examples illustrate some key tensions within the disability and survivor movements regarding issues such as 'welfare dependency' and ideals of 'independence'. Some disability scholars and activists, highlighting conflicting approaches to the defence of disability rights, have called for the disabled people's movement to discuss political strategy more openly (see, for example, Williams-Findlay, 2011). There is a need for this within the survivor/mental health service user movement too. It seems that more sophisticated forms of dialogue are necessary in order to air and discuss these issues more fully. We hope, through this chapter, to contribute to their development.

The case for deliberative democracy

Representative democracy, as the dominant form of democracy in western societies, can be criticised as merely the intermittent control of leadership elites; utilising largely reactionary accounts of rational choice; and constructing the citizenry as passive consumers. Deliberative democracy offers an alternative that starts from a standpoint of valuing public participation (Bohman and Rehg, 1997). Deliberative democracy is based on the idea that the way we talk about issues can help or hinder collective action and the chances of achieving positive social change. Deliberative democracy is often presented as an 'ideal-type' of communication (or 'communicative action') to facilitate effective social change (Habermas, 1986; 1987).

Deliberative democracy requires a number of conditions to be met to ensure that the best ideas for social change and action result. Democratic forums must insist on equalised power relations between contributors to the discussion and respect for difference. Reason and persuasion are privileged and participants must be prepared to enter any debate ready to change their mind in the face of persuasive argumentation. Lengthy, considered discussions are often required, to explore more fully issues and different points of view, rather than a rush to achieve dominance or a too easy consensus.

Some commentators have advocated deliberative processes as a means to ensure that the voices of subordinate groups, especially service users, are included in social policy delivery (Barnes, 2002; Elstub, 2006). Such communicative interactions are more likely to emerge within the organisational forms of newer social movements, typified by prefigurative ideals,[2] flattened hierarchies and more horizontal democracies. Indeed the growth of new social movements can be seen as resulting from public discontent with mainstream democracy and its lack of meaningful participation. To some extent then, deliberative democracy has already been adopted within social movements and disability groups, especially with regard to their relations with the state and social policy formation. Barnes (2002) lists a number of forums, including citizens' juries, disability coalitions and participatory approaches to strategy and policy that offer varied, if imperfect, forms of deliberation and participation. Latterly, there has been a growth of citizens' movements and people's assemblies which also offer alternatives to official democratic processes. Social movements such as *Occupy* have notably attempted to perform deliberative and inclusive internal decision-making and debating (Maeckelbergh, 2012). They have also included specific forums to discuss health and welfare issues (see *Asylum: the magazine for democratic psychiatry*, 2013). However, these have not always been experienced as inclusive of survivor perspectives (see for example, Ronny, 2013).

On one level, processes of deliberation have potential as a means to navigate some of the complexities and tensions within disability and mental health politics. Deliberative democracy is not, however, without its critics, and ought not to be uncritically adopted as a panacea. In the following section we outline these critiques, especially as they play out in relation to mental health and disability movement politics.

Difficulties applying deliberative democracy

Deliberative democracy, on the surface at least, seems well placed to achieve the demands of disabled people, rather than mental health activists, because of its emphasis on reason. Disability activists' demands (for ramps, adjustments etc) may seem more inherently 'reasonable' than those of mental health activists (which may seem 'unreasonable', if they are articulated at all). Habermas talks about communicative competence as a pre-requisite for meaningful dialogue and his concept of 'systematically disordered communication' relies upon notions of psycho-pathology and psychoanalysis (Habermas, 1979; 1990), which complicates the appeal of these theories for survivor movement activists. Requirements for 'competence' can also extend to privileging well-articulated speech, which can work against people with speech difficulties and people whose ability to be articulate has been affected by various impairments and treatments (especially medication). Such criticisms extend to other forms of disability. Deliberative democracy has specifically been criticised in relation to the position of learning disabled individuals in a context of user involvement (Weinberg, 2007). Clifford (2009) goes further – to suggest that embodied communication, including non-verbal expression, is excluded from the deliberative ideal.[3] In addition, Barnes (2002) notes how deliberative practices can exclude people deemed not to be legitimate participants or whose emotional expression can be used to call into question their rationality (see also Church, 1996; Gardiner, 2004).

The privileging of rationality is certainly problematic when considering the psychiatric survivor movement (members of which have been deemed inherently irrational within psychiatric processes of diagnosis and treatment). Psychiatric survivors have a long history of being silenced on grounds of their irrationality and Mary O'Hagan noted how mad people are silenced, their views effectively 'seized by the reality regulators' (1986, 32). Of course, the survivor movement does not have a monopoly on this kind of silencing of protesting voices. Disability activists will recognise the myriad institutional tactics used against the free expression of their views (Scott-Hill, 2002). The denial of reason, however, is uniquely deployed against survivor voices. Indeed, one of the rhetorical strategies of the survivor movement has been to challenge boundaries between the sane and the insane; the normal and abnormal; and the rational and irrational.

Notwithstanding these concerns, we do not think it is advisable to completely discount notions of rationality and reason. Dialogue within movements must achieve some clarity of expression and comprehensibility if ideas are to be taken forward. Moreover, arguably, it is equally oppressive to deny capacity for rationality to people deemed irrational by others. Coleman charts the extent to which psychiatric survivor activists have 'significantly contributed to a reconfiguring of the relationship between madness and rationality' and 'forcefully nullified entrenched stereotypes of their incapacity through vibrant political expression' (2008, 341). She concludes that users of mental health services must be seen as holding 'a rational capacity to speak credibly about their condition and their treatment and...the science of psychiatry' (Coleman, 2008, 341).

In this way, the psychiatric survivor/service user movement has often developed 'collectively reasonable' demands (Pilgrim and Tomasini, 2012). What might appear irrational or unreasonable on an individual level can be articulated differently when issues are discussed openly and collectively. This relates to the function of many new social movements in translating personal troubles into public issues. For example, individuals who demanded the right to harm themselves may have initially been considered irrational. However, the self-harm movement collectively developed the idea that self-harm may be a valid coping strategy and pioneered 'harm minimisation' strategies which have become increasingly accepted within practice (Spandler and Warner, 2007; *Asylum: the magazine for democratic psychiatry*, 2013).

It could also be argued that neither consensus nor rationality is necessary for positive social action or change to take place. This might especially be the case for mental health activism where the complexity of available perspectives means consensus can be difficult to achieve and rationality itself is contested. Indeed mental health activism may often be characterised as much by emotional as rational discussion, as is probably the case with other movements seeking redress for perceived disadvantage or oppression (Barker, 2001; Taylor and Whittier, 1995; Jasper, 1997). People's experiences of oppression and being discredited can fuel powerful feelings of anger and frustration, leading to recalcitrant behaviour in meetings, and this can complicate any idealised notions of communicative action (Hodge, 2005a). This urges modifications to Habermas's idealistic notion of the public sphere, to include alternative, perhaps 'wilder' counter-publics. In this vein, Gardiner (2004, 45) invokes the work of Bakhtin which 'strives to grasp the experiential and affective qualities of human embodiment within diverse lived contexts, and is sensitive to the full range of human relations that are not simply cognitive or narrowly "rational"'.

In this vein, feminist critiques of deliberative democracy contend that the emphasis on *reason* is masculinist and downplays the importance of factors such as care or kindness. As a result of these concerns, feminists such as Iris Young have argued for a more nuanced consideration of factors such as difference, emotionality *and* reason (Young, 1997; 2001). She sees difference as a resource 'for a discussion based politics in which participants aim to co-operate, reach understanding and do justice' (1997, 383).

Indeed, despite the negative consequences of being denied opportunities to communicate freely in the mainstream, there may be certain advantages to being an oppressed group because: 'the oppressed are free to know differently' (O'Hagan 1986, 40). Bringing together the different forms of knowing of both survivors and disabled people may be unsettling but ultimately helpful to us all. Moreover, perhaps democrats should broaden the scope of reasonableness at the same time as engineering more inclusive spaces for deliberants to occupy (Drake, 2007). In this vein, noisy forms of dissent and protest, raucous recalcitrance and rebellion can be conceived as *implicitly* reasonable as long as we make the time to properly attend both to the message and the motivation, seeking a deeper understanding of each other's experiences and wishes. Of course, this requires everyone present to be patient and make concerted efforts at understanding, even if others' contributions provoke disagreement or negative reactions in the first instance.

Therefore, deliberative democracy still offers possibilities, as long as we take on board these concerns. After all, positive change is more likely to occur when emotion and reason come together. Rational debate and deliberation is still important, but needs to be engaged in more ethically and sensitively, through what Barnes calls 'care-full deliberation' (Barnes, 2012, 160). This idea is especially important given the very real welfare consequences of these debates for individual disabled people and service users. This means attending equally to relational as well as rational forms of deliberation (Ryfe, 2002).

Relational forms of organising

Scott-Hill (2002) has advocated relational politics in a context of disability activism as a means to avoid the trap of reinventing forms of power and dominance in the course of challenging oppression. She argues for more relational approaches which tackle 'reified notions of impairment and disability, *and policy and politics*' (Scott-Hill, 2002, 407 emphasis in original). Effectively, this boils down to recognising that the oppression and disadvantage experienced by disabled people always has a social-relational aspect; it is *people* who oppress each other. It is worth noting that this also resonates with the 'relational' social model of disability advanced by Carol Thomas and the notion of psycho-emotional disablement (Reeve, 2004; Thomas, 2007), as discussed elsewhere in this book. Therefore, transforming our social relations – the way we are with each other – can be an important prefigurative dimension to tackling wider structural inequalities.

More relational organising may help the active participation of particular oppressed groups and enhance the quality of their involvement experience. For example, the appeal of deliberative democracy for disability activists and mental health survivors could be enhanced if it were to bring in notions of inter-dependence and shared vulnerability as counterpoints to simplistic ideals of autonomy and rationality (Barnes, 2012). Equally, these ideas could also help inform new ways of organising, and more care-full deliberative practices. For example, Ng (2011, 10) argues that, in essence, organising should be framed by positive emotions towards comrades: 'love that is steeped in the collective sense of justice, solidarity and hopefulness'. This connects with Barnes' (2008; 2012) plea for deliberative forums more fully to accommodate participants' emotions, such that aspirations for social justice reflect an ethical caring for each other. In this way, the relationship between the personal and political is revisited, drawing on feminist ideas for relational organising models which should ultimately be supportive of deliberative communication.

Arguably, more relational types of organising may thrive in smaller protected spaces, and political activism often emerges out of the cooperation and peer resources evident in support groups and self-help settings (Parr, 2008; Noorani, 2013). However, while this is important and necessary, an argument can also be made for cross-sectional alliances that seek more directly to influence the state and its institutions. Trade unions are one set of organisations that retain a commitment to wider influence and also hold the possibility of organising deliberative mass-participation alongside smaller, more contained forums. Unfortunately, while there has been a longstanding concern with participative and workplace democracy among trade unions (Voss, 2010), there has been little work considering the applicability of deliberative forums and relational organising as discussed here. The next section addresses their potential in more detail.

Alliances between workers and disability movements

There are many areas of common interest between unions and disability/survivor movements, such as the defence of services and welfare provision; a commitment to equality and rights; a shared interest in better living standards and in the inequities of precarious labour for disabled people. These common interests offer key opportunities to develop and deepen solidarity. Contemplating the experiences of service users *and* staff within services, reveals the ways in which both may feel constrained and alienated, and provides 'ways in' to identifying other mutual concerns. These discussions may also break down the (often) artificial division between 'workers' and 'service users', given that many service users will have worked in services and many workers will have suffered mental health problems (McKeown et al, 2014)

Recently, groups like Disabled People against the Cuts and Black Triangle have worked with the Scottish Trade Union Congress (TUC) on joint campaigning, and this led to trade union funding to support disabled activists from further afield to engage in protests, such as attending the large TUC anti-cuts demonstration in London in November 2011 (Scott, 2014). Another benefit of public sector trade unions is that they bring together workers from across different service sectors (such as mental health and disability) and can potentially develop forums to discuss, and take action about, common issues of shared humanity. Indeed alliances are more likely to happen in the first place, and then to be effective, if workers' and users' interests coincide. For example, trade union activists and local user groups mobilised a successful campaign to defend threatened day care services in Salford, Greater Manchester, England in 2013 (Salford against the Cuts, 2013).

These kinds of (more defensive) struggles, however, rarely engage with more radical critiques of the mental health system, or systems of care in general. What solidarity there has been has rarely been harnessed towards truly transformative ends. When such alliances do occur, they highlight some of the tensions between worker and service user standpoints and suggest opportunities for deeper solidarity, grounded in more critical understandings of each other's politics. For example, while day care services are valued by many individual local service users and user groups, these systems of care have often been criticised by more radical mental health and disability organisations for being pseudo-institutionalising, controlling and paternalistic. In addition, there is a long history within the disability movement of critiquing professional practice as well as division over issues such as 'care' and paternalism. This is not dissimilar to differences in the psychiatric survivor movement between people who want to abolish psychiatry and people who want a transformed/much better psychiatry.

While struggles to defend services often unite (at least some sections of) the care workforce and service users, in other contexts workers and service users may have different (often conflicting) perspectives. Take the following example. Disabled people have campaigned against the use of impersonal devices, such as 'hoists' for lifting, as disregarding their human rights and personal dignity. On the other hand, public sector unions have defended care workers from having manually to lift clients, because of long-term back problems among workers (Spandler, 2004). Both perspectives may be 'right' and 'reasonable' in their own terms. Workers should not have to incur back problems in the course of their work and disabled people should not have to suffer undignified procedures. However, it is only when these perspectives are brought into dialogue that such issues can be aired, people can appreciate each other's position, and create mutually beneficial solutions. This is why we have previously advanced the idea of 'paradoxical spaces' that is, social spaces where seemingly conflicting positions, which may both be right, can co-exist in dialogue (Spandler, 2009). It is precisely because of the need to work through these tensions that sustained and open dialogue is necessary, rather than the creation of simplistic 'for or against' solutions which ultimately create divisions and splits, within and between movements.

Limitations of union democracy

In our experience, despite the many positive features of union democracy, current organising deficits mean that union meetings involve activists talking to activists only, missing out grass-roots members (let alone wider communities of interest) entirely. The labour movement has delegate conferences and Trade Councils; though the former are now increasingly stage-managed or debate a fairly narrow range of issues, and the latter are arguably a pale shadow of their former selves, prone to domination by the ultra-left. Furthermore, unions often engage in simple representative democracy, voting 'for or against' motions where consensus actually masks the complex deliberation of members. Of course, these strategies are sometimes necessary when taking decisive action, but time is rarely spent deliberating over tricky issues and their nuances. Such tricky matters might include the complexities of disability and distress; the 'asymmetrical' nature of solidarity between workers and service users; or the ways in which worker focused employment relations might be a turn-off for community allies, many of whom are worse off than the public sector workforce (McKeown et al, 2014).

A case can certainly be made that the traditional 'left' and trade unions have failed to fully appreciate the sheer depth of the critique of professional practice mounted by disabled people and psychiatric survivors (Sedgwick, 1982; Foster and Fosh, 2010; McKeown et al, 2014). As a result, unions have often taken for granted levels of support for action in defence of welfare institutions. In addition, disabling barriers and attitudes may still exist in traditional trade unions and labour politics (Williams-Findlay, 2011). One of the problems with public sector unions is that they tend to separate workers' interests from those of service users; even if the outcome of their disputes would arguably benefit service users (for example, better trained, supported and valued workers are likely to be more motivated and better at their job). This means that ill thought-out union inspired action, which does not meaningfully engage with wider communities of interest, could damage unity. Moreover, with the increasing focus on welfare consumerism and user involvement, service user action might be equally as powerful (at least rhetorically) as workers' actions. In addition, there may be alternative forums to bring together workers, disabled people and survivors; for example, multi-stakeholder cooperatives and other kinds of 'mutuals', or, more obliquely, critical pedagogy or action research projects (McKeown and Jones, 2012). In addition, social movements do not necessarily require trade unions to be effective, although they are more effective and influential when they work together.

Notwithstanding these caveats, trade unions – if they can reinvigorate and re-position themselves – are still well-placed to wield effective power to secure the rights of disabled people. They are, for example, able to mobilise both financial and human resources into campaigns, and can wield political and economic power through negotiation or industrial action. Assessment of the power of the public sector workforce needs to take into account ways in which employment relations are complicated by practical and ethical concerns regarding industrial action and strikes. In some sense, this renders the public sector unions uniquely powerful. Despite workers in this sector being relatively disinclined to take industrial action, the very threat of action has historically proven to be a very potent strategy. In the UK context, the employer is ultimately the government who are also responsible for wider welfare reform and, despite a relative decline in influence, unions are still present in many key national and international forums close to government. Therefore, industrial relations in this territory are always intensely politicised.

Union revitalising strategies

Ideas about developing alliances with trade unions have intermittently figured in the strategic thinking of disability movement activists and scholars. For example, the veteran disability rights activist, Vic Finkelstein (1999) argued that care workers would be better seeing themselves as 'professions allied to the community' and he also called for a trade union to represent disabled people. Other disability activists envisaged a role for trade unions in supporting disability struggles (Campbell and Oliver, 1996; Hales, 1996). In addition, the Mental Patients Union in the UK called itself a 'union' and some of the early membership sought to get official union recognition, although the TUC weren't interested (Spandler, 2006). Similarly, two highly influential publications – *In and Against the State* (London Edinburgh Weekend Return Group, 1979) and *Beyond the Fragments* (Rowbotham et al, 1980) – arose out of grass-roots organising initiatives involving trade unionists, both of which attempted to reconcile the interests of public sector workers and service users in a context of promoting participation (Beresford, 2002b).

More recently, various unions have embarked upon a range of renewal tactics aimed at union growth and revitalisation of organising. Arguably, the best of these strategies aim to rebuild a sense of community within the union and to mobilise union resources and interests into local communities. Such initiatives have been referred to as 'reciprocal community trade unionism' or 'social movement unionism' (Tattersall, 2010). Some of these emphasise distinctly relational and rational methods of connecting with union members and community activists. For example, Unison[4] activists in the UK have taken up relational approaches to strengthening social ties between union members (Saundry and McKeown, 2013); Unite[5] has developed community membership branches; and some unions have been involved in broad-based coalitions such as London Citizen's and Living Wage campaigns (Wills and Simms, 2006). These have a direct bearing on the disability and mental health constituency through mutual interest in the defence of welfare, but also in terms of a general social justice mission to tackle inequalities and address the concerns of people at the margins of the economy and labour market.

It is not too much of a stretch for union revitalisation to reach out from public service industries into communities with relational and deliberative democracy as its goal; that is, the development of democratic structures and processes, inclusive of worker *and* service user voices, to discuss how public sector work is organised (McKeown et al, 2014). Alliances forged between unions and disability/survivor groups could bring in more care-full deliberation that moves beyond simple economistic or workplace concerns (such as workers' pay and conditions, important though they are) to embrace critical thinking and diverse perspectives and how this might relate to strategising and campaigning.

Some unions already have in place strong foundations for recognising and supporting difference and attending to diversity and the voice of the marginalised in their own internal structures; such as self-organised groupings within the UK public sector union, Unison (Colgan and Ledwith, 2002). Union renewal strategies are typically linked with critiques of representative versus participatory forms of democracy, and have increasingly brought forward issues of diversity; notably gender and race, but also sexuality and latterly disability (Humphrey, 1998; 1999; 2000a; 2000b). The growth of local resistance to neoliberal policies, for example people's assemblies and increasing union interest in models of community unionism, are of particular interest because they potentially prefigure new forms of deliberative democracy within trade union cultures of participation.

The member-led Edge Fund[6] offers another potential democratic alternative – funding radical community activism through disbursing grants to community organisations and campaigns which would not ordinarily receive funding from mainstream sources. Key constituencies include the health and disability sectors, and members typically also affiliate to other social movement groups. Recently the Edge Fund has supported movement activism by Disabled People Against the Cuts, Black Triangle and the WOW Petition (all campaigning around the impact of welfare reforms for disabled people); Shafted (an HIV performance group); Quiet Riot (a militant campaigning group led by people without speech); and ReVision (a radical mental health group based in Liverpool). The latter group will be working on a creative writing initiative which will bring local trade union and survivor activists together. Organisations like the Edge Fund could be in a position to forge arm's-length alliances with trade unions that could begin to mobilise union resources to the support of disability and survivor-led causes. Such an alliance, for example, could democratically 'crowdsource' donations from affiliated union branches to disability and survivor groups who may be potential allies. Although such funding would be proportionally small for each branch, it would effectively align trade unionists with local activists and develop foundations for future solidarity. Better still, these links need not stop at merely funding transactions; instead they could be the starting point for more deeply relational alliances (Cresswell, 2009; McKeown et al, 2014).

Conclusions

We have argued that alliances between disability, survivor movements and trade unions represent one possibility for more dialogue and action. We suggest that these alliances could be based on deliberative practices which take on board more emotional communications (via the expansion of notions of reason/rationality) and develop more relational types of organising. Currently, it would be naïve to pretend that such alliances are ideal, fully-formed, or that communication therein is completely open. Any solidarity developed between health and social care workers and service user groups is probably best described as imperfect, and any cooperation between them will likely precipitate unsettling conversations. However, the vicissitudes of neoliberalism makes these forms of alliance building ever more necessary. This context is arguably becoming a more hostile one for both workers *and* service users, whose standards and conditions of conditions of living are worsening (Clarke, 2007). This situation is likely to have an increasingly disabling impact on both and may ultimately undermine any fixed differences between workers and service users. In this context, health and social care workplaces are increasingly becoming places where industrial action and community activism come together to resist the burgeoning hegemony of neoliberalism: challenging specific policies which disproportionately affect our lives. This situation will inevitably afford further possibilities to stand together and the means for establishing deeper solidarity is possible through the forms of organising dialogue we have discussed here.

If developing these social spaces is a work in progress, then, arguably, they should flourish where survivor and disability activism coincides with willing trade unionists, critically engaged in their communities. Bringing together alliances of disabled/survivor activists, workers and trade unions does not have to be derailed by contradictory forces, as long as these tensions are acknowledged and faced up to. Moreover, these endeavours may also help forge new understandings of madness and disability.

Notes

[1] See Elementalists website: www.elemental.org.uk/#!__human-rights

[2] In this context, 'prefigurative' refers to the ideal that social movements often try to embody (in their organisation and social relationships) the changes which they want to see in the world

[3] In this regard, it is notable that recent 'occupy' movements explicitly utilised hand gestures as a way of enabling people to contribute in different ways to discussions. See, for example, occupytogether.wikispot.org/Hand_Gestures.

[4] Large public sector trade union representing mainly health and local government workforce, see www.unison.org.uk/

[5] Large general union, representing workers across the public and private sector workforce, see www.unitetheunion.org/

[6] For more information about the Edge Fund, see http://edgefund.org.uk/ and the on-line article 'Edge Fund: a new grassroots fund for social justice' on the Open Democracy website, www.opendemocracy.net/ourkingdom/edge-fund/edge-fund-new-grassroots-fund-for-social-justice

TWENTY

Beyond the horizon: the landscape of madness, distress and disability

Jill Anderson, Helen Spandler and Bob Sapey

This book has explored the distinctions and boundaries between madness/distress and disability, and has highlighted some potential bridges between them. Through bringing together key scholars and activists, from the disabled people's and survivor movements, and from disability studies and mad studies, we wanted to build on established knowledge to generate fresh learning, support the formation of alliances and even inspire action. Our project seemed both timely and considerably overdue.

We were conscious that engagement at these boundaries brings risks: of talking at cross purposes, of semantic entanglements, intellectualisations and the fuelling of misunderstandings and misperceptions. Common words like madness or disability resonate differently in diverse contexts and are interconnected, so that 'using one particular word leads more easily to some words than to others' (Biesta, 2010, 540); impairment to mental illness, for example. We were aware that our attempts, and those of our contributors, to articulate complex issues, especially where there is disagreement, might sow the seeds of conflict, confusion or inertia. Rather than bringing people closer, there was a danger of reaping greater distance and division.

Yet we wanted to promote understanding and appreciation of each other's positions and perspectives, and we felt that highlighting these complexities would ultimately be helpful. As we have seen, differences and disagreements exist not only between people in the mental health user/survivor movements on the one hand, and the disabled people's movement on the other, but within those movements too. Moreover, these debates take on a different flavour and importance as they are refracted through diverse welfare contexts. For example, this book includes reflections on the impact of psychiatric colonialism in India; welfare collectivist traditions in Western Europe; and the individual rights focus which has characterised activism in the US.

We have tried to build on earlier initiatives (Plumb, 1994; Sayce, 2000; Beresford et al, 2010; Anderson et al, 2012) to create new opportunities for learning in the borderlands of madness, distress and disability. Consciously inhabiting that territory while pulling this book together, we are left with many unanswered questions. Each and every chapter has significantly increased our understanding of the issues. Yet we remain profoundly ambivalent about some of the issues we originally set out to resolve in this book. For example, we still haven't decided whether we think it is helpful to situate madness/distress within a disability framework and we still can't decide whether we should 'apply' the social model of disability to madness/distress; whether it needs adapting to a mental health context; or whether users/survivors need to develop their own specific and complementary framework. Indeed we are beginning to think, paradoxically, that all of these may be necessary.

We are attracted by the pragmatism offered by Tina Minkowitz's and David Webb's contributions, which effectively incorporate users/survivors into a disability rights framework. At the same time, we find ourselves drawn back to the challenges articulated by Anne Plumb, and by Nev Jones and Timothy Kelly, who express a concern that, until mental health/survivor specific issues have been fully attended to, such efforts are premature. We, like Kathryn Church, Peter Beresford and other contributors, are encouraged by the emergence of 'mad studies'. Yet, reflecting on the core concerns of this book, questions remain about the place of mad studies within disability studies. As mad studies gradually orientates itself – within, beside and outside of disability studies – resolving that is also perhaps neither desirable nor (yet) possible.

Such questions continue to gnaw away at us, and not just in our waking hours. Sometimes we have found ourselves thinking, or dreaming, in metaphors about the 'problem of impairment' and we often felt that we were going round in circles. On occasion, we have come away from meetings and conversations more confused than when we started. We didn't want to iron these confusions out, pretend they don't exist, or to impose a premature closure. We assume that some of our own confusions will be shared by others, and look forward to further dialogue. Therefore, rather than offering a summary or conclusion to this book, we wanted to set the scene for that ongoing conversation.

Although our ultimate aim was to inspire greater engagement and solidarity, it is worth noting that certainty and resolution are not requirements for taking the struggle forward in a positive direction.

After all, activists don't have to wait around for the 'right' or 'correct' theory – one that solves all the challenges that they face – before they act to defend or advance their collective interests. Indeed some of the most powerful learning takes place in the process of articulating the struggle against oppression or initiating social change – when people attempt to make sense of what is happening to them and to formulate a plan for action (Foley, 1999).

Contributors to this book have drawn on thinking developed in the disabled people's movement, the mental health survivor movements and both 'disability studies' and 'mad studies'; which have their origins in the above movements, and continue to engage with movement politics. Each of those might be conceived of as an individual 'community of practice' (Wenger, 1998), characterised by mutual engagement, a joint enterprise, and a developing shared repertoire of experiences, tales, tools and approaches to recurrent challenges, such as the social model of disability (see Lawthom with Chataika, 2012). If these are distinct communities of practice, then the concerns of this book might be characterised as the broader 'landscape of practice' within which they are located, and through which each of us wends our own way (Wenger-Trayner and Wenger-Trayner, 2014).

Within such a landscape each diverse practice has its own way of knowing and, crucially, no one practice should subsume another (Wenger-Trayner and Wenger-Trayner, 2014). Boundaries between practices, which reflect sustained histories of shared learning, have to be approached with sensitivity because knowledge can be colonised or misused. Yet boundaries can be places of unanticipated learning too, where a community can expand or even challenge what it perceives to be important. In that sense it can be fruitful to create 'intentional moments of boundary crossing and boundary encounters' (Wenger-Trayner and Wenger-Trayner, 2014, 7).

We think that there is ample evidence of that kind of learning in this book, as contributors have sought to bring the social model of disability into a dialogue with new areas such as sexuality or trauma studies: developing arguments which cast light back on the social model of disability itself, applying ideas about psycho-social disablism, introducing news ideas about attributed impairments and highlighting bridging practices (as exemplified by the neurodiversity movement).

For each of us, on our trajectory through a landscape of practice, our learning is influenced by practices with which we identify, as well as those about which we are in two minds, or intentionally bypass. We made efforts – especially in our first chapter – to engage with some tricky issues which we might have been tempted to skirt around;

what Sibbett and Thompson (2008) term *nettlesome knowledge* which, if grasped, might 'sting'. That said, there may be other points where perspectives have seemed too far apart to be engaged with; as the boundaries were still too obscured. So, inevitably, there are absences in this book – places where we have not gone – through active choice, lack of space or ambivalence; some we are aware of, others may be apparent only to others.

Obvious omissions include, for example, a range of other boundary 'conditions' such as learning disabilities, dementia and chronic illness. In relation to the latter, medically unexplained symptoms, and other 'syndromes' – such as myalgic encephalomyelitis (ME) and chronic fatigue syndrome (CFS) – are worth exploring as potential bridging concepts and experiences. These conditions are often seen as occupying another part of this borderland between the physical and the mental, especially as people with these experiences have often been inappropriately psychiatrised. Exploring related struggles around these issues would arguably have brought even more of the landscape of practice into view. It would also have highlighted other boundary issues, tensions and challenges; developing the discussion in new and unique ways; and potentially enriching our understanding of madness/distress, disability *and* illness. This seems to be an important next step.

The chapters in this book highlight three distinct modes of inhabiting a landscape of practice, and developing our identities in it: engagement, imagination and alignment (Wenger-Trayner and Wenger-Trayner, 2014). Individual contributions bear witness to the power of direct *engagement*: with ideas, with each other and with wider social movements and policies. They also shed light on the power of *imagination* – identifying with a group of people on the other side of the world or in the twittersphere, for example – to see the landscape, and one's role in it, through a new lens. Finally, central to what we have been grappling with here, is the question of *alignments* (across movements, fields of study and nations), in relation to evolving law and policies. We have been writing for a readership which will include those who identify as disabled, mad, distressed, mentally ill; as all, some, or maybe none of these.

This final section has drawn on a social theory of learning. Traditional education can conspire to hide the importance of boundaries 'under an illusion of seamless applicability across contexts' (Wenger-Trayner and Wenger-Trayner, 2014, 7). While this approach can feel reassuring – both to learners and to educators – it fails to harness the power of boundaries as learning assets. Arguably, it also fails to reflect the times in which we live: 'a pedagogy for uncertain times has itself to be uncertain. It is open, it is daring, it is risky, it is itself, unpredictable' (Barnett, 2007, 137). If this book has functioned as a boundary encounter, perhaps it can move forward in the role of a boundary object, supporting a kind of 'boundary-oriented pedagogy' (Wenger-Trayner and Wenger-Trayner, 2014) and creating a focus for the on-going engagement of perspectives. The knowledge generated may be *unsettling* (Church, 1995) or *troublesome* (Perkins, 1999). Our efforts will be worth it, however, if these discussions increase our collective understanding of the issues at stake. There is much still to do: engagements not yet entered; identities not yet imagined; and alignments still to be negotiated and explored.

References

American Psychiatric Association, 2013, *Diagnostic and Statistical Manual of Mental Disorders*, 5th edn, Washington, DC: American Psychiatric Association

Anderson, J, Sapey, B, Spandler, H (eds), 2012, Distress or Disability?, Lancaster: Centre for Disability Research, www.lancaster.ac.uk/fass/centres/cedr/publications/Anderson_Sapey_and_Spandler_eds_2012.pdf

Angell, M, 2011, The epidemic of mental illness: Why?, *New York Review of Books* 58, 11, www.nybooks.com/issues/2011/jun/23/

Angermeyer, M, Matschinger, H, 2005, Causal beliefs and attitudes to people with schizophrenia: Trend analysis based on data from two population surveys in Germany, *British Journal of Psychiatry* 186, 3, 331–4

Antonetta, S, 2005, *A Mind Apart: Travels in a Neurodiverse World*, New York: Tarcher/Penguin

Arciniegas, D, Topkoff, J, Held, K, Frey, L, 2001, Psychosis due to neurologic conditions, *Current Treatment Options in Neurology* 3, 4, 347–64

Arya, S, 2007, Govt to study DNA link to suicides, *Times of India*, 27 September 27

AS-IF (Asperger Syndrome Information and Features), 2007, Neurodiversity now, http://web.archive.org/web/20070526035709/http://www.as-if.org.uk/ndn/index.htm

Asylum: the magazine for democratic psychiatry (2012) *Anti-capitalism and Mental Health* Autumn, 19, 3

Asylum: the magazine for democratic psychiatry (2013) *Self harm: Minimising Harm, Maximising Hope* Summer, 20, 2

Babiak, P, Hare, R, 2006, *Snakes in Suits: When Psychopaths Go to Work*, New York: Regan Books

Baggs, A, 2006, *Things We learned From Therapy and Doctors (by the Amorpha Household)*, ballastexistenz.wordpress.com

Baker, A, 1991, Madness the forgotten way, *Asylum: An International Magazine for Democratic Psychiatry* 5, 2, 32–3

Baker, A, 2004, *Invisible at the End of the Spectrum: Shadows, Residues, 'BAP', and the Female Asperger's Experience*, www.avaruthbaker.com

Bakhtin, M, 1981, *The dialogic imagination: Four essays by MM Bakhtin*, M Holquist (ed) Austin, TX: Texas University Press

Bapu Trust, 2010, *Mad lives India*, Kavita Nair (ed), Pune, India: Published by the Bapu Trust

Barker, C, 2001, Fear, laughter and collective power: The making of solidarity at the Lenin shipyard in Gdansk, Poland, August 1980, in J Goodwin, J Jasper, F Polletta (eds) *Passionate Politics*, 175–94, Chicago, IL: University of Chicago Press

Barker, M, 2011a, Existential sex therapy, *Sexual and Relationship Therapy* 26, 1, 33–47

Barker, M, 2011b, De Beauvoir, Bridget Jones' pants and vaginismus, *Existential Analysis* 22, 2, 203–16

Barker, M, 2013a, Consent is a grey area? A comparison of understandings of consent in *50 Shades of Grey* and on the BDSM blogosphere, *Sexualities* 16, 8, 896–914

Barker, M, 2013b, *Rewriting the Rules: An Integrative Guide to Love, Sex and Relationships*, London: Routledge

Barker, M, 2013c, What can we all learn about sex from The Sessions?, *Rewriting the Rules*, rewritingtherules.wordpress.com

Barker, M, in press, Mindfulness in sex therapy, in Z Peterson (ed) *Handbook of Sex Therapy*, Hoboken, NJ: Wiley-Blackwell

Barker, M, Langdridge, D, 2013, Sexuality and embodiment in relationships, in S Iacovou, E Van Deurzen (eds) *Existential Perspectives on Relationship Therapy*, 54–67, Basingstoke: Palgrave Macmillan

Barker, M, Richards, C, 2013, Brief report: What does Bancroft's *Human Sexuality and its Problems* tell us about current understandings of sexuality?, *Feminism and Psychology* 23, 2, 243–51

Barker, M, Richards, C, Jones, R, Bowes-Catton, H, Plowman, T, 2012, *The Bisexuality Report: Bisexual Inclusion in LGBT Equality and Diversity*, Milton Keynes: The Open University, Centre for Citizenship, Identity and Governance

Barker, M, Gill, R, Harvey, L, in press, *Mediated Intimacy: Sex Advice in Media Culture*, London: Polity Press

Barnes, C, 2000, A working social model? Disability, work and disability politics in the 21st century, *Critical Social Policy* 20, 4, 441–57

Barnes, C, Mercer, G (eds), 1997, *Doing Disability Research*, Leeds: The Disability Press

Barnes, C, Mercer, G, 2004, *Disability Policy and Practice: Applying the Social Model*, Leeds: The Disability Press

Barnes, C, Mercer, G, Shakespeare, T, 1999, *Exploring Disability: A Sociological Introduction*, Cambridge: Polity

Barnes, C, Oliver, M, Barton, L (eds), 2002, *Disability Studies Today*, Cambridge: Polity

Barnes, M, 2002, Bringing difference into deliberation? Disabled people, survivors and local governance, *Policy and Politics* 30, 3, 319–31

Barnes, M, 2008, Passionate participation: Emotional experiences and expressions in deliberative forums, *Critical Social Policy* 28, 4, 461–81

Barnes, M, 2012, *Care in Everyday Life: An Ethic of Care in Practice*, Bristol: Policy Press

Barnes, M, Harrison, S, Mort, M, Shardlow, P, 1999, *Unequal Partners: User groups and community care*, Bristol: Policy Press

Barnett, R, 2007, *A Will To Learn: Being a Student in an Age of Uncertainty*, Milton Keynes: Open University Press

Barton, L (ed), 1997, *Disability Studies: Past, Present and Future*, Leeds: Disability Press

Bateson, G, Jackson, D, Haley, J, Weakland, J, 1956, Towards a theory of schizophrenia, *Behavioral Science* 1, 4, 251–64

BCODP (British Council of Disabled People), 1981, *The Social Model of Disability*, Derby: BCODP, www.bcodp.org.uk

Belgrave, L, Celaya, A, Gurses, S, Boutwell, A, Fernandez, A, 2012, Meaning of political controversy in the classroom: A dialogue across the podium, *Symbolic Interaction*, 25, 1, 68–87

Bentall, R, 2003, *Madness Explained: Psychosis and Human Nature*, London: Penguin

Bentall, R, 2006, Madness explained: Why we must reject the Kraepelinian paradigm and replace it with a complaint oriented approach to understanding mental illness, *Medical Hypotheses* 66, 2, 220–33

Bentall, R, Fernyhough, C, 2008, Social predictors of psychotic experiences: Specificity and psychological mechanisms, *Schizophrenia Bulletin* 34, 6, 1012–20

Beresford, P, 2000, What have madness and psychiatric system survivors got to do with disability and disability studies?, *Disability and Society* 15, 1, 167–72

Beresford, P, 2002a, Thinking about 'mental health': Towards a social model, *Journal of Mental Health* 11, 6, 581–84

Beresford, P, 2002b, Participation and social policy: Transformation, liberation or regulation?, *Social Policy Review* 14, 265–87

Beresford, P, 2004, Madness, distress, research and a social model, in C Barnes, G Mercer (eds) *Implementing the Social Model of Disability: Theory and Research*, 208–22, Leeds: The Disability Press

Beresford, P, Gifford, G, 1996, Psychiatric system survivors and the Disabled People's Movement, in B Walker (ed) *Disability Rights Symposium: A Symposium of the European Regions*, pp 83–4, Hampshire: Hampshire Coalition of Disabled People

Beresford, P, Wilson, A, 2002, Genes spell danger: Mental health service users/survivors, bioethics and control, *Disability and Society* 17, 5, 541–53

Beresford, P, Gifford, G, Bowden, J, 1995, Psychiatric system survivors and the Disabled People's Movement, *Disability Awareness In Action* 23, 4

Beresford, P, Gifford, G, Harrison, C, 1996, What has disability got to do with psychiatric survivors?, in J Reynolds, J Read (eds) *Speaking Our Minds: Personal Experience of Mental Distress and its Consequences*, pp 209–14, Basingstoke: Palgrave

Beresford, P, Harrison, C, Wilson, A, 2002, Mental health, service users and disability: Implications for future strategies, *Policy and Politics* 30, 3, 387–96

Beresford, P, Nettle, M, Perring, R, 2010, *Towards a Social Model of Madness or Distress? Exploring What Services Users Say*, York: Joseph Rowntree Foundation

Berghs, M, 2011, Embodiment and emotion in Sierra Leone, *Third World Quarterly* 32, 8, 1399–417

Berman, L, 2011, *Loving Sex: The Book of Joy and Passion*, London: Dorling Kindersley

Berne, P, 2008, Disability, dancing, and claiming beauty, in R Solinger, M Fox, K Irani (eds) *Telling Stories to Change the World: Global Voices on the Power of Narrative to Build Community and Make Social Justice Claims*, pp 201–12, New York: Routledge

Berry, M, Barker, M, 2015, Sex therapy, in C Richards, M Barker (eds) *Handbook of the Psychology of Sexuality and Gender*, Basingstoke: Palgrave Macmillan

Biesta, G, 2010, Learner, student, speaker: Why it matters how we call those we teach, *Educational Philosophy and Theory* 42, 5–6, 540–52

Blume, S, 2009, *The Artificial Ear: Cochlear Implants and the Culture of Deafness*, Rutgers: Rutgers University Press

Bohman, J, Rehg, W, 1997, Introduction, in J Bohman, W Rehg (eds) *Deliberative Democracy: Essays on Reason and Politics*, Cambridge, MA: MIT Press, ix–xxx

Bondi, L, 2014, Feeling insecure: A personal account in a psychoanalytic voice, *Social and Cultural Geography* 15, 3, 332–50

Bouchard, D, 2012, *A Community of Disagreement: Feminism in the University*, New York: Lang

Boundy, K, 2008, 'Are you sure, sweetheart, that you want to be well?': An exploration of the neurodiversity movement, *Radical Psychology* 7, 2, radicalpsychology.org

Bousquet, M, 1998, The institution as false horizon, *Workplace: A Journal for Academic Labor*, 1, 1–8

Bowman, M, 1997, *Individual Differences in Traumatic Response: Problems with the Adversity–Distress Connection*, Mahweh, NJ: Lawrence Erlbaum Associates

BPS (British Psychological Society), 2013, *DSM-5: The Future of Psychiatric Diagnosis, 2012 – Final Consultation): British Psychological Society Response to the American Psychiatric Association*, Leicester: British Psychological Society

Bracken, P, Thomas, P, 2001, Postpsychiatry: A new direction for mental health?, *British Medical Journal* 322, 724–27

Brady, SM, 2001, Sterilization of girls and women with intellectual disabilities past and present justifications, *Violence Against Women* 7, 4, 432–61

Brannan, M, Pearson, G, Worthington, F, 2007, Ethnographies of work and the work of ethnography, *Ethnography* 8, 4, 395–402

Breggin, P, 1990, Brain damage, dementia and persistent cognitive dysfunction associated with neuroleptic drugs: Evidence, etiology, implications, *The Journal of Mind and Behavior* 11, 3–4, 425–64

Breggin, P, 1994, *Toxic Psychiatry*, New York: St Martin's Press

Breggin, P, 1997, *Brain-Disabling Treatments in Psychiatry: Drugs, Electroshock, and the Psychopharmaceutical Complex*, New York: Springer

Breggin, P, 2002, *The Ritalin Fact Book: What Your Doctor Won't Tell You*, Cambridge: Perseus Books

Breggin, PR, 2007, ECT damages the brain: Disturbing news for patients and shock doctors alike, *Ethical Human Psychology and Psychiatry* 9, 83–6

Breggin, P, 2008, *Brain-Disabling Treatments in Psychiatry: Drugs, Electroshock and the Psychopharmaceutical Complex*, 2nd edn, New York: Springer

Briggs, C, 2004, Theorizing modernity conspiratorially: Science, scale, and the political economy of public discourse in explanations of a cholera epidemic, *American Ethnologist* 31, 2, 164–87

Broderick, A, Ne'eman, A, 2008, Autism as metaphor: Narrative and counter-narrative, *International Journal of Inclusive Education* 12, 5/6, 459–76

Brown, J, Hanlon, P, Turok, I, Webster, D, Arnott, J, MacDonald, E, 2009, Mental health as a reason for claiming incapacity benefit: A comparison of national and local trends, *Journal of Public Health* 31, 74–80

Brown, T, 2003, Critical race theory speaks to the sociology of mental health: Mental health problems produced by racial stratification, *Journal of Health and Social Behavior* 44, 3, 292–301

Bumiller, K, 2008, Quirky citizens: Autism, gender, and reimagining disability, *Signs* 33, 4, 967–91

Burnham, A, 2012, *Rethinking mental health in the twenty-first century, speech to the Centre for Social Justice,* www.archive.labour.org.uk

Burstow, B, 2013, A rose by any other name: Naming and the battle against psychiatry, in B LeFrançois, R Menzies and G Reaume (eds) *Mad Matters: A Critical Reader in Canadian Mad Studies,* pp 79–90, Toronto: Canadian Scholars' Press

Burstow, B, LeFrançois, B, Diamond, S (eds), 2014, *Psychiatry Disrupted: Theorising Resistance and Crafting the Revolution,* Quebec: McGill-Queen's University Press

Cameron, C, 2008, Further towards an affirmation model, in T Campbell, F Fontes, L Hemingway, A Soorenian, C Till (eds) *Disability Studies: Emerging Insights and Perspectives,* pp 14–30, Leeds: The Disability Press

Cameron, C, 2011, Not our problem: Impairment as difference, disability as role, *Journal of Inclusive Practice in Further and Higher Education* 3, 2, 10–24

Campbell, J, Oliver, M, 1996, *Disability Politics: Understanding Our Past, Changing Our Future,* London: Routledge

Campbell, P, 1993, Spiritual Crisis *OpenMind* 61 pp 10–11

Campbell, P, 1996, The history of the user movement in the United Kingdom, in T Heller, J Reynolds, R Gomm, R Muston, S Pattison (eds) *Mental Health Matters,* pp 218–25, Basingstoke: Macmillan/Open University

Campbell, P, 2009, The service user/survivor movement, in J Reynolds, R Muston, T Heller, J Leach, M McCormick, J Wallcraft, M Walsh (eds) *Mental Health Still Matters,* pp 46–52, Basingstoke: Palgrave/Open University Press

Campbell, P, nd, A survivor speaks out, *Health Rights' Report: Consumerism in the NHS*

Canguilhem, G, 1950, *On the Normal and the Pathological,* New York: Zone, 1989

Care Quality Commission, National Mental Health Development Unit, 2011, *Count me in 2010,* London: CQC

Care Services Improvement Partnership, Royal College of Psychiatrists, Social Care Institute for Excellence, 2007, *A Common Purpose: Recovery in Future Mental Health Services,* London: SCID

Cattrell, A, Harris, E, Palmer, K, Kim, M, Aylward, M, Coggon, D, 2011, Regional trends in awards of incapacity benefit by cause, *Occupational Medicine* 61, 3, 148–51

Chamberlin, J, 1987, The case for separatism: Ex-patient organising in the United States, in I Barker, D Peck (eds) *Power in Strange Places: User Empowerment in Mental Health Services*, pp 24–6, London: Good Practices in Mental Health

Chamberlin, J, 1997, A working definition of empowerment, *Psychiatric Rehabilitation Journal* 20, 4, 43–6

Church, K, 1995, *Forbidden Narratives: Critical Autobiography as Social Science*, Amsterdam: International Publishers Distributors; reprinted by Routledge, London

Church, K, 1996, Beyond 'bad manners': The power relations of 'consumer participation' in Ontario's community mental health system, *Canadian Journal of Community Mental Health* 15, 2, 27–44

Church, K, 2012, Making madness matter in academic practice, in B LeFrançois, R Menzies, G Reaume (eds) *Mad Matters: A Critical Reader in Canadian Mad Studies*, pp 181–90, Toronto: Canadian Scholars' Press

Clark, L, 2003, *Leonard Cheshire vs The Disabled People's Movement: A Review*, http://disability-studies.leeds.ac.uk/library/author/clark.laurence

Clarke, J, 2007, Citizen-consumers and public service reform: At the limits of neo-liberalism?, *Policy Futures in Education* 5, 239–48

Clifford, S, 2009, Disabling democracy: How disability reconfigures deliberative democratic norms, proceedings of the *American Political Science Association 2009 Annual Meeting*, http://papers.ssrn.com/sol3/papers.cfm?abstract_id=1451092

Coleman, E, 2008, The politics of rationality: Psychiatric survivors' challenge to psychiatry, in B Da Costa, K Philip (eds) *Tactical Biopolitics: Art, Activism, and Technoscience*, pp 341–63, Cambridge, MA: MIT Press

Coleman, E, Elders, J, Satcher, D, Shindel, A, Parish, S, Kenagy, G, Light, A, 2013, Summit on medical school education in sexual health: Report of an expert consultation, *The Journal of Sexual Medicine* 10, 4, 924–38

Coleman, R, Smith, M, 1997, *Working with Voices: From Victim to Victor*, Gloucester: Handsell

Coles, S, Keenan, S, Diamond, B (eds), 2013, *Madness Contested: Power and Practice*, Ross-on-Wye: PCCS Books

Colgan, F, Ledwith, S, 2002, Gender diversity and mobilisation in UK trade unions, in F Colgan, S Ledwith (eds) *Gender, Diversity and Trade Unions: International Perspectives*, pp 154–85, London : Routledge

Collins, P, 1998, It's all in the family: Intersections of gender, race, and nation, *Hypatia* 13, 3, 62–82

Collins, P, Patel, V, Joestl, S, March, D, Insel, T, Daar, A, 2011, Grand challenges in global mental health, *Nature* 475, 27–30

Commons Treloar, A, Lewis, A, 2008, Professional attitudes towards deliberate self harm in patients with borderline personality disorder, *Australian and New Zealand Journal of Psychiatry* 42, 578–84

Connell, R, 2011, Southern bodies and disability: Re-thinking concepts, *Third World Quarterly* 32, 8, 1369–81

Conte, J, O'Neil, M, 2007, Studying power: Qualitative methods and the global elites, *Qualitative Research* 7, 1, 63–82

Cooklin, A, 2006, Children as carers of parents with mental illness, *Psychiatry* 5, 1, 32–5

Corbett, S, Walker, A, 2013, The big society: Rediscovery of 'the social' or rhetorical fig-leaf for neo-liberalism?, *Critical Social Policy* 33, 3, 451–72

Corker, M, French, S (eds), 1999, *Disability Discourse*, Disability, Human Rights and Society series, Buckingham: Open University Press

Corrigan, P, Watson, A, 2004, Stop the stigma: Call mental illness a brain disease, *Schizophrenia Bulletin* 30, 3, 477–79

Corrigan, P, Roe, D, Tsang, H, 2011, *Challenging the Stigma of Mental Illness*, Chichester: Wiley

Corstens, D, May, R, Longden, D (nd) *Talking with Voices*, Maastricht, hearingvoicesmaastricht.eu

Costa, L, Voronka, J, Landry, D, Reid, J, McFarlane, B, Reville, D, Church, K, 2012, Recovering our stories: A small act of resistance, *Studies in Social Justice* 6, 1, 86–101

Crenshaw, K, 1989, Demarginalizing the intersection of race and sex: A black feminist critique of antidiscrimination doctrine, feminist theory and antiracist politics, *The University of Chicago Legal Forum*, pp 139–67

Crenshaw, K, 1991, Mapping the margins: Intersectionality, identity politics, and violence against women of color, *Stanford Law Review* 43, 6, 1241–99

Cresswell, M, 2009, Deeply engaged relationships? Community trade unionism and mental health movements in the UK, Lead address to fringe meeting, *Unison in the Community: Mutuality and Solidarity*, Unison Health Conference, Harrogate, April 20–22

Cresswell, M, Spandler, H, 2009, Psychopolitics: Peter Sedgwick's legacy for the politics of mental health, *Social Theory and Health* 7, 2, 129–47

Cresswell, M, Spandler, H, 2012, The engaged academic: Academic intellectuals and the psychiatric survivor movement, *Social Movement Studies: Journal of Social Cultural and Political Protest* 11, 4, 138–54

Cross-Government Strategy: Mental Health Division, 2009, *New Horizons: A Shared Vision for Mental Health*, http://webarchive.nationalarchives.gov.uk

Crow, L, 1996a, All of our lives: Renewing the social model of disability, in C Barnes, G Mercer (eds) *Exploring the Divide: Illness and Disability*, pp 55–72, Leeds: The Disability Press

Crow, L, 1996b, Renewing the social model of disability, *Coalition*, July, 5–9

CRPD (Committee on the Rights of Persons with Disabilities), 2012, *Concluding Observations on the Initial Report of China, Adopted by the Committee at its Eighth Session (CRPD/C/CHN/CO/1)*, Geneva: Office of the United Nations High Commissioner for Human Rights

Curtis, T, Dellar, R, Leslie, E, Watson, B (eds), 2000, *Mad Pride: A Celebration of Mad Culture*, London: Spare Change Books

Davar, B, 2008a, Our mind our madness, in M John (ed) *Women's Studies in India: A Reader*, pp 395–99, New Delhi: Penguin Books India

Davar, B, 2008b, From mental illness to psychosocial disability: Choices of identity for women users and survivors of psychiatry, *Indian Journal of Gender Studies* 15, 2, 261–90

Davar, B, 2012, Legal frameworks for and against people with psychosocial disabilities, *Economic and Political Weekly* 47, 52, 123–31

Davar, B, 2014, Globalizing psychiatry and the case of 'vanishing' alternatives in a neo-colonial state, *Disability and the global south* 1, 2, pp 266–84

Davar, B, 2015a, Delivering justice, withdrawing care: The norms and etiquettes of being 'mentally ill' in India, in B Davar, S Ravindran (eds) *Gendering mental health: Knowledges, identities, institutions*, New Delhi: Oxford University Press

Davar, B, 2015b, Identity constructions for 'mentally disturbed' women: Identities versus institutions in B Davar, S Ravindran (eds) *Gendering mental health: Knowledges, identities, institutions* Oxford University Press: New Delhi

Davar, B, Lohokare, M, 2008, Recovering from psychosocial traumas: The place of Dargahs in Maharashtra, *Economic and Political Weekly* 44, 16, 60–8

Davar, B, Ravindran, S (eds), 2015, *Gendering mental health: Knowledges, Identities, Institutions*, Oxford University Press: New Delhi

Davis, L, 1995, *Enforcing Normalcy: Disability, Deafness and the Body*, London: Verso

Davis, K, Mullender, A, 1993, *Ten turbulent years: A review of the work of the Derbyshire Coalition of Disabled People*, Nottingham: Centre for Social Action, Nottingham University

De Wet, P, 2014, Oscar Pistorius tests new limits of disability, *Mail and Guardian*, 10 April, http://mg.co.za/article/2014-04-10-oscar-pistorius-tests-new-limits-of-disability

Deal, M, 2003, Disabled people's attitudes toward other impairment groups: a hierarchy of impairments, *Disability and Society* 18, 7, 897–910

Deegan, P, 1990, Spirit breaking: When the helping professions hurt, *The Humanistic Psychologist* 18, 3, 301–13

Deegan, P, 1992, The independent living movement and people with psychiatric disabilities: Taking back control over our own lives, *Psychosocial Rehabilitation Journal* 15, 3, 3–19

Deem, R, 1998, 'New managerialism' and higher education: The management of performances and cultures in universities in the United Kingdom, *International Studies in Sociology of Education* 8, 1, 47–70

Dekker, M, 2004, *On Our Own Terms: Emerging Autistic Culture*, http://web.archive.org/web/20061111053135/http://trainland.tripod.com/martijn.htm

Delgado, R, Stefancic, J, 2003, *Critical Race Theory: An Introduction*, New York: New York University Press

Denman, C, 2004, *Sexuality: A Biopsychosocial Approach*, Basingstoke: Palgrave Macmillan

Department of Health, 2002, *A Sign of the Times: Modernising Mental Health Services for people who are Deaf*, London: Department of Health

Department of Health, 2005, *Mental Capacity Act*, London: The Stationery Office

Derrida, J, 1978, *Writing and Difference*, Chicago, IL: University of Chicago Press

Dewan, V, 2001, Life support, in J Read (ed) *Something Inside So Strong: Strategies for Surviving Mental Distress*, pp 44–9, London: Mental Health Foundation

Dhanda, A, 2000, *Legal Order/Mental Disorder*, New Delhi: Sage

Dietrich, S, Matschinger, H, Angermeyer, M, 2006, The relationship between biogenetic causal explanations and social distance toward people with mental disorders: results from a population survey in Germany, *International Journal of Social Psychiatry* 52, 2, 166–74

Dillon, J, 2010, The tale of an ordinary little girl, *Psychosis* 2, 1, 79–3

Doe, T, 2011, The hell of living with a schizophrenic, *Salon*, 12 January www.salon.com/2011/01/12/schizophrenic_mother_tucson_reaction_open2011/

Doucet, M, Rovers, M, 2010, Generational trauma, attachment, and spiritual/religious interventions, *Journal of Loss and Trauma* 15, 93–105

Drake, A, 2007, Group difference and institutional accommodation: deliberative resources and activist challenges, *Printemps* 2, 1, 41–6

Edwards, P, Belander, J, 2008, Generalizing from workplace ethnographies: From induction to theory, *Journal of Contemporary Ethnography* 37, 3, 291–313

Elstub, S, 2006, Towards an inclusive social policy for the UK: The need for democratic deliberation in voluntary and community associations, *Voluntas: International Journal of Voluntary and Nonprofit Organizations* 17, 1, 17–39

ENUSP (European Network of (ex) Users and Survivors of Psychiatry), 1994, *Report of the Second European Conference of Users and ex-Users in Mental Health in Elsinore, Denmark*, www.enusp.org/enusp-events-dates/congresses/elsinore.pdf

ENUSP (European Network of (ex) Users and Survivors of Psychiatry), 1997, *Report of the Third Conference in Reading*, www.enusp.org/index.php/events-dates/142-third-conference-3-6-january-1997

ENUSP (European Network of (ex) Users and Survivors of Psychiatry), 2009, *Nothing About Us Without Us: How to Make This a Reality?*, www.enusp.org/enusp-events-dates/congresses/luxembourg/empow-seminar2009.pdf?phpMyAdmin=f62c3a4496df92b2798ee4de97870d4d

ENUSP (European Network of (ex) Users and Survivors of Psychiatry), 2010, *Determining our Own Future: The Way Forward for all European Users and Survivors of Psychiatry*, http://enusp.org/enusp-events-dates/congresses/thessaloniki/thessaloniki_report.pdf

Erevelles, N, Minear, A, 2010, Unspeakable offenses: Untangling race and disability discourses of intersectionality, *Journal of Literary and Cultural Disability Studies* 4, 2, 127–45

Ernst, W, 1991, *Mad tales from the Raj: The European insane in British India 1800-1858*, London: Routledge

Eyerman, A, 2000, *Women in the Office: Transitions in a Global Economy*, Toronto: Sumach Press

Fabris, E, 2011, *Tranquil Prisons: Chemical Incarceration under Community Treatment Orders*, Toronto: University of Toronto Press

Fanon, F, 1967, *Black Skin, White Masks*, New York: Grove Press Inc

Farber, S, 2012, *The Spiritual Gift of Madness: The Failure of Psychiatry and the Rise of the Mad Pride Movement*, Rochester, VT: Inner Traditions

Farmer, P, 2005, *Pathologies of Power: Health, Human Rights and the New War on the Poor*, Berkeley, CA: University of California Press

Faulkner, A, Layzell, S, 2000, *Strategies For Living: A Report of User-led Research into People's Strategies for Living with Mental Distress*, London, The Mental Health Foundation

Faulkner, A, Nicholls, V, 1999, *The DIY Guide To Survivor Research*, London, The Mental Health Foundation

Fernando, S, 2014, *Mental Health Worldwide: Culture, Globalization and Development*, London: Palgrave Macmillan

Fernando, S, Weerackody, C, 2009, Challenges in Developing Community Mental Health Services in Sri Lanka, *Journal of Health Management* 11, 1, 195–208

Feyerabend, P, 1975, *Against Method*, 4th edn, London: Verso

Finkelstein, V, 1975, Phase 2: Discovering the person in 'disability' and 'rehabilitation', *The Magic Carpet* 27, 1, 31–8

Finkelstein, V, 1980, *Attitudes and Disabled People: Issues for Discussion*, New York: World Rehabilitation Fund

Finkelstein, V, 1999, A profession allied to the community: The Disabled People's Trade Union, in D Stone (ed) *Disability and Development: Learning from Action and Research on Disability in the Majority World*, Leeds: The Disability Press, 21–4

Foley, G, 1999, *Learning in Social Action: A Contribution to Understanding Informal Education*, London: Zed books

Foster, D, Fosh, P, 2010, Negotiating 'difference': Representing disabled employees in the British workplace, *British Journal of Industrial Relations* 48, 560–82

Fotaki, M, 2013, Woman is like a man (in academia): The masculine symbolic order and the unwanted female body, *Organization Studies* 34, 9, 1251–75

Foucault, M, 1967, *Madness and Civilisation: A History of Insanity in the Age of Reason*, London: Tavistock

Foucault, M, 1971, Nietzsche, genealogy, history, in P Rabinow (ed) *The Foucault Reader*, pp 76–100, London: Penguin

Foucault, M, 1991, *Discipline and Punish: The Birth of the Prison*, London: Penguin

Foucault, M, 2006, *History of Madness*, New York: Routledge

Foucault, M, 2008, *Psychiatric Power: Lectures at the Collège De France 1973–1974*, Basingstoke: Palgrave Macmillan

Foucault, M, 2010, *The Birth of the Clinic*, London: Routledge

Fox, N, 2012, *The Body*, Cambridge: Polity Press

Fraser, N, Honneth, A, 2003, *Redistribution or Recognition?: A Political–Philosophical Exchange*, London: Verso

Freeman, S, 2014, "Original position", in EN Zalta (ed) *The Stanford encyclopedia of philosophy* (Fall 2014 Edition), http://plato.stanford.edu/archives/fall2014/entries/original-position/

Freire, P, 1972, *Pedagogy Of The Oppressed*, London: Penguin

Garcia, I, Kennett, C, Quraishi, M, Durcan, G, 2005, *Acute Care 2004: A National Survey of Adult Psychiatric Wards in England*, London: The Sainsbury Centre for Mental Health

Gardiner, M, 2004, Wild publics and grotesque symposiums: Habermas and Bakhtin on dialogue, everyday life and the public sphere, *The Sociological Review* 52, supp 1, 28–48

Gardos, G, Cole, J, 1978, Withdrawal syndromes associated with antipsychotic drugs, *American Journal of Psychiatry* 135, 1321–24

Gee, M, 2010, The Ryerson revolution, *Toronto Life*, April Issue, 54–60

Geekie, J, 2004, Listening to the voices we hear: Clients' understandings of psychotic experiences, in J Read, L Mosher, R Bentall (eds) *Models of Madness: Psychological, Social and Biological Approaches to Schizophrenia*, pp 147–60, Hove: Brunner-Routledge

Gill, R, 2009, Breaking the silence: The hidden injuries of neo-liberal academic, in R Flood, R Gill (eds) *Secrecy and Silence in the Research Process: Feminist Reflections*, pp 228–44, London: Routledge

Ginsburg, F, Rapp, R, 2013, Disability worlds, *Annual Review of Anthropology* 42, 53–68

Goghari, V, Harrow, M, Grossman, L, Rosen, C, 2012, A 20-year multi-follow-up of hallucinations in schizophrenia, other psychotic, and mood disorders, *Psychological Medicine* 43, 1151–60

Goldberg, JF, Harrow, M, 2004, Consistency of remission and outcome in bipolar and unipolar mood disorders: A 10-year prospective follow-up, *Journal of Affective Disorders* 81, 2, 123–31

Gombos, G, Dhanda, A, 2009, *Catalyzing Self Advocacy: An Experiment in India*, Pune, India: Bapu Trust for Research on Mind and Discourse

Goodley, D, 2012, Is disability theory ready to engage with the politics of mental health?, In J Anderson, B Sapey, H Spandler, *Distress or Disability: Proceedings of a Symposium Held at Lancaster University, 15–16 November 2011*, Lancaster: Centre for Disability Research, 24–9

Gopikumar, V, Parsuraman, S, 2013, Mental illness, care and the Bill: A simplistic interpretation, *Economic and Political Weekly* 48, 9, 48–9

Gorman, R, 2013, Mad nation? Thinking through race, class, and mad identity politics, in B LeFrançois, R Menzies, G Reaume (eds) *Mad matters: A critical reader in Canadian Mad Studies*, pp 269–80, Toronto: Canadian Scholars' Press

Gould, M, 2012, *Service Users Experiences of Recovery Under The Care Programme Approach: A Research Study*, London: NSUN (National Survivor User Network) and Mental Health Foundation

Gray, P (ed), 2006, *The Madness of Our Lives: Experiences of Mental Breakdown and Recovery*, London: Jessica Kingsley

Grech, S, 2009, Disability, poverty and development: Critical reflections on the majority world debate, *Disability and Society* 24, 6, 771–84

Grech, S, 2011, Recolonising debates or perpetuated coloniality? Decentring the spaces of disability, development and community in the global south, *International Journal of Inclusive Education* 15, 1, 87–100

Griffiths, R, Allen, R, 2007, *Whose Health, Whose Care, Whose Say?: The Opportunities and Challenges of Contemporary Policy for People with Complex Mental Health Needs*, London: Social Perspectives Network

Gross, Z, 2012, Metaphor stole my autism: The social construction of autism as separable from personhood, and its effect on policy, funding and perception, in J Bascom (ed) *Loud Hands: Autistic People Speaking*, pp 179–90, Washington, DC: The Autistic Press

Habermas, J, 1979, *Communication and the Evolution of Society*, Heinemann: London

Habermas, J, 1986, *The Theory of Communicative Action: Volume 1 Reason and the Rationalization of Society*, Cambridge: Polity

Habermas, J, 1987, *The Theory of Communicative Action, Volume 2 The Critique of Functionalist Reason*, Cambridge: Polity

Habermas, J, 1990, *Moral Consciousness and Communicative Action*, Cambridge: Polity

Hales, G (ed), 1996, *Beyond Disability: Towards an Enabling Society*, London: Sage

Hall, W, 2013, *Living with Suicidal Feelings*, Address to the Scottish Recovery Network, 24 April

Hanivsky, O, 2002, Women's health, men's health, and gender and health: Implications of intersectionality, *Social Science and Medicine* 74, 1712–20

Harper, D, Speed, E, 2012, Uncovering recovery: The resistible rise of recovery and resilience, *Studies in Social Justice* 6, 1, 9–25

Hasler, F, 1993, Developments in the Disabled People's Movement, in J Swain, V Finkelstein, S French, M Oliver (eds) *Disabling Barriers, Enabling Environments*, pp 278–84, London: Sage Publications

Hemmingson, H, Jonsson H, 2005, An occupational perspective on the concept of participation in the International Classification of Functioning, Disability and Health: Some critical remarks, *The American Journal of Occupational Therapy* 59, 5, 569–76

Herman, J, 1992, Complex PTSD: A syndrome in survivors of prolonged and repeated trauma, *Journal of Traumatic Stress* 5, 337–91

Herman, J, 1997, *Trauma and Recovery: The Aftermath of Violence from Domestic Abuse to Political Terror*, London: Basic Books.

Higashida, N, 2013, *The Reason I Jump*, London: Sceptre

HMHAG (Hackney Mental Health Action Group), 1986, *Charter of Rights for People in Mental Distress*, London: HMHAG

Hodge, S, 2005, Participation, discourse and power: A case study in service user involvement, *Critical Social Policy*, 25, 164–79

Hollinsworth, D, 2013, Decolonizing indigenous disability in Australia, *Disability and Society* 28, 5, 601–15

Hopper, K, 2006, Redistribution and its discontents: On the prospects of committed work in public mental health and like settings, *Human Organization* 65, 218–26

Hopper, K, 2007, Rethinking social recovery in schizophrenia: What a capabilities approach might offer, *Social Science and Medicine* 65, 868–79

Hopper, K, 2012, Reframing early psychiatric crises: A capabilities perspective, *Journal of Human Development, Disability and Social Change* 20, 23–39

Hornstein, G, 2002, Narratives of madness as told from within, *The Chronicle of Higher Education*, 25 January, http://chronicle.com/article/Narratives-of-Madness-as-Told/30189

Hornstein, G, 2009, *Agnes's Jacket: A Psychologist's Search for the Meanings of Madness*, New York: Rodale

Horton-Salway, M, 2007, The 'ME bandwagon' and other labels: Constructing the genuine case in talk about a controversial illness, *British Journal of Social Psychology* 46, 4, 895–914

Hoskins, T, 2011, Protests as Bhopal massacre company sponsors Olympics, *Counterfire*, 4 December, www.counterfire.org/international/15290-bhopal-massacre-company-sponsors-olympics

Hulette, A, Kaehler, L, Freyd, J, 2011, Intergenerational associations between trauma and dissociation, *Journal of Family Violence* 26, 217–25

Human Rights Watch, 2011, Sterilization of women and girls with disabilities: A briefing paper, www.hrw.org/news/2011/11/10/sterilization-women-and-girls-disabilities

Humphrey, J, 1998, Self-organise and survive: Disabled people in the British trade union movement, *Disability and Society* 13, 587–602

Humphrey, J, 1999, Disabled people and the politics of difference, *Disability and Society* 14, 173–88

Humphrey, J, 2000a, Researching disability politics, or, some problems with the social model in practice, *Disability and Society* 15, 63–86

Humphrey, J, 2000b, Self-organisation and trade union democracy, *The Sociological Review* 48, 262–82

Humphreys, A, 2014, Tony Blair has finally gone mad: The meteoric rise and fall of Britain's most unpopular ex-PM ever, *National Post*, June 27, http://news.nationalpost.com/2014/06/27/tony-blair-has-finally-gone-mad-the-meteoric-rise-and-fall-of-britains-most-unpopular-ex-pm-ever/

Hunt, P (ed), 1966, *Stigma: The Experience of Disability*, London: Geoffrey Chapman

Hyman, S, Nestler, E, 1996, Initiation and adaptation: A paradigm for understanding psychotropic drug action, *American Journal of Psychiatry* 153, 151–61

Iantaffi, A, 2009, Disability and polyamory: Exploring the edges of interdependence, gender and queer issues in non-monogamous relationships, in M Barker, D Langdridge (eds) *Understanding Non-Monogamies*, pp 160–5, New York: Routledge

Iantaffi, A, 2013, Sexuality and disability, in F Attwood, C Bale, M Barker (eds) *The Sexualization Report*, https://senseaboutsex.files.wordpress.com/2012/08/thesexualizationreport.pdf

Iantaffi, A, Mize, S, 2015, Disability, in C Richards, M Barker (eds) *Handbook of the Psychology of Sexuality and Gender*, Basingstoke: Palgrave Macmillan

Inckle, K, 2010, *Flesh Wounds: New Ways of Understanding Self-injury*, Ross-on-Wye: PCCS Books

Irvine, J, 2005, *Disorders of Desire*, Philadelphia, PA: Temple University Press

Jackson, V, 2002, In our own voice: African-American stories of oppression, survival and recovery in mental health systems, *International Journal of Narrative Therapy and Community Work* 2002, 2, 11–31

Jacob, K, Sharan, P, Mirza, I, Garrido-Cumbrera, M, Seedat, S, Mari, J, Sreenivas, V, Saxena, S, 2007, Mental health systems in countries: Where are we now?, *Lancet* 370, 9592, 1061–77

Jasper, J, 1997, *The Art of Moral Protest: Culture, Biography and Creativity in Social Movements*, Chicago, IL: University of Chicago Press

Johnson, M, 1994, A test of wills: Jerry Lewis, Jerry's Orphans, and the Telethon, in B Shaw (ed) *The Ragged Edge: The Disability Experience from the Pages of the First Fifteen Years of the Disability Rag*, pp 120–30, Louisville, KY: The Advocado Press

Johnstone, L, 1997, Self-injury and the psychiatric response, *Feminism and Psychology* 7, 3, 421–26

Johnstone, L, 2011, Can traumatic events traumatize people? Trauma, madness and 'psychosis', in M Rapley, J Moncrieff, J Dillon (eds) *De-Medicalizing Misery: Psychiatry, Psychology and the Human Condition*, pp 99–109, Basingstoke: Palgrave Macmillan

Johnstone, L, 2013, Time to abolish psychiatric diagnosis?, *Mad in America: Science, Psychiatry and Community*, www.madinamerica.com/2013/01/time-to-abolish-psychiatric-diagnosis/

Jolly, D, Novak, S, 2012, A French film takes issue with the psychoanalytic approach to autism, *New York Times*, 19 January 19

Jones, N, 2014, *Redefining Research*, Interviewed by Will Hall, Madness Radio, 4 January, www.madnessradio.net/madness-radio-diversity-voices-nev-jones/

Jones, N, Shattell, M, 2014, Beyond easy answers: Facing the entanglements of violence and psychosis, *Issues in Mental Health Nursing* 35, 10, 809–11

Jordan, B, Dalal, B, 2006, Persuasive encounters: Ethnography in the corporation, *Field Methods* 18, 4, 359–81

Kannabiran, K, Singh, R, 2008, *Challenging the rules of law: Colonialism, criminology and human rights*, New Delhi: Sage

Kapp, S, Gillespie-Lynch, K, Sherman, L, Hutman, T, 2013, Deficit, difference, or both? Autism and neurodiversity, *Developmental Psychology* 49, 1, 59–71

Karlsen, S, 2007, *Ethnic Inequalities in Health: The Impact of Racism*, London: Race Equality Foundation

Karlsen, S, Nazroo, J, McKenzie, K, Bhui, K, Wiech, S, 2005, Racism, psychosis and common mental disorder among ethnic minority groups in England, *Psychological Medicine* 35, 1–9

Katsakou, C, Rose, D, Amos, T, Bowers, L, McCabe, R, Oliver, D, Wykes, T, Priebe, S, 2012, Psychiatric patients views on why their involuntary hospitalisation was right or wrong: A qualitative study, *Social Psychiatry Psychiatric Epidemiology* 47, 1169–79

Kaufman, M, Silverberg, C, Odette, F, 2007, *The Ultimate Guide to Sex and Disability: For All of Us Who Live With Disabilities, Chronic Pain, and Illness*, Berkeley, CA: Cleis Press

Kawachi, I, Berkman, L, 2001, Social ties and mental health, *Journal of Urban Health* 78, 3, 458–67

Keating, F, 2007, *African and Caribbean Men and Mental Health*, London: Race Equality Foundation

Keating, F, Robertson, D, Francis, F, McCulloch, A, 2002, *Breaking the Circles of Fear: A Review of the Relationship Between Mental Health Services and African and Caribbean Communities*, London: The Sainsbury Centre for Mental Health

Kennedy, J, 1963, Special message on mental illness and mental retardation, John F Kennedy Presidential Library Digital archive, www.jfklibrary.org/Asset-Viewer/Archives/JFKPOF-052-012.aspx

Killaspy, H, Dalton, J, McNicholas, S, Johnson, S, 2000, Drayton Park, an alternative to hospital admission for women in acute mental health crisis, *Psychiatric Bulletin* 24, 101–4

Kim, E, 2011, Asexuality in disability narratives, *Sexualities* 14, 4, 479–93

Kleinplatz, P (ed), 2012, *New Directions in Sex Therapy: Innovations and Alternatives*, London: Routledge

Kras, J, 2010, The 'ransom notes' affair: When the neurodiversity movement came of age, *Disability Studies Quarterly* 30, 1, http://dsq-sds.org/article/view/1065/1254

Krishnakumar, A, 2001, Deliverance in Erwady, *Frontline* 18, 17, 18–31

Kristiansen, K, 2004, Madness, badness, and saneness: Ontology control in 'mental health land', in K Kristiansen, R Traustadóttir (eds) *Gender and Disability Research in the Nordic Countries*, pp 365–93, Lund, Sweden: Studentlitteratur

Krumer-Nevo, M, Benjamin, 0, 2010, Critical poverty knowledge: Contesting othering and social distancing, *Current Sociology* 58, 5, 693–714

Kumar, S, Kumar, R, 2008, Institute of mental health and hospital, Agra: Evolution in 150 years, *Indian Journal of Psychiatry* 50, 308–12

Kutchins, H, Kirk, S, 1997, *Making Us Crazy: DSM: The Psychiatric Bible and the Creation of Mental Disorders*, London: Constable

Lacasse, J, 2014, After DSM-5: A critical mental health research agenda for the 21st century, *Research on Social Work Practice* 24, 5–10

Lakoff, A, 2005, *Pharmaceutical Reason: Knowledge and Value in Global Psychiatry*, Cambridge: Cambridge University Press

Lampei, J, Honig, B, Drori, I, 2014, Organizational ingenuity: Concept, processes and strategies, *Organization Studies* 35, 4, 465–82

Lancet Global Mental Health Group, 2007, Scale up services for mental disorders: A call for action, *The Lancet* 370, 9594, 87–98

Laurance, J, 2003, *Pure madness: How fear drives the mental health system*, London: Routledge

Lawson, W, 2005, *Sex, Sexuality and the Autism Spectrum*, London: Jessica Kingsley Publishers

Lawthom, R with Chataika, T, 2012, Lave and Wenger, communities of practice and disability studies, in D Goodley, B Hughes, L Davis (eds) *Disability and Social Theory: New Developments and Directions*, pp 233–51, Basingstoke: Palgrave Macmillan

LDC (London Development Centre), SPN (Social Perspectives Network), 2006, *Meeting the Mental Health Needs of Refugees, Asylum Seekers and Immigration Detainees*, London: SPN

Leamy, M, Slade, M, Le Boutillier, C, Williams, J, Bird, V, 2011, A conceptual framework for personal recovery in mental health: Systematic review and narrative synthesis, *British Journal of Psychiatry* 199, 445–52

Leavy, J, Howard, J, 2013, *What Matters Most? Evidence from 84 Participatory Studies with Those Living with Extreme Poverty and Marginalisation*, London: Institute of Development Studies

Lefevre, S, 1996, *Killing me softly. Self-harm: survival not suicide*, Gloucester: Handsell

LeFrançois, B, Menzies, R, Reaume, G (eds), 2013, *Mad Matters: A Critical Reader in Canadian Mad Studies*, Toronto: Canadian Scholars Press

Lehmann, P (ed), 2004, *Coming off Psychiatric Drugs: Successful Withdrawal from Neuroleptics, Antidepressants, Lithium, Carbamazepine and Tranquilizers*, Berlin: Peter Lehmann Publishing

Leitch, V, 2005, Work theory, *Critical Inquiry* 31, 2, 286–301

Lerner, G, 2010, Activist: Farmer suicides in India linked to debt, globalization, CNN, 5 January, http://edition.cnn.com/2010/WORLD/asiapcf/01/05/india.farmer.suicides/

Levy, S, 2011, Innovation and entrepreneurship: A new direction for universities, speech to the Economic Club of Canada, Toronto

Levy, S, 2012, Investing in youth and innovation, speech to the Empire Club of Canada, Toronto

Liddiard, K, 2014, (Re)Producing Pistorius: Patriarchy, prosecution and the problematics of disability, *The Sociological Imagination*, http://sociologicalimagination.org/archives/15144

Link, B, Phelan, J, 2001, Conceptualising stigma, *Annual Review of Sociology* 27, 363–65

Linstead, S, Marechal, G, Griffin, R, 2014, Theorizing and researching the dark side of organization, *Organization Studies* 35, 2, 165–88

Linton, S, 1998, *Claiming Disability: Knowledge and Identity*, New York: NYU Press

Lister, R, 2008, Inclusive citizenship, gender and poverty: Some implications for education for citizenship, *Citizenship, Teaching and Learning* 4, 1, 5–19

Littlewood, R, 1988, From vice to madness: The semantics of naturalistic and personalistic understandings in Trinidad local medicine, *Social Science and Medicine* 27, 129–48

Littlewood, R, 2006, Mental health and intellectual disability: Culture and diversity, *Journal of Intellectual Disability Research* 50, 8, 555–60

London Edinburgh Weekend Return Group, 1979, *In and Against the State*, London: CSE Books/Pluto

Lord, J, Nelson, G, Ochocka, J, 2001, *Shifting the Paradigm of Community Mental Health: Toward Empowerment and Community*, Toronto: University of Toronto Press

Lorenz, C, 2012, If you're so smart, why are you under surveillance? Universities, neoliberalism, and new public management, *Critical Inquiry* 38, 3, 599–629

Lumb, K, 1990, The drama of disability in charity fundraising, *Coalition*, December

Lysaker, P, Roe, D, Yanos, P, 2006, Toward understanding the insight paradox, *Schizophrenia Bulletin* 33, 1, 192–9

McCarthy-Jones, S, 2012, *Hearing Voices: The Histories, Causes and Meanings of Auditory Verbal Hallucinations*, Cambridge: Cambridge University Press

McCaskill, D, 2012, Discrimination and public perceptions of Aboriginal people in Canadian cities, Urban Aboriginal Knowledge Network, http://uakn.org/wp-content/uploads/2014/08/2012-UAKN-Research-Paper-Series_Discrimination-and-Public-Perceptions-of-Aboriginal-People-in-Canadian-Cities_Dr.-Don-McCaskill.pdf

MacDonald, D, Wilson, D, 2013, *Poverty or Prosperity: Indigenous Children in Canada*, Ottawa: Canadian Centre for Policy Alternatives, www.policyalternatives.ca/publications/reports/poverty-or-prosperity

McKeown, M, Jones, F, 2012, Can universities be radical places?, *Asylum: An International Magazine for Democratic Psychiatry* 19, 1, 20–22

McKeown, M, Cresswell, M, Spandler, H, 2014, Deeply engaged relationships? Trade unionism and the organized Left's alliance building with psychiatric survivors in the UK, in B Burstow, S Diamond, B LeFrançois (eds) *Psychiatry Disrupted: Theorizing Resistance and Crafting the (R)evolution*, pp 145–62, Montreal: McGill/Queen's University Press

McNamara, J, 1996, Out of order: Madness is a feminist and a disability issue, in J Morris (ed) *Encounters with Strangers: Feminism and Disability*, pp 194–205, London: The Women's Press

McRuer, R, 2006, *Crip Theory: Cultural Signs of Queerness and Disability*, New York: New York University Press

McRuer, R, 2011, Disabling sex: Notes for a crip theory of sexuality, *GLQ: A Journal of Lesbian and Gay Studies* 17, 1, 107–17

Madhok, S, Rae, S, 2012, Agency, injury and transgressive politics in neoliberal times, *Signs* 37, 3, 645–69

Maeckelbergh, M, 2012, *Experiments in Democracy and Diversity within the Occupy Movement(s)*, www.opendemocracy.net/marianne-maeckelbergh/experiments-in-democracy-and-diversity-within-occupy-movements

Mari, J, Thornicroft, G, 2010, Principles that should guide mental health policies in low- and middle-income countries, *Reista Brasileira de Psiquiatria* 32, 3, 210–11

Meekosha, H, 2011, Decolonising disability: Thinking and acting globally, *Disability and Society* 26, 6, 667–82

Meekosha, H, Soldatic, S, 2011, Human rights and the global south: The case of disability, *Third World Quarterly* 32, 8, 1383–97

Méndez, J, 2013, *Report of the Special Rapporteur on Torture and Other Cruel, Inhuman or Degrading Treatment or Punishment*, A/HRC/22/53, Geneva: OHCHR

Mental Health Policy Group, 2012, *How Mental Health Loses Out in the NHS*, London: The Centre for Economic Performance, LSE (The London School of Economics)

Metzl, J, 2009, *The Protest Psychosis: How Schizophrenia Became a Black Disease*, Boston, MA: Beacon Press

Meyerding, J, 2002, *Thoughts on Finding Myself Differently Brained*, www.planetautism.com/jane/diff.html

MHSS (Mental Health System Survivors), 1987, Second revised draft policy statement for mental health system survivors, *Recovery and Re-emergence* 4, 4–16

Michelson, E, 1996, 'Auctoritee' and 'experience': Feminist epistemology and the assessment of experiential learning, *Feminist Studies* 22, 3, 627–55

Miettinen, R, Samra-Fredericks, D, Yanow, D, 2009, Return to practice: An introductory essay, *Organization Studies* 30, 2, 1309–27

Miller, A, 1991, *Banished Knowledge: Facing Childhood Injuries*, New York: Anchor Books

Millett, K, 1990, *The Loony Bin Trip*, London: Virago

Mills, C, 2014, *Decolonizing Global Mental Health: The Psychiatrization of the Majority World*, London: Routledge

Mills, J, 2000, *Madness, Cannabis and Colonialism: The 'Native Only' Lunatic Asylums of British India, 1857–1900*, Basingstoke: Macmillan

Mills, J, 2004, Body as target, violence as treatment: Psychiatric regimes in colonial and post-colonial India, in J Mills, S Sen (eds) *Confronting the Body: The Politics of Physicality in Colonial and Post-colonial India*, pp 80–101, London: Anthem South Asian Studies

Mind, 2004, *Ward Watch: Mind's Campaign to Improve Hospital Conditions for Mental Health Patients*, London: Mind

Mind, 2007, *Another Assault: Mind's Campaign for Equal Access to Justice for People with Mental Health Problems*, London: Mind

Minkowitz, T, 2011, *Why Mental health Laws Contravene the CRPD: An Application of Article 14 with Implications for the Obligations of State Parties*, Chestertown, NY: Centre for the Human Rights of Users and Survivors of Psychiatry

Minkowitz, T, 2012, CRPD Advocacy by the World Network of Users and Survivors of Psychiatry: The emergence of a user/survivor perspective in human rights, www.addc.org.au/documents/resources/120814-the-emergence-of-an-usersurvivor-perspective-in-human-rights_1422.pdf

Minkowitz, T, Dhanda, A (eds), 2006, *First Person Stories on Forced Treatment and Legal Capacity*, Pune, India: World Network of Users and Survivors of Psychiatry and Bapu Trust

Mitchell, K, Mercer, C, Ploubidis, G, Jones, K, Datta, J, Field, N, Copas, A, Tanton, C, Erens, B, Sonnenberg, P, Clifton, S, Macdowall, W, Phelps, A, Johnson, A, Wellings, K, 2013, Sexual function in Britain: Findings from the third National Survey of Sexual Attitudes and Lifestyles (Natsal-3), *The Lancet* 382, 9907, 1817–29

Mitra, S, 2003, *The Capabilities Approach of Disability*, New Brunswick, NJ: Rutgers University

Mitra, S, 2006, The capability approach and disability, *Journal of Disability Policy Studies* 16, 4, 236–47

Mize, S, Iantaffi, A, 2013, The place of mindfulness in a sensorimotor psychotherapy intervention to improve women's sexual health, *Sexual and Relationship Therapy* 28, 1/2, 63–76

Moncrieff, J, 2007, Diagnosis and drug treatment, *The Psychologist* 5, 5, 296–7

Moncrieff, J, 2009, *The Myth of the Chemical Cure: A Critique of Psychiatric Drug Treatment*, Basingstoke: Palgrave Macmillan

Moncrieff, J, 2010, Psychiatric diagnosis as a political device, *Social Theory and Health* 8, 4, 370–82

Moncrieff, J, Cohen, D, 2006, Do anti-depressants cure or create abnormal brain states?, *PLoS Medicine* 3, 7, e240

Morrill, C, Fine, G, 1997, Ethnographic contributions to organizational sociology, *Sociological Methods and Research* 25, 4, 424–51

Morris, J, 1991, *Pride against Prejudice: Transforming Attitudes to Disability*, London: Women's Press

Morris, J, 1992, Personal and Political: A Feminist Perspective on Researching Physical Disability, *Disability, Handicap and Society* 7, 2, 157–66

Morris, J, 1993, *Independent Lives? Community Care and Disabled People*, Basingstoke: Macmillan

Morris, J (ed), 1996, *Encounters with strangers: Feminism and Disability*, London: Women's Press

Morris, J, 2004a, *One Town For My Body, Another For My Mind: Services For People With Physical Impairments and Mental Health Support Needs*, York: Joseph Rowntree Foundation

Morris, J, 2004b, *People with Physical Impairments and Mental Health Support Needs: A Critical Review of the Literature*, York: Joseph Rowntree Foundation

Morris, J, 2011, *Rethinking Disability Policy*, York: Joseph Rowntree Foundation

Morrison, A, Frame, L, Larkin W, 2003, Relationship between trauma and psychosis: A review and integration, *British Journal of Clinical Psychology* 42, 4, 331–53

Morrison, L, 2005, *Talking Back to Psychiatry: The Consumer/Survivor/ Ex-patient Movement*, New York: Routledge

Mosher, L, Hendrix, V, Fort, D, 2004, *Soteria: Through Madness to Deliverance*, Philadelphia, PA: Xlibris Corporation

Mulvany, J, 2000, Disability, impairment or illness? The relevance of the social model of disability to the study of mental disorder, *Sociology of Health and Illness* 22, 5, 582–601

Murthy, R, 2001, Lessons from the Erwady tragedy for mental health care in India, *Indian Journal of Psychiatry* 43, 4, 362–77

Myers, N, 2009, *Culture of Recovery? Schizophrenia, the United States' Mental Health System, and the American Ethos of the Self-made Man*, Chicago, IL: University of Chicago

Myers, N, 2010, Culture, stress and recovery from schizophrenia: Lessons from the field for global mental health, *Culture, Medicine, and Psychiatry* 34, 3, 500–28

NAAJMI, 2009, *Insights of a Mad Pride Campaign, 2005–08*, Pune, India: Bapu Trust for Research on Mind and Discourse

NAAJMI and Bapu Trust, 2010, *Bill of rights: Insights from a mad pride campaign*, 2005-2010, Published by National Alliance on Access to Justice for persons living with a Mental Illness and Bapu Trust, Pune

Nabbali, E, 2009, A 'mad' critique of the social model of disability, *International Journal of Diversity in Organizations, Communities and Nations* 9, 4, 1–12

Nagi, S, 1965, Some conceptual issues in disability and rehabilitation, in M Sussman (ed) *Sociology and Rehabilitation*, pp 100–13, Washington, DC: American Sociological Association

Nagi, S, 1991, Disability concepts revisited: Implications for prevention, in A Pope, A Tarlov (eds) *Disability in America: Toward a National Agenda for Prevention*, pp 307–27, Washington, DC: The National Academies Press

Nazroo, J, 2003, The structuring of ethnic inequalities in health: Economic position, racial discrimination and racism, *American Journal of Public Health* 93, 2, 277–84

Nelson, C, 2006, Of eggshells and thin skins: A consideration of racism-related mental illness impacting women, *International Journal of Law and Psychiatry* 29, 2, 112–36

Ng, W, 2011, *The spirit of our movement: Celebrating Toronto labour in the 21st century*, Toronto: Toronto and York Region Labour Council

NIMHE (National Institute for Mental Health in England), 2003, *Personality Disorder: No Longer a Diagnosis of Exclusion*, Leeds: NIMHD

Niven, J, 2011, *The Second Coming*, London: Vintage

Nizamie, S, Goyal, N, 2010, History of psychiatry in India, *Indian Journal of Psychiatry* 52, 7–12

Noorani, T, 2013, Service user involvement, authority and the 'expert-by-experience' in mental health, *Journal of Political Power* 6, 1, 49–68

Norman, R, Windell, D, Manchanda, R, 2012, Examining differences in the stigma of depression and schizophrenia, *International Journal of Social Psychiatry* 58, 1, 69–78

Nosek, M, Foley, C, Hughes, R, Howland, C, 2001, Vulnerabilities for abuse among women with disabilities, *Sexuality and Disability* 19, 3, 177–89

Nussbaum, M, 2000, *Women and Human Development: The Capabilities Approach*, Cambridge: Cambridge University Press

Nussbaum, M, Sen, A (eds), 1993, *The Quality of Life*, Oxford: Clarendon Press

O'Brien, C, 2005, Benzodiazepine use, abuse, and dependence, *Journal of Clinical Psychiatry* 66, supp 2, 28–33

ODI (Office for Disability Issues), 2008, *Independent Living: A cross-government strategy about independent living for disabled people*, London: TSO

O'Hagan, M, 1986, From taking snapshots to making movies, *Community Mental Health in New Zealand* 3, 1, 31–49

O'Hagan, M, 1993, *Stopovers on My Way Home from Mars: A Journey into the Psychiatric Survivor Movement in the USA, Britain, and the Netherlands*, London: Survivors Speak Out

Okoro, C, Strine, T, Balluz, L, Crews, J, Dhingra, S, Berry, J, Mokdad, A, 2009, Serious psychological distress among adults with and without disabilities, *International Journal of Public Health* 54, 1, 52–60

Oliver, M, 1994, *Capitalism, Disability and Ideology: A Materialist Critique of the Normalization Principle*, http://disability-studies.leeds.ac.uk/files/library/Oliver-cap-dis-ideol.pdf

Oliver, M, 1996, *Understanding Disability*, Basingstoke: Macmillan

Oliver, M, 2004, If I had a hammer: The social model in action, in J Swain, S French, C Barnes, C Thomas (eds) *Disabling barriers: Enabling environments*, 2nd edn, London: Sage, pp 7–12

Oliver, M, 2009, The social model in context, in T Titchkosky, R Michalko (eds) *Rethinking Normalcy: A Disability Studies Reader*, pp 19–30, Toronto: Canadian Scholars' Press

Oliver, M, 2010, Preface, in P Beresford, M Nettle, R Perring, *Towards a Social Model of Madness and Distress? Exploring what Service Users Say*, p 5, York: Joseph Rowntree Foundation

Oliver, M, 2013, The social model of disability: Thirty years on, *Disability and Society* 28, 7, 1024–6

Oliver, M, Barnes, C, 1998, *Disabled People and Social Policy: From Exclusion to Inclusion*, London: Longman

Olsson, M, 2012, The digital revolution: Disability and social media, *The McNair Scholars Journal* 11, 179–202

ONS (Office of National Statistics), 2012, *Ethnicity and National Identity in England and Wales*, London: ONS

Ortega, F, 2009, The cerebral subject and the challenge of neurodiversity, *BioSocieties* 4, 4, 425–45

Panitch, M, 2008, *Disability, Mothers and Organization: Accidental Activists*, Abingdon: Routledge

PANUSP, 2012, *Press Package*, www.panusp.org/wp-content/uploads/2013/02/28-June-Press-Package-WHO-Toolkit-Launch-1.pdf

PANUSP, 2014, The Cape Town Declaration (16th October 2011), *Disability and the Global South* 1, 2, 385–86

Papakostas, G, 2007, Tolerability of modern antidepressants, *The Journal of Clinical Psychiatry* 69, 8–13

Parker, I, Georgaca, E, Harper, D, McLaughlin, T, Stowell-Smith, M, 1995, *Deconstructing Psychopathology*, London: Sage

Parker, M, 2014, University, Ltd: Changing a business school, *Organization* 21, 2, 281–92

Parr, H, 2008, *Mental health and social space: Towards inclusionary geographies?*, Oxford: Wiley-Blackwell

Parsons, T, Fox, R, 1952, Illness, therapy and the modern urban American family, *Journal of Social Issues* 8, 31–44

Patel, N, Fatimilehin, I, 1999, Racism and mental health, in C Newnes, G Holmes, C Dunn (eds) *This is Madness: A Critical Look at Psychiatry and the Future of Mental Health Services*, pp 51–73, Ross-on-Wye: PCC Books

Patel, V, 2013, Legislating the right to care for mental illness, *Economic and Political Weekly* 48, 9, 49

Patel, V, Araya, R, Chatterjee, S, Chrisholm, D, Cohen, A, De Silva, M, Hosman, C, McGuire, H, Rajas, G, van Ommeren, M, 2007, Treatment and prevention of mental disorders in low-income and middle-income countries, *The Lancet* 370, 9590, 44–58

Patel, V, Boyce, N, Collins, PY, Saxena, S, Horton, R, 2011, A renewed agenda for global mental health, *The Lancet* 378, 1441–2

Pathare, S, Sagade, J, 2013, *Mental Health: A Legislative Framework to Empower, Protect and Care. A Review of Mental Health Legislation in Commonwealth Member States*, commissioned by Commonwealth Health Professions Alliance, Pune, India: Center for Mental Health Law and Policy

Peck, J, 2010, *Constructions of Neoliberal Reason*, Oxford: Oxford University Press

Penson, W, 2011, Reappraising the social model of disability: A Foucauldian reprise, in D Moore, A Gorra, H Smith, J Reaney (eds) *Disabled Students in Education: Technology, Transition and Inclusivity*, pp 171–90, Hershey: IGI Global

Perkins, D, 1999, The many faces of constructivism, *Educational Leadership* 57, 3, 6–11

Perkins, R, Farmer, P, Litchfield, P, 2009, *Realising Ambitions: Better Mental Health Support for People with a Mental Health Condition*, London: Department for Work and Pensions

Perkins, R, Repper, J, Rinaldi, M, Brown, H, 2012, *Recovery Colleges*, London: Centre for Mental Health

Perspectives Team, The, 2009, *Harvesting Despair: Agrarian Crisis in India*, Delhi: Perspectives

Pescosolido, B, Martin, J, Long, J, Medina, T, Phelan, J, Link, B, 2010, 'A disease like any other'? A decade of change in public reactions to schizophrenia, depression, and alcohol dependence, *American Journal of Psychiatry* 167, 11, 1321–30

Phillips, M, 2013, Can China's new mental health law substantially reduce the burden of illness attributable to mental disorders?, *The Lancet* 381, 9882, 1964–66

Pilgrim, D, 2008, 'Recovery' and current mental health policy, *Chronic Illness* 4, 295–304

Pilgrim, D, 2009, *Key Concepts in Mental Health*, 2nd edn, London: Sage

Pilgrim, D, Tomasini, F, 2012, On being unreasonable in modern society: Are mental health problems special?, *Disability and Society* 27, 5, 631–46

Pinfold, V, Thornicroft, G, Huxley, P, Farmer, P, 2005, Active ingredients in anti-stigma programmes in mental health, *International Review of Psychiatry* 17, 2, 123–31

Pinikahana, J, Happell, B, Hope, J, Keks, N, 2002, Quality of life in schizophrenia: A review of the literature from 1995 to 2000, *International Journal of Mental Health Nursing* 11, 2, 103–11

Plumb, A, 1989, Survivors speak out, *Cahoots*, March/April/May, Survival Issue

Plumb, A, 1993, The challenge of self-advocacy, *Feminism and Psychology* 3, 2, 169–87

Plumb, A, 1994, Distress or disability? A discussion paper, Manchester: GMCDP (Greater Manchester Coalition of Disabled People)

Plumb, A, 1999, New mental health legislation: A lifesaver? Changing paradigm and practice, *Social Work Education* 18, 4, 459–78

Plumb, A, 2012a, Incorporation, or not, of MH survivors into the disability movement, in J Anderson, B Sapey, H Spandler (eds) *Distress or Disability? Proceedings of a Symposium Held at Lancaster University, 15–16 November 2011*, pp 18–23, Lancaster: Centre for Disability Research

Plumb, A, 2012b, Demons in the age of light: A memoir of psychosis and recovery, by Whitney Robinson, Book Review, *Asylum: An International Magazine for Democratic Psychiatry* 19, 1, 28–9

Plumb, A, 2013, Szasz's unsettling legacy, *Asylum: An International Magazine for Democratic Psychiatry* 20, 1, 26

Plumb, S, 2005, The social/trauma model: Mapping the mental health consequences of childhood sexual abuse and similar experiences, in J Tew (ed) *Social Perspectives in Mental Health: Developing Social Models to Understand and Work with Mental Distress*, pp 112–28, London: Jessica Kingsley

Poole, R, Higgo, R, Robinson, C, 2013, *Mental Health and Poverty*, Cambridge: Cambridge University Press

Prince, M, Patel, V, Saxena, S, Maj, M, Maselko, J, Phillips, M, Rahman, A, 2007, Health without mental health, *The Lancet* 370, 9590, 859–77

Rahnema, M, 1992, Poverty, in W Sachs (ed) *The Development Dictionary: A Guide to Knowledge as Power*, pp 174–94, London: Zed Books

Ramon, S, Williams, J (eds), 2005, *Mental Health at the Crossroads: The promise of the psychosocial approach*, Farnham: Ashgate

Rawls, J, 1971, *A Theory of Justice*, Cambridge, MA: Harvard University Press

Read, J, Van Os, J, Morrison, A, Ross, C, 2005, Childhood trauma, psychosis and Schizophrenia: A literature review with theoretical and clinical implications, *Acta Psychiatrica Scandinavica* 112, 330–50

Read, J, Haslam, N, Sayce, L, Davies, E, 2006a, Prejudice and schizophrenia: A review of the 'mental illness is an illness like any other' approach, *Acta Psychiatrica Scandanavica* 114, 303–18

Read, J, Rudegeair, T, Farrelley, S, 2006b, The relationship between child abuse the psychosis: Public opinion, evidence, pathways and implications, in W Larkin, A Morrison (eds) *Trauma and Psychosis: New Directions for Theory and Therapy*, pp 23–57, London: Routledge

Read, J, Fosse, R, Moskowitz, A, Perry, B, 2014, The traumagenic neurodevelopmental model of psychosis revisited, *Neuropsychiatry* 4, 1, 65–79

Reeve, D, 2004, Psycho-emotional dimensions of disability and the social model, in C Barnes, G Mercer (eds) *Implementing the Social Model of Disability: Theory and Research*, pp 83–100, Leeds: The Disability Press

Reeve, D, 2006, Towards a psychology of disability: The emotional effects of living in a disabling society, in D Goodley, R Lawthom (eds) *Disability and Psychology: Critical Introductions and Reflections*, pp 94–107, London: Palgrave

Reeve, D, 2008, *Negotiating Disability in Everyday Life: The Experience of Psycho-Emotional Disablism*, PhD Thesis, Lancaster: Lancaster University

Reeve, D, 2012a, Psycho-emotional disablism in the lives of people experiencing mental distress, in J Anderson, B Sapey, H Spandler (eds) *Distress or Disability? Proceedings of a Symposium Held at Lancaster University, 15–16 November 2011*, pp 24–9, Lancaster: Centre for Disability Research

Reeve, D, 2012b, Psycho-emotional disablism: The missing link?, in N Watson, A Roulstone, C Thomas (eds) *Routledge Handbook of Disability Studies*, pp 78–92, London: Routledge

Repper, J, Perkins, R, 2003, *Social Inclusion and Recovery: A Model for Mental Health Practice*, London: Bailliere Tindall

Reville, D, 2012, Is Mad Studies emerging as a new field of inquiry?, in B LeFrançois, R Menzies, G Reaume (eds) *Mad Matters: A Critical Reader in Canadian Mad Studies*, pp 170–80, Toronto: Canadian Scholars Press

Richards, C, Barker, M (eds), 2013, *Sexuality and Gender for Mental Health Professionals: A practical guide*, London: Sage.

Ridge, D and Ziebland, S, 2006, 'The old me could not have done that': How people give meaning to recovery following depression, *Qualitative Health Research* 16, 1038–53

Robinson, M, Keating, F, Robertson, S, 2011, Ethnicity, gender and mental health, *Diversity in Health and Care* 8, 81–92

Robinson, W, 2011, *Demons in the Age of Light: A Memoir of Psychosis and Recovery*, Port Townsend, WA: Process

Rogers, A, Pilgrim, D, 2010, *A Sociology of Mental Health and Illness*, 4th edn, Milton Keynes: Open University Press

Romme, M, Escher, S, 1993, The new approach: A Dutch experiment, in M Romme, S Escher (eds) *Accepting Voices*, pp 11–27, London: MIND

Ronald, A, 2014, The times they are a-changin', *The Psychologist* 23, 3, 164–6

Ronny, 2013, Bigots amongst the anti-capitalists, *Asylum: An International Magazine for Democratic Psychiatry* 20, 3, 15

Rose, D, Willis, R, Brohan, E, Sartorius, N, Villares, C, Wahlbeck, K, Thornicroft, G, 2011, Reported stigma and discrimination by people with a diagnosis of schizophrenia, *Epidemiology and Psychiatric Sciences* 20, 2, 193–204

Rosenfield, S, 2012, Triple jeopardy? Mental health at the intersection of gender, race, and class, *Social Science and Medicine* 74, 1791–801

Rowbotham, S, Segal, L, Wainwright, H, 1980, *Beyond the Fragments: Feminism and the Making of Socialism*, London: Merlin

Rubin, G, 1984, Thinking sex: Notes for a radical theory of the politics of sexuality, in C Vance (ed), 1992, *Pleasure and Danger: Exploring Female Sexuality*, pp 267–319, London: HarperCollins

Ruger, J, 2012, Global health justice and governance, *The American Journal of Bioethics* 12, 12, 35–54

Rusch, N, Lieb, K, Bohus, M, Corrigan, P, 2006, Self-stigma, empowerment and perceived legitimacy of discrimination among women with mental illness, *Psychiatric Services* 57, 3, 399–402

Russo, J, 2009, Reclaiming a life written off: Survivor perspectives on first breakdown, working paper for *INTAR/Center to Study Recovery in Social Contexts Conference, Rethinking Psychiatric Crisis: Alternative Responses to 'First Breaks'*, 23 November, New York: New York University

Ryfe, D, 2002, The practice of deliberative democracy: A study of 16 deliberative organisations, *Political Communication* 19, 359–77

Salford Against the Cuts, 2013, *Cuts Can be Beaten: How Mental Health Services Users Took on Salford Council...and Won*, Salford: Salford Against the Cuts

Sandahl, C, 2003, Queering the crip or cripping the queer? Intersections of queer and crip identities in solo autobiographical performance, *GLQ: A Journal of Lesbian and Gay Studies* 9, 1, 25–56

Sapey, B, Bullimore, P, 2013, Listening to Voice hearers, *Journal of Social Work* 13, 6, 616–32

Sargant, W, 1967, *The Unquiet Mind*, Boston, MA: Little, Brown

Sargant, W, Slater, E, Kelly, D, 1963, *An Introduction to Physical Methods of Treatment in Psychiatry*, 4th edn, Edinburgh and London: E and G Livingstone Ltd

Saundry, R, McKeown, M, 2013, Relational union organising in a healthcare setting: a qualitative study, *Industrial Relations Journal* 44, 533–47

Savage, M, Devine, F, Cunningham, N, Taylor, M, Li, Y, Hjellbrekke, J, Le Roux, B, Friedman, S, Miles, A, 2013, A new model of social class? Findings from the BBC's Great British Class Survey Experiment, *Sociology* 47, 219–52

Savarese, E, Savarese, R, 2010, 'The superior half of speaking': An Introduction, *Disability Studies Quarterly* 30, 1, http://dsq-sds.org/article/view/1062/1230

Sayce, L, 2000, *From Psychiatric Patient To Citizen: Overcoming discrimination and social exclusion*, Basingstoke: Macmillan

Sayer, A, 2011, *Why Things Matter to People*, Cambridge: Cambridge University Press

Schizophrenia Commission, 2012, *The Abandoned Illness: A Report from the Schizophrenia Commission*, London: Rethink Mental Illness

Schomerus, G, Schwahn, C, Holzinger, A, Corrigan, P, Grabe, H, Carta, M, Angermeyer, M, 2012, Evolution of public attitudes about mental illness: A systematic review and meta-analysis, *Acta Psychiatrica Scandinavica* 125, 6, 440–52

Scott, B, 2014, The broadest shoulders? Disabled people and 'welfare reform', *Concept: The Journal of Contemporary Community Education Practice Theory* 5, 1, 1–10

Scott-Hill, M, 2002, Policy, politics and the silencing of voice, *Policy and Politics* 30, 3, 397–409

Sedgwick, P, 1982, *Psychopolitics*, London: Pluto Press

Seikkula, J, Olson, M, 2003, The open dialogue approach to acute psychosis: Its poetics and micropolitics, *Family Process* 42, 403–18

Sen, A, 1979, Utilitarianism and welfarism, *The Journal of Philosophy* 76, 9, 463–89

Sen, A, 1985a, *Commodities and Capabilities*, Oxford: Oxford University Press

Sen, A, 1985b, *Women, Technology and Sexual Division*, New York: United Nations Trade and Development

Sen, A, 1989, Development as capability expansion, *Journal of Development Planning* 19, 1, 41–57

Sen, A, 1999, *Development as freedom*, Oxford: Oxford University Press

Sen, A, Nussbaum, M, 1993, Capability and well-being, *The Quality of Life* 1, 30–54

Sequenzia, A, 2012, Why Autism Speaks hurts us, in J Bascom (ed) *Loud Hands: Autistic People Speaking*, pp 192–4, Washington, DC: The Autistic Press

Shakespeare, T, 2006, *Disability: Rights and Wrongs*, London: Routledge

Shakespeare, T, 2007, Disability rights and wrongs, *Scandinavian Journal of Disability Research* 9, 3, 278–81

Shakespeare, T, Watson, N, 2002, The social model of disability: An outdated ideology?, *Research in Social Science and Disability* 2, 9–28

Shakespeare, T, Gillespie-Sells, K, Davies, D (eds), 1996, *The Sexual Politics of Disability: Untold Desires*, London: Cassell

Sharma, D, 2004, India's agrarian crisis: No end to farmers' suicides, *Share the World's Resources*, www.eduardhiebert.com/corporations/Devinder%20Sharma%20on%20farmer%20suicides.htm

Shaw, G , 1903, *Maxims for Revolutionists*, Project Gutenberg, www.gutenberg.org/ebooks/26107

Shimrat, I, 2013, The tragic farce of 'community mental health care', in B LeFrançois, R Menzies, G Reaume (eds) *Mad Matters: A Critical Reader in Canadian Mad Studies*, pp 144–57, Toronto: Canadian Scholars' Press

Shneidman, E, 1993, Suicide as psychache, *Journal of Nervous and Mental Disease*, 181, 147–49

Shore, C, 2010, Beyond the multiversity: Neoliberalism and the rise of the schizophrenic university, *Social Anthropology* 18, 1, 15–29

Shukla, A, Philip, A, Zachariah, A, Phadke, A, Suneetha, A, Davar, B, CEHAT, Srinivasan, C, Mankad, D, Qadeer, I, Kalathil, J, Lalita, K, Sajaya, K, Jacob, K, Balimahabal, K, Gupte, M, Rao, M, Salie, M, Prakash, P, Chatterjee, P, Baru, R, Melkote, R, Shukla, R, Gaitonde, R, Bisht, R, Duggal, R, Khanna, R, Priya, R, Srivatsan, R, Timimi, S, Sarojini, N, Sathyamala, C, Ashtekar, S, Fernando, S, Tharu, S, Shatrugna, V, 2012, Critical perspectives on the NIMH initiative 'Grand challenges to global mental health', *Indian Journal of Medical Ethics* 9, 4, 292–3

Shulkes, D, 2013, *Notes after psychiatry*, Unpublished manuscript

Sibbett, C, Thompson, W, 2008, Nettlesome knowledge, liminality and the taboo in cancer and art therapy experiences: Implications for teaching and learning, in R Land, J Meyer, J Smith (eds) *Threshold Concepts Within the Disciplines*, pp 227–42, Rotterdam: Sense Publishers

Sibitz, I, Unger, A, Woppman, A, Zidek, T, Amering, M, 2009, Stigma resistance in patients with schizophrenia, *Schizophrenia Bulletin* 37, 2, 316–23

Sin, C, Hedges, A, Cook, C, Mguni, N, Comber, N, 2009, Disabled people's experiences of targeted violence and hostility, *Research Report* 21, Manchester: Office for Public Management

Sinclair, J, 2012a, Don't mourn for us, in J Bascom (ed) *Loud Hands: Autistic People Speaking*, pp 13–16, Washington, DC: The Autistic Press

Sinclair, J, 2012b, Why I dislike 'person first' language', in J Bascom (ed) *Loud Hands: Autistic People Speaking*, pp 152–3, Washington, DC: The Autistic Press

Singer, J, 1999, 'Why can't you be normal for once in your life?' From a 'problem with no name' to the emergence of a new category of difference, in M Corker, S French (eds) *Disability Discourse*, pp 59–67, Buckingham: Open University Press

Singh, S, Burns, T, 2006, Race and mental health: There is more to race than racism, *British Medical Journal* 333, 648–51

Slade, M, Amering, M, Farkas, M, Hamilton, B, O'Hagan, M, Panther, G, Perkins, R, Shepherd, G, Tse, S, Whitley, R, 2014, Uses and abuses of recovery: Implementing recovery-oriented practices in mental health systems, *World Psychiatry* 13, 12–20

Smith, D, 1987, *The Everyday World as Problematic: A Feminist Sociology*, Toronto: University of Toronto Press

Snyder, S, Mitchell, D, 2006, *Cultural Locations of Disability*, Chicago, IL: University of Chicago Press

Somasundaram, O, 2008, The Government mental hospital, Kilpauk, Madras: Memoirs of the fifties, *Indian Journal of Psychiatry* 50, 224–6

Spandler, H, 1996, *Who's Hurting Who? Young People, Self Harm and Suicide*, Manchester: 42nd Street

Spandler, H, 2004, Friend or foe? Towards a critical assessment of direct payments, *Critical Social Policy* 24, 2, 187–209

Spandler, H, 2006, *Asylum to Action: Paddington Day Hospital, Therapeutic Communities and Beyond*, London: Jessica Kingsley

Spandler, H, 2009, Spaces of psychiatric contention: A case study of a therapeutic community, *Health and Place* 15, 672–78

Spandler, H, 2012, Setting the scene, in J Anderson, B Sapey, H Spandler (eds) *Distress or Disability? Proceedings of a Symposium Held at Lancaster University, 15–16 November 2011*, pp 14–17, Lancaster: Centre for Disability Research

Spandler, H, 2014, Letting madness breathe?: Critical challenges facing mental health social work today, in J Weinstein (ed) *Mental Health: Critical and Radical Debates in Social Work*, pp 29–38, Bristol: Policy Press

Spandler, H, Calton, T, 2009, Psychosis and human rights: Conflicts in mental health policy and practice, *Social Policy and Society* 8, 2, 245–56

Spandler, H, Stickley, T, 2011, Hope without compassion: The importance of compassion in recovery-focused mental health services, *Journal of Mental Health* 20, 6, 555–66

Spandler, H, Warner, S (eds), 2007, *Beyond Fear and Control: Working with Young People who Self-harm*, Ross-on-Wye: PCCS Books

Spivak, G, 1988). 'Can the subaltern speak?', in C Nelson, L Grossberg (eds) *Marxism and the Interpretation of Culture*, pp 271–313, Chicago, IL: University of Illinois Press

Staddon, P (ed), 2013, *Mental Health Service Users In Research: Critical Sociological Perspectives*, Bristol: Policy Press

Staniland, L, 2011, *Public Perceptions of Disabled People: Evidence from the British Social Attitudes Survey 2009*, London: ODI

Stefánsdóttir, G, Hreinsdóttir, E, 2013, Sterilization, intellectual disability, and some ethical and methodological challenges: It shouldn't be a secret, *Ethics and Social Welfare* 7, 3, 302–8

Stuart, O, 1992, Race and disability: Just a double oppression?, *Disability, Handicap and Society* 7, 2, 177–88

Stuart, O, 2012, Not invited to the party? Black and minority ethnic adults and the personalisation of social care, in C Craig, K Atkin, S Chattoo, R Flynn (eds) *Understanding 'Race' and Ethnicity: Theory, History, Policy, Practice*, pp 133–50, Bristol: The Policy Press

Sullivan, P, Daly, M, O'Donovan, M, 2012, Genetic architectures of psychiatric disorders: The emerging picture and its implications, *Nature Reviews Genetics* 13, 8, 537–51

Summerfield, D, 2008, How scientifically valid is the knowledge base of global mental health?, *British Medical Journal* 336, 992–94

Summerfield, D, 2012, Afterword: Against 'global mental health', *Transcultural Psychiatry* 49, 3, 519–30

Susser, M, Watson, W, Hopper, K, 1985, Social class and disorders in health, in M Susser, W Watson, K Hopper (eds) *Sociology in Medicine*, 3rd edn, pp 213–75, New York: Oxford University Press

Swain, J, French, S, 2000, Towards and affirmative model of disability, *Disability and* Society 15, 4, 569–82

Szasz, T, 1960, The myth of mental illness, *American Psychologist* 15, 113–18

Szasz, T, 1973, *Ideology and Insanity: Essays on the Psychiatric Dehumanisation of Man*, London: Calder and Boyers

Tam, L, 2013, Whither indigenizing the mad movement? Theorizing the social relations of race and madness through conviviality, in B LeFrançois, R Menzies, G Reaume (eds) *Mad Matters: A Critical Reader in Canadian Mad Studies*, pp 281–97, Toronto: Canadian Scholars' Press

Tang, L, 2013, *Recovery from What to Where? A Case Study of Chinese Mental Health Service Users in the UK*, PhD thesis, University of Warwick

Tarsy, D, Baldessarini, R, 2006, Epidemiology of tardive dyskinesia: Is risk declining with modern antipsychotics?, *Movement Disorders* 21, 5, 589–98

Tattersall, A, 2010, *Power in Coalitions: Strategies for Strong Unions and Social Change*, Sydney: Allen and Unwin

Taylor, V, Whittier, N, 1995, Analytical Approaches to Social Movement Culture: The Culture of the Women's Movement, in H Johnston, B Klandermans (eds) *Social Movements and Culture*, pp 163–87, Minneapolis/London: University of Minnesota Press/UCL Press

Tew, J, 2005a, Power relations, social order and mental distress, in J Tew (ed) *Social Perspectives and Mental Health: Developing Social Models to Understand and Work with Mental Distress*, pp 71–89, London, Jessica Kingsley

Tew, J (ed), 2005b, *Social Perspectives In Mental Health: Developing Social Models to Understand and Work with Mental Distress*, London, Jessica Kingsley

Tew, J, 2011, *Social Approaches to Mental Distress*, Basingstoke: Palgrave Macmillan

Tew, J, 2012, Recovery capital: What enables a sustainable recovery from mental health difficulties?, *European Journal of Social Work* 16, 3, 360–74

Tew, J, Ramon, S, Slade, M, Bird, V, Melton, J, Le Boutillier, C, 2012, Social factors and recovery from mental health difficulties: A review of the evidence, *British Journal of Social Work* 42, 3, 443–60

The Centre for Social Justice, 2011, *Completing the Revolution. Transforming Mental Health and Tackling Poverty*, www.centreforsocialjustice.org.uk

Thomas, C, 1999, *Female Forms: Experiencing and Understanding Disability*, Buckingham: Open University Press

Thomas, C, 2007, *Sociologies of Disability and Illness: Contested Ideas in Disability Studies and Medical Sociology*, Basingstoke: Palgrave Macmillan

Thomas, C, 2008, Disability: Getting it 'right', *Journal of Medical Ethics* 34, 1, 15–17

Thomas, P, 2013, 'Soteria: Contexts, practice and philosophy' in S Coles, S Keenan, B Diamond (eds) *Madness contested: Power and practice*, Ross-on-Wye: PCCS Books, pp 141–57

Thomas, C, Corker, M, 2002, A journey around the social model, in M Corker, T Shakespeare (eds) *Disability/Postmodernity: Embodying Disability Theory*, pp 18–31, London: Continuum

Thomas, P, Bracken, P, Cutler, P, Hayward, R, May, R, Yasmeen, S, 2005, Challenging the globalisation of biomedical psychiatry, *Journal of Public Mental Health*, 4, 3, 23–32

Thornicroft, G, 2006a, *Actions Speak Louder: Tackling Discrimination against People with Mental Illness*, London: Mental Health Foundation

Thornicroft, G, 2006b, *Shunned: Discrimination against People with Mental Illness*, Oxford: Oxford University Press

Tiefer, L, 1995, *Sex is Not a Natural Act*, Boulder, CO: Westview Press

Tilley, E, Walmsley, J, Earle, S, Atkinson, D, 2012, 'The silence is roaring': Sterilization, reproductive rights and women with intellectual disabilities, *Disability and Society* 27, 3, 413–26

Timimi, S, 2002, *Pathological Child Psychiatry and the Medicalization of Childhood*, Hove: Brunner Routledge

Timimi, S, 2011, *More Psychiatric Labels*, www.criticalpsychiatry.net/wp-content/uploads/2011/05/CAPSID12.pdf

Tomasini, F, 2012, Disability 'and' distress: Towards understanding the vulnerable body-subject, in J Anderson, B Sapey, H Spandler, *Distress or Disability: Proceedings of a Symposium Held at Lancaster University, 15–16 November 2011*, pp 24–29, Lancaster: Centre for Disability Research

Tregaskis, C, 2002, Social model theory: The story so far…, *Disability and Society* 17, 4, 457–70

Tremain, S, 2002, On the subject of impairment, in M Corker, T Shakespeare (eds) *Disability/Postmodernity: Embodying Disability Theory*, pp 32–47, London: Continuum

Tremain, S, 2006, On the government of disability: Foucault, power, and the subject of impairment, in L Davis (ed) *The Disability Studies Reader*, 2nd edn, pp 185–96, London: Routledge

Trueman, J, 2013, The mirage of mental health reform, in S Walker (ed) *Modern Mental Health: Critical Perspectives on Psychiatric Practice*, pp 128–43, St Albans: Critical Publishing

Tuohy, B, Cooper, G, 2007, Listening to deaf people, *Mental Health Today*, July/August, 27–9

United Nations, 1948, *The Universal Declaration of Human Rights*, New York: UN

United Nations, 2006, *Convention on the Rights of Persons with Disabilities*, New York, UN

UPIAS, 1974, *Policy Statement*, London: The Union of the Physically Impaired Against Segregation

UPIAS, 1981, *Disability Challenge Number 1*, London: The Union of the Physically Impaired Against Segregation

UPIAS/Disability Alliance, 1976, *Fundamental Principles of Disability: Being a Summary of the Discussion Held on 22nd November, 1975 and Containing Commentaries from Each Organization*, London, The Union of the Physically Impaired Against Segregation and the Disability Alliance

Vassilev, I, Pilgrim, D, 2007, Risk, trust and the myth of mental health services, *Journal of Mental Health* 16, 3, 347–57

Venkatapuram, S, 2012, *Health Justice*, Cambridge: Polity

Ventura33, 2005, *Ventura33's Neurodiversity Page*, www.ventura33.com/neurodiversity/

Viruell-Fuentes, E, Miranda, P, Abdulrahim, S, 2012, More than culture: Structural racism, intersectionality theory, and immigrant health, *Social Science and Medicine* 75, 2099–106

Voss, K, 2010, Democratic dilemmas: Union democracy and union renewal, *Transfer: European Review of Labour and Research* 16, 369–82

Wadham, H, Warren, R, 2013, Telling organizational tales: The extended case method in practice, *Organizational Research Methods* 17, 1, 5–20

Walker, C, Johnson, K, Cunningham, L, 2012, *Community Psychology and the Socio-economics of Mental Distress: International Perspectives*, Basingstoke: Palgrave Macmillan

Walker, N, 2012, Throw away the master's tools: Liberating ourselves from the pathology paradigm, in J Bascom (ed) *Loud Hands: Autistic People Speaking*, pp 154–62, Washington, DC: The Autistic Press

Wallcraft, J, 2002a, We should abolish the Mental Health Act, *Survivors United Network Newsletter*, January

Wallcraft, J, 2002b, *Turning Towards Recovery?*, PhD thesis, London: South Bank University

Wallcraft, J, 2010, The capabilities approach in mental health, presentation at Nottingham University, www.nottingham.ac.uk/ sociology/pdfs/qrmh/keynote-addresses/jan-wallcraft.ppt

Wallcraft, J, 2011, Service users' perceptions of quality of life measurement in psychiatry, *Advances in Psychiatric Treatment* 17, 266–74

Wallcraft, J, Michaelson, J, 2001, Developing a survivor discourse to replace the 'psychopathology' of breakdown and crisis, in C Newnes, G Holmes, C Dunn (eds) *This is Madness Too: Critical Perspectives on Mental Health Services*, pp 177–90, Ross on Wye: PCCS Books

Waltz, M, 2013, *Autism: A Social and Medical History*, Basingstoke: Palgrave Macmillan

Ware, N, Hopper, K, Tugenberg, T, Dickey, B, Fisher, D, 2007, Connectedness and citizenship: Redefining social integration, *Psychiatric Services* 58, 469–74

Warner, M (ed), 1993, *Fear of a Queer Planet: Queer Politics and social theory*, Chicago, IL: University of Minnesota Press

Warner, R, 2004, *Recovery from Schizophrenia: Psychiatry and Political Economy*, London: Routledge

Warner, S, 2009, *Understanding the Effects of Child Sexual Abuse: Feminist Revolutions in Theory, Research and Practice*, London: Routledge

Webb, D, 2010, *Thinking about Suicide: Contemplating and Comprehending the Urge to Die*, Ross-on-Wye: PCCS Books

Weinberg, D, 2007, Habermas, rights, and the learning disabled citizen, *Social Theory and Health* 5, 70–87

Welch, P, 2002, *Applying the Capabilities Approach in Examining Disability, Poverty, and Gender*, proceedings of the conference Promoting Women's Capabilities: Examining Nussbaum's Capabilities Approach, Cambridge: St Edmund's College

Wendell, S, 1996, *The Rejected Body: Feminist Philosophical Reflections on Disability*, London: Routledge

Wendell, S, 2001, Unhealthy Disabled: Treating Chronic Illnesses as Disabilities, *Hypatia* 16, 4, 17–33

Wenger, E, 1998, *Communities of Practice: Learning, Meaning and Identity*, Cambridge: Cambridge University Press

Wenger-Trayner, E, Wenger-Trayner, B, 2014, Learning in a landscape of practice: a framework, in D Wenger-Trayner, M Fenton-O'Creevy, S Hutchinson, C Kubiak, B Wenger-Trayner (eds) *Learning in Landscapes of Practice: Boundaries, Identity, and Knowledgeability in Practice-based Learning*, pp 13–30, Abingdon: Routledge

West, K, 2013, Following in North Carolina's footsteps: California's challenge in compensating its victims of compulsory sterilization, *Santa Clara Law Review* 53, 301–27

Westcott, H, Cross, M, 1996, *This Far and No Further: Towards Ending the Abuse of Disabled Children*, Birmingham: Venture Press

Whitaker, R, 2010, *Anatomy of an Epidemic: Magic Bullets, Psychiatric Drugs, and the Astonishing Rise of Mental Illness in America*, New York: Random House

WHO (World Health Organization), 1994, *International Classification of Diseases*, 10th edn, Geneva: WHO

WHO (World Health Organization), 2001a, *International Classification of Functioning Disability and Health (ICF)*, Geneva: WHO

WHO (World Health Organization), 2001b, *World Health Report 2001: Mental Health: New Understanding, New Hope*, Geneva: WHO

WHO (World Health Organization), 2003, *Investing in Mental Health*, Geneva: WHO

WHO (World Health Organization), 2005, *Promoting the Rights of People with Mental Disabilities*, Mental Health, Human Rights and Legislation Information Sheet, 1, Geneva: WHO

WHO (World Health Organization), 2008, *Closing the gap in a generation: health equity through action on the social determinants of health. Final report of the Commission on the Social Determinants of Health*, Geneva: WHO

WHO (World Health Organization), 2010, *mhGAP Intervention Guide for Mental, Neurological and Substance Use Disorders in Non-Specialized Health Settings*, Geneva: WHO

WHO (World Health Organization), 2011a, *Global Burden of Mental Disorders and the Need for a Comprehensive, Coordinated Response from Health and social sectors at the Country Level: Report by the Secretariat*, Geneva: WHO

WHO (World Health Organization), 2011b, *Model List of Essential Medicines for Adults*, 17th edn, Geneva: WHO

WHO (World Health Organization), 2011c, *Model List of Essential Medicines for Children*. 3rd edn, Geneva: WHO

WHO (World Health Organization), World Bank, 2011, *World Report on Disability*, Geneva: WHO

Williams-Findlay, R, 2011, Lifting the lid on disabled people against cuts, *Disability and Society* 26, 6, 773–78

Wills, J, Simms, M, 2006, Building reciprocal community unionism in the UK, *Capital and Class* 82, 59–84

Wilson, A, Beresford, P, 2002, Madness, distress and postmodernity: Putting the record straight, in M Corker, T Shakespeare (eds) *Disability/Postmodernity: Embodying Disability Theory*, pp 143–58, London: Continuum

Withers, A, 2012, *Disability Politics and Theory*, Halifax and Winnipeg: Fernwood Publishing

Withers, A, 2014, Disability, Divisions, Definitions, and Disablism: When Resisting Psychiatry is Oppressive, in B Burstow, B LeFrancois, S Diamond (eds) *Psychiatry disrupted. Theorizing resistance and crafting the (R)evolution*, Montreal and Kingston: McGill Queen's University Press, pp 114–28

WNUSP (World Network of Users and Survivors of Psychiatry), 2008, *Implementation Manual for the United Nations Convention on the Rights of People with Disabilities*, www.wnusp.net/documents/WNUSP_CRPD_Manual.pdf

WNUSP (World Network of Users and Survivors of Psychiatry), 2011, *Position Paper on the Implications of the CRPD*, www.wnusp.net/index.php/newsletters/

WNUSP (World Network of Users and Survivors of Psychiatry), Bapu Trust, 2013, *Human Rights of Persons with Psychosocial Disabilities in the Post 2015 Inclusive Development Agenda: Towards HLMDD*, Pune, India: World Network of Users and Survivors of Psychiatry and Bapu Trust

WNUSP (World Network of Users and Survivors of Psychiatry), CHRUSP (Centre for the Human Rights of Users and Survivors of Psychiatry), 2013, *Comments to the Committee against Torture on Standards Applicable to Psychiatric Institutions and Mental Health Services*, www.wnusp.net/documents/2013_WNUSPcommentsCAT.pdf

Woolford, A, Nelund, A, 2013, The responsibilities of the poor: Performing neoliberal citizenship within the bureaucratic field, *Social Service Review* 87, 2, 292–318

Wyatt, R, 2012, *Thomas Szasz on Freedom and Psychotherapy*, www.psychotherapy.net/interview/thomas-szasz

Xanthos, C, 2012, Racializing mental illness: Understanding african-caribbean schizophrenia in the UK, *Critical Social Work* 9, 1, 1–8

Young, I, 1997, Difference as a resource for democratic communication, in J Bohman, W Rehg (eds) *Deliberative Democracy: Essays on Reason and Politics*, pp 383–406, Cambridge MA: MIT Press

Young, I, 2001, *Inclusion and Democracy*, New York: Oxford University Press

Index